NEUROSCIENCE RESEARCH PROGRESS

HALLUCINATIONS: TYPES, STAGES AND TREATMENTS

NEUROSCIENCE RESEARCH PROGRESS

Additional books in this series can be found on Nova's website under the Series tab.

Additional E-books in this series can be found on Nova's website under the E-books tab.

NEUROSCIENCE RESEARCH PROGRESS

HALLUCINATIONS: TYPES, STAGES AND TREATMENTS

MEREDITH S. PAYNE
EDITOR

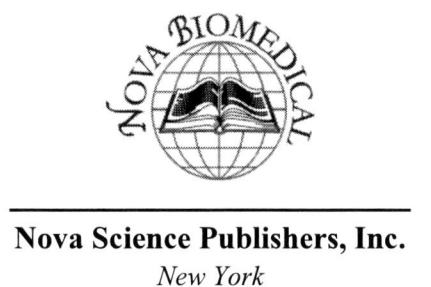

Nova Science Publishers, Inc.
New York

Copyright © 2011 by Nova Science Publishers, Inc.

All rights reserved. No part of this book may be reproduced, stored in a retrieval system or transmitted in any form or by any means: electronic, electrostatic, magnetic, tape, mechanical photocopying, recording or otherwise without the written permission of the Publisher.

For permission to use material from this book please contact us:
Telephone 631-231-7269; Fax 631-231-8175
Web Site: http://www.novapublishers.com

NOTICE TO THE READER

The Publisher has taken reasonable care in the preparation of this book, but makes no expressed or implied warranty of any kind and assumes no responsibility for any errors or omissions. No liability is assumed for incidental or consequential damages in connection with or arising out of information contained in this book. The Publisher shall not be liable for any special, consequential, or exemplary damages resulting, in whole or in part, from the readers' use of, or reliance upon, this material. Any parts of this book based on government reports are so indicated and copyright is claimed for those parts to the extent applicable to compilations of such works.

Independent verification should be sought for any data, advice or recommendations contained in this book. In addition, no responsibility is assumed by the publisher for any injury and/or damage to persons or property arising from any methods, products, instructions, ideas or otherwise contained in this publication.

This publication is designed to provide accurate and authoritative information with regard to the subject matter covered herein. It is sold with the clear understanding that the Publisher is not engaged in rendering legal or any other professional services. If legal or any other expert assistance is required, the services of a competent person should be sought. FROM A DECLARATION OF PARTICIPANTS JOINTLY ADOPTED BY A COMMITTEE OF THE AMERICAN BAR ASSOCIATION AND A COMMITTEE OF PUBLISHERS.

Additional color graphics may be available in the e-book version of this book.

Library of Congress Cataloging-in-Publication Data

Hallucinations : types, stages, and treatments / editor, Meredith S. Payne.
    p. ; cm.
Includes bibliographical references and index.
ISBN 978-1-61728-275-1 (hardcover)
1. Hallucinations and illusions. I. Payne, Meredith S.
 [DNLM: 1. Hallucinations. WM 204 H1938 2010]
RC553.H3H38 2010
615'.7883--dc22
                                              2010022883

Published by Nova Science Publishers, Inc. † New York

Contents

Preface		vii
Chapter 1	About the Origin of Hallucinations: From a Phenomenological, Cognitive and Neurophysiological Point of View *Viola Oertel-Knoechel*	1
Chapter 2	Auditory Verbal Hallucination in Schizophrenic Patients and the General Population: The Sense of Agency in Speech *Tomohisa Asai, Eriko Sugimori and Yoshihiko Tanno*	33
Chapter 3	The Roles of Negative Affect in Auditory Hallucinations *Georgie Paulik and Johanna C. Badcock*	61
Chapter 4	Hallucinations and Intrusive Thoughts *M. F. Soriano and Teresa Bajo*	79
Chapter 5	Charles Bonnet Syndrome *Chris Plummer*	97
Chapter 6	Assessing Anomalous Perceptions in Youths: A Preliminary Validation Study of the Cardiff Anomalous Perceptions Scale (CAPS) *Martin Debbané, Maude Schneider, Stephan Eliez and Martial Van der Linden*	113
Chapter 7	Psychotic-like Experiences in Nonclinical Adolescents *Eduardo Fonseca-Pedrero, Serafín Lemos-Giráldez, Mercedes Paino and Susana Sierra-Baigrie*	131
Chapter 8	Nonpharmacological Inhibition of Cerebral Dopaminergic Activity May Be an Option for Medication-Resistant Hallucinations *Nikolai A. Shevchuk*	147

Chapter 9	Hallucinations and Suicide Risk: Future Directions for Research and Clinical Implications *Maurizio Pompili, Gianluca Serafini, Marco Innamorati, S. Diletta Del Bono, Eleonora Piacentini, David Lester and Roberto Tatarelli*	163
Chapter 10	Behavioral Symptoms of Dementia *Ladislav Volicer and Elizabeth Vongxaiburana*	179
Chapter 11	Analysis and Relevance of Psychotic-Like Experiences: Repercussions on the Continuity Model of Hallucinations *J. Adolfo Cangas and I. Álvaro Langer*	195
Chapter 12	Hallucinatory Disorder: A Clinical Entity? *Massimo Carlo Mauri, Filippo Dragogna, Isabel Valli, Giancarlo Cerveri, Lucia S. Volonteri and Giorgio Marotta*	207
Chapter 13	The Neurobiological Basis of Hallucinations *Jitka Bušková*	219
Chapter 14	Social Variables Related to the Origin of Hallucinations *Adolfo J. Cangas, Álvaro I. Langer, José M. García-Montes, José A. Carmona and Luz Nieto*	225
Index		235

Preface

A hallucination, in the broadest sense, is a perception in the absence of a stimulus. In a stricter sense, hallucinations are defined as perceptions in a conscious and awake state in the absence of external stimuli which have qualities of real perception, in that they are vivid, substantial, and located in external objective space. The latter definition distinguishes hallucinations from the related phenomena of dreaming, which does not involve wakefulness. This new book gathers and presents research from around the globe in the study of hallucinations including the origin of hallucinations, auditory verbal hallucinations in schizophrenic patients, Charles Bonnet Syndrome, as well as hallucinations and suicide risk and the neurobiological basis of hallucinations.

Chapter 1- The main interest of this chapter is the investigation of the underpinnings of hallucinations, including phenomenological descriptions (Bentall, 1990; Oertel et al., 2009), cognitive models (Frith, 1992) and neurophysiological evidence (e.g., Dierks et al., 1999; Oertel et al., 2007; Sireteanu et al., 2008). The term *hallucination* was introduced in the psychiatric literature by Esquirol (1832), who first distinguished it from other disorders of perception. Hallucinations can occur in all sensory modalities, under several conditions (e.g., sensory deprivation) and pathological processes (e.g., epilepsy, Manford & Andermann, 1998; schizophrenia, Hahlweg, 1998), but can even occur in normal individuals in non-psychiatric environments (Johns & van Os, 2001).

A certain vividness of mental imagery is generally regarded as contributing to, if not the cause of, hallucinations. We investigated the occurrence and form of appearance of hallucinations (Aggernaes, 1972) and phenomenological issues and found no evidence for a linear relationship between vividness of mental imagery and predisposition to hallucinate (Oertel et al., 2009). Studies of cognitive biases, however, showed that hallucinating individuals failed to distinguish between internal and external phenomena (Bentall et al., 1991; Van de Ven & Merckelbach, 2003).

Important findings come from functional magnetic resonance imaging (fMRI) studies (Dierks et al., 1999; Lennox et al., 2000; Linden et al., 2002; Shergill et al., 2004; Van de Ven et al., 2005). They detected neurological evidence for a similar processing of auditory verbal hallucinations and real auditory perception in the brain. Studies regarding the visual modality of hallucinations found associations in the visual association cortex (Silbersweig et al., 1995; Oertel et al., 2007; Sireteanu et al., 2008), but not in the primary visual area, and an association between the locations of activity within specialized cortex and the contents of visual hallucinations (ffytche et al., 1998; Oertel et al., 2007). Surprisingly, memory-related areas were found involved during schizophrenia-induced hallucinations (Oertel et al., 2007), but not when they were artificially induced, e.g., by blindfolding (Sireteanu et al., 2008).

In general, attempts to define the distinctive features of hallucinations have drawn attention to the variety of hallucinatory phenomena and the difficulty in distinguishing between these phenomena and other normal or abnormal mental states. It is proposed that individual differences in psychopathology, as well as neuropsychological and psychosocial functioning may provide further means to understand the complex and highly dynamic aspects of hallucinations specifically and schizophrenia in general.

Chapter 2- Recently, boundaries between "normal" and "abnormal," even with regard to mental disorders like schizophrenia, have blurred. Thought auditory verbal hallucinations (AVH) are a cardinal feature of schizophrenia, recent studies have suggested that even healthy general population might experience the AVH (i.e., auditory verbal hallucination like experiences) (e.g., Barrett et al., 1992), indicating the continuum of schizophrenic symptoms. In this chapter, we reviewed the results of the studies about AVH both in schizophrenic patients and general population with AVH in terms of self-monitoring or sense of agency in speech, including our own studies. A perspective that situates schizophrenia on a continuum implies that this disorder constitutes a potential risk for everyone and, thus, helps in promoting understanding and correcting misunderstandings that contribute to prejudice within communities.

We first reviewed the phenomenology of AVH in general population including quality and quantity, compared with patients with AVH. According to these previous studies, we developed the auditory hallucination experience scale (AHES) for general population because a scale for directly measuring AVH was needed. What causes AVH even in general population? Recent studies have suggested the relationship with the sense of agency in speech.

The sense of agency is the feeling of causing our own actions, in this case, speech (Gallagher, 2000). One's own speech could seem to be AVH (McGuigan, 1966). The activation of Broca's area, which can produce but cannot listen to speech, has been associated with AVH (McGuire et al., 1993). Therefore, these people might produce speech but not think that they actually spoke. As a result, they may hear their own voices as the voices of others. Indeed, schizophrenic patients with AVH tend to misattribute their own speech (self-speech recognition task: e.g., Johns et al., 1999; 2001). To measure the subjective aspect of the sense of agency, we developed a scale to measure the sense of agency in a general population.

The sense of agency approach to AVH could be a key not only to understand schizophrenic cardinal symptom but to understand the sense of "self" in healthy general population in the sense that even general population could experience AVH. We finally discussed on the neurocognitive model of the sense of agency in speech and its potential disturbance in people with AVH.

Chapter 3- You hear a voice saying "Everyone is looking at you. You're making a fool of yourself *again*. You're pathetic". It's the voice of a young man, he sounds angry and he seems to be close by. You start to reply, then look around. No one is there.

Auditory hallucinations (AHs) are frequently pessimistic in content and intrusive in nature, and – not surprisingly – they are most often perceived by the individual as confronting and distressing. This potentially explains the high co-occurrence of AHs with depression, anger, fear, anxiety, low self-esteem, and suicide. However, in recent years it has become increasingly evident that negative affect plays more than one role in an hallucinatory event: it may be a trigger, a maintenance mechanism, a determinant of content, and an outcome. This chapter will start by briefly defining and describing the phenomenology of AHs in different populations, and then proceed to review the literature pertaining to each of the roles of negative affect in an hallucinatory event, and make recommendations for the treatment of AHs according to this multifaceted relationship.

Chapter 4- Hallucinations have traditionally been conceptualized as a perceptual disorder. However, several lines of research have recently highlighted the similarity between hallucinations and intrusive thoughts. For example, Morrison and Baker (2000) have shown that patients who experience hallucinations also have more intrusive thoughts than patients who do not hallucinate. Similarly, Moritz and Laroi (2008) examined the cognitive and sensory characteristics of thoughts, intrusions and hallucinations, and they did not find a specific profile for hallucinations, compared to intrusions and normal thoughts. From this view, perceptual abnormalities would not be central to the experience of hearing voices, but an interpretation of cognitive intrusions.

Recently, we have found (Soriano, Román, Jiménez & Bajo, 2009) that schizophrenic patients with hallucinations showed impairments in intentional inhibition in memory, compared to schizophrenics without hallucinations, and healthy controls. We have hypothesized that both hallucinations and intrusive thoughts could be partly due to difficulties to inhibit mental events, so that unwanted or repetitive thoughts or images intrude into consciousness. Consistent with this idea, Verwoerd, Wessel and de Jong (2009) have found a relationship between individual differences in inhibitory control and the frequency of experiencing intrusive memories. Interestingly, intrusive thoughts and images were only related to cognitive inhibition (measured as resistance to proactive interference), but not to response inhibition. Therefore, we suggest that inhibitory difficulties may underlie the frequency of intrusions, whereas the interpretation of these intrusions might lead to the experience of them as voices, intrusions-obsessions, or normal thoughts. As Morrison (2001) has proposed, in hallucinating patients, metacognitive beliefs would induce the erroneous attribution of intrusions to external sources, producing the hallucinatory experience.

This view has important consequences in the conceptualization of mental disorders. Hallucinations have been considered a cardinal symptom in schizophrenia, while intrusions are a common symptom of various mental disorders, such as obsessive-compulsive disorder, generalized anxiety, or post-traumatic stress disorder. The parallelism between hallucinations and intrusions may support the idea that differences between schizophrenia and other anxiety disorders are more quantitative than qualitative, and that certain common basic cognitive dysfunctions underlie mental disorders in general.

Chapter 5- Charles Bonnet Syndrome (CBS) is a fascinating disorder that is generally defined as the presence of visual hallucinations (simple or complex) in patients who meet two additional clinical criteria i) visual impairment is due to eye disease and ii) higher cognitive function is intact. The condition is most commonly encountered in elderly patients with advanced, age-related macular degeneration. The prevalence of the disorder is almost certainly under-estimated; this is because patients are typically reluctant to reveal their symptoms for fear of being labelled insane or demented. This underscores the importance of improved patient and physician awareness of CBS as its incidence is only likely to rise in an ever increasingly aged population. It is perhaps ironic that despite the major advances in neuroimaging technology over recent years, we have not moved so far from Bonnet's original insightful discourse on the possible pathogenesis of the disorder – the first recognized account of hallucinatory phenomena in the scientific literature. CBS still has much to teach us about the complexity of the visual association cortex in man.

Chapter 6- Survey studies indicate that hallucinations and other anomalous perceptions constitute relatively common mental events in adults, yet they remain poorly characterized in younger individuals. Information about the factor structure of anomalous perceptions or information on their frequency in the general and clinical youth populations are still incomplete. Recent epidemiological studies have provided the most consistent data, suggesting that some early anomalous perceptions such as auditory hallucinations can be predictive of later psychiatric illness during adulthood. Would this be true of other anomalous perceptions? Longitudinal studies also observe that the intrusive quality of early hallucinations combined to emotional distress in young voice-hearers sustain the expression and development of auditory hallucinations. If perceived distress and intrusiveness contribute to the potential unfolding of hallucinations, how do they relate to other anomalous perceptions? The first step to answer these questions is to provide a psychometric instrument that could assess the variety of anomalous perceptions in youths, combined with subjective ratings of frequency, distress and intrusiveness. This chapter presents preliminary data on the validation of a self-report instrument shown to reliably measure anomalous perceptions and their experiential dimensions in adults. The current study introduces a validation of the Cardiff Anomalous Perception Scale adapted for francophone youths. The results demonstrate its usefulness in characterizing the multifactorial nature of anomalous perceptions in youths. Further, the analyses support the pertinence of this instrument as an assessment tool for psychosis-proneness in young samples. Finally, the study highlights significant associations between specific anomalous perceptions and self-reported anxiety and depression ratings. The CAPS adaptation for youths thus contains the features required for the advancement of research on anomalous perceptions in young individuals.

Chapter 7- Interest in psychotic-like experiences (PLEs), such as magical thinking, delusional ideation or hallucinatory experiences, in general and clinical populations has recently increased in the scientific community. Psychotic symptoms, particularly in the context of schizophrenia-spectrum disorders, have traditionally been viewed as categorical phenomena (i.e., either present or absent in an individual). However, the literature shows that PLEs can be found in the general population, even during adolescence, becoming in this way even more prevalent than the clinical phenotype itself. Thus, PLEs are understood as alterations in how one perceives and thinks about reality, in such a way that the individuals who experience these would present a certain bizarreness of thought, characterized by non-conventional logic. This group of experiences, also known as positive schizotypy, can be found, therefore, below the clinical threshold without necessarily being associated to a psychological, medical or any other type of alteration (Nelson & Yung, 2009; Scott, Chant, Andrews, & McGrath, 2006; Verdoux & van Os, 2002). From a dimensional point of view, it is assumed that the psychotic phenotype is distributed in the general population along a *continuum* of severity, with the psychotic disorder at its extreme end (van Os, Hanssen, Bijl, & Ravelli, 2000; van Os, Linscott, Myin-Germeys, Delespaul, & Krabbendam, 2009). In this regard, the expression of the psychotic phenotype would fluctuate from a normal state of functioning, going from the apparition of intermediate transitory states that precede the development of subsyndromal psychotic symptoms, toward its clinical manifestation in the form of psychosis. PLEs would be, therefore, located on a point of the continuum next to the transitory intermediate states, being understood as subclinical processes. In this manner, PLEs could be seen as an "intermediate" phenotype qualitatively similar to the symptomatology found in patients with psychosis, but quantitatively less severe, showing lower intensity, persistence, frequency of symptoms and associated impairment (Dominguez, Wichers, Lieb, Wittchen, & van Os, in press; Scott, Martin, Welham, Bor, Najman, O'Callaghan et al., 2009; Yung, Nelson, Baker, Buckby, Baksheev, & Cosgrave, 2009).

From an epidemiological perspective, the presence of psychotic experiences in nonclinical populations may represent the phenotypic expression of the increased proneness or risk for the development of psychotic disorders. Follow up studies conducted in nonclinical adolescents and adults selected from the general population have shown that the presence of PLEs increases the future risk of transiting toward a schizophrenia-spectrum disorder (Chapman, Chapman, Raulin, & Eckblad, 1994; Gooding, Tallent, & Matts, 2005; Poulton, Caspi, Moffitt, Cannon, Murray, & Harrington, 2000; Welham et al., 2009) or predicts delusional-like experiences in adulthood (Scott, Martin, Welham, Bor, Najman, O'Callaghan et al., 2009). A continuous dose-response risk function exists between subclinical psychotic experiences and later clinical disorder (van Os et al., 2009). However, it is equally true that most of the participants who report PLEs may be experiencing a transitory state or may never progress to clinical psychotic disorder, or may develop other types of disorders (e.g., depression or substance abuse) (Dhossche, Ferdinand, van der Ende, Hofstra, & Verhulst, 2002; Hanssen, Bak, Bijl, Vollebergh, & Van Os, 2005; Verdoux, van Os, & Maurice-Tison, 1999). Specifically, between 10 and 25% of these subclinical psychotic experiences can interact synergetically or additively with other environmental factors (i.e., genetic, trauma, cannabis, urbanicity, victimization, etc.) increasing the persistence of psychotic experiences and consequently becoming abnormally persistent, clinically relevant and in need of care (Bendall, Jackson, Hulbert, & McGorry 2008; Cougnard et al., 2007; Freeman & Fowler, 2009; Kelleher, Harley, Lynch, Arseneault, Fitzpatrick, & Cannon, 2008; Kelly, O'Callaghan, Waddington, Feeney, Browne, Scully, et al., 2010; Larkin & Morrison, 2006; Morgan & Fisher 2007; Spauwen, Krabbendam, Lieb, Wittchen, & van Os, 2006; van Os, Hanssen, Bak, Bijl, & Vollebergh, 2003; van Os & Poulton, 2009). In this regard, the prompt detection of these individuals with PLEs, and subsequent implementation of prophylactic treatments in early prevention programs is of particular interest. Likewise, their study allows us to explore and improve the comprehension of the risk or vulnerability markers toward psychosis and its related disorders and offer more evidence in support of the dimensional models of psychosis.

Chapter 8- Some percentage of patients experience hallucinations that are not responsive to different classes of neuroleptic drugs and to electroconvulsive therapy. Interestingly, some nonpharmacological treatments can inhibit dopaminergic activity in the brain and produce physiological effects that are similar to those of neuroleptic medication, suggesting that these approaches may potentially be useful as a therapeutic option for medication-resistant hallucinations. Two examples are temporary hyperthermia and low-protein diets.

A temporary increase in core body temperature via external heating, such as immersion in hot water (39-40 degrees Celsius), can increase the plasma and brain level of serotonin and the plasma level of prolactin. Hyperthermia typically induces fatigue and can cause lethargy and loss of motivation. All of these changes are consistent with increased serotonergic and reduced dopaminergic activity in the brain. It is also noteworthy that cerebral serotonergic neurons, for the most part, have inhibitory projections to dopaminergic neurons.

Low-protein diets lower the plasma levels of tyrosine and phenylalanine, which are metabolic precursors of cerebral dopamine. Experiments on laboratory rats have shown that low-protein diets can lower the total concentration of dopamine in the striatum and reduce the density of dopamine D2 receptors in this brain region. Low protein diets are also known to impair the coping ability of laboratory animals in experimental models of depression such as Porsolt swim test. These changes are consistent with reduced dopaminergic activity in the brain and are similar to the effects of neuroleptic drugs. It should be noted that neuroleptics inhibit most dopamine receptors and tend to reduce dopaminergic transmission overall, although these drugs typically cause a compensatory increase in the density of D2 receptors and a temporary increase in the level of extracellular dopamine due to inhibition of presynaptic D2 receptors.

The two aforementioned treatments cannot be used on a permanent basis, but each of them can be used intermittently, for example, 30-minutes of whole-body hyperthermia per day or alternation of one week of very-low-protein diet with two weeks of a balanced diet. Although the proposed treatments are temporary, they may produce lasting changes in the dopaminergic system due to neural plasticity. Clinical effectiveness of these approaches is currently unknown. The dietary approach is likely to be safe to use in combination with pharmacotherapy, whereas hyperthermic treatments are known to be dangerous for patients taking neuroleptics.

Chapter 9- Suicide has taken lives around the world and across the centuries, and it accounts for about one million deaths annually, with devastating socioeconomic costs and consequences (Mann, 2003). It's one of the world's largest public health problems and has multiple causes in which, according to a stress-diathesis model, both genetic make up and acquired susceptibility contribute to a person's predisposition to suicidal acts in stressful situations (Mann, 2003; Wasserman, 2001). Suicide is a complex phenomenon resulting from various factors, including psychiatric, biological and environmental factors. Mental disorders (particularly depression and schizophrenia) are associated with suicide, and over 90% of suicide attempters and 60% of completed suicides have mood disorders (Beautrais et al., 1996; Shaffer et al., 1996), and between 70-95% of suicide victims have some form of diagnosable mental illness (Conwell et al., 2002; Conwell et al., 2002; American Psychiatric Association, 2003). Depression and schizophrenia, no doubt, both play a critical role in suicidal behaviour. Suicide is the leading cause of death among people with schizophrenia (Allebeck and Wistedt, 1986; Caldwell and Gottesman, 1990; Pompili et al, 2007; Pompili et al, 2008; Roy and Pompili, 2009), and people with schizophrenia have an 8.5-fold greater risk for suicide than those in the general population (Harris and Barraclough, 1997).

Nearly half of schizophrenic individuals report suicidal ideation at some point during their lives, while 20-50% have a history of suicide attempts (Breier and Pickar, 1991; Roy, 1986) and 4-13% of them eventually take their own lives (Allebeck, 1989; Drake et al., 1985; Inskip et al., 1998; Meltzer and Okayli, 1995; Miles, 1977; American Psychiatric Association, 2003).

Schizophrenia often leads to decreased social support (Drake et al., 1985; Caldwell and Gottesman, 1992; Pinikahana et al., 2003; Siris, 2001; Raymont, 2001), lower levels of occupational and daily functioning, decreased insight, and maladaptive coping skills (Raymont, 2001; Modestin et al., 1992). Additionally, people with schizophrenia have two or more of the following indicators: (a) delusions, (b) hallucinations, (c) disorganized speech, (d) grossly disorganized behavior, and (e) negative symptoms (American Psychiatric Association, 1994).

Hallucinations may be auditory, visual or tactile and may include highly idiosyncratic content (e.g., threats, suggestions, affirmations) (American Psychiatric Association, 1994; World Health Organization, 1973). Command hallucinations are a particular subtype of auditory hallucination in which the patient is instructed to "act, making a gesture or grimace to committing suicidal or homicidal acts" (Hellerstein, Frosch, & Koenigsberg, 1987, p. 219). Patients with schizophrenia may hear voices that instruct them to engage in suicidal acts or to proceed with violent acts toward others.

Command hallucinations in schizophrenic individuals may be common but often ignored by psychiatrists (Rogers, 1988). The prevalence of this symptom is reported to vary from 18-50% (Harkavy-Friedman, et al, 2003), and several studies have reported rates between 30-50% (Zisook et al., 1995; McNiel et al., 2000; Kasper et al., 1996; Rogers et al., 1990). The presence of hallucinations, especially command hallucinations, in schizophrenic patients may increase the risk of suicide.

This chapter investigates whether hallucinations may impact on suicidal behaviour in schizophrenia. We review the literature, citing the most relevant studies about the association between hallucinations and suicidal behaviour. We also report the most common indicators of treatment adherence and treatment options in people with schizophrenia having hallucinations, and we emphasize research in this field and provide clinical implications for future research.

Chapter 10- Behavioral symptoms of dementia are often more difficult to manage than consequences of cognitive impairment. They may lead to caregiver burn-out or need for institutionalization. It is important to distinguish two types of behavioral symptoms: those which occur when the patient is solitary and those which occur when the patient is interacting with others. When patients are solitary they may develop agitation or apathy; very often these symptoms alternate in the same patient. When the patients are interacting with their caregivers, they may resist their care efforts because they do not understand why they need the care. If the caregiver persists in providing care despite patient's resistiveness, the patients may defend themselves, become combative and their behavior may be called abusive. Behaviors labeled abusive are often the most difficult behaviors of nursing home residents to manage. Resistiveness to care, related to lack of understanding, depression, hallucinations and delusions, are strongly related to abusive behaviors. Presence of depressive symptoms and delusions is also related to abusive behaviors independent of resistiveness to care. Very few residents who understand others and are not depressed are abusive. Behavioral interventions preventing escalation of resistiveness to care into combative behavior and the treatment of depression can be expected to decrease or prevent abusive behavior of many nursing home residents with dementia. Therefore, antidepressants should be used initially when non-pharmacological interventions are not effective.

Chapter 11- There are currently many works that focus on the possible continuity of psychotic symptoms, that is, on the consideration of behaviors traditionally associated with schizophrenia (such as hallucinations and delusions) as not being exclusive to this condition, and being related to other alterations, and even manifesting in an attenuated form in the general population.

Many studies confirm the presence of psychotic symptoms in various psychopathological disorders (depression, dissociative disorders, posttraumatic stress disorder, etc.) (Altman, Collins, & Mundy, 1997; Dhossche, Ferdinand, van der Ende, Hostra, & Verhulst, 2002; Romme & Escher, 1996; Ohayon, 2000; Tien, 1991) and also in the general population

(Baker & Morrison, 1998; Barret & Etheridge, 1992; Bentall & Slade, 1985; Johns & van Os, 2001; Kot & Serper, 2002; Morrison, 2001; Morrison & Wells, 2003; Ohayon, 2000; Pearson et al., 2008; Serper, Dill, Chang, Kot, & Elliot, 2005; Slade & Bentall, 1988; Tien, 1991; Verdoux & van Os, 2002). Likewise, diverse laboratory investigations have shown that hallucinatory or pseudohallucinatory experiences can be generated by means of mechanisms that include suggestion, sensory deprivation, or classic conditioning (Barber & Calverley, 1964; Bryant & Mallard, 2003; Zukerman & Cohen, 1964).

In some people from the general population, this type of experience may lead to mental disorders or, contrariwise, hallucinatory experiences may become pseudohallucinatory experiences (they are not assigned the same meaning, the people disagree with their "authenticity", etc.) as time goes by.

However, in the literature, there are diverse models of continuity and the changeover in these types of experiences is not clear. Likewise, there is some debate about the mechanisms that are common to these behaviors in diverse populations (clinical and nonclinical) and their essential differences. The analysis of these aspects is the goal of this chapter.

Chapter 12- Chronic Hallucinatory Psychosis (CHP) is a disease that has long been considered in the French literature, but is neglected by the current Anglo-Saxon classification systems, which generally classify it among the atypical forms of Schizophrenia.

Various authors have described the disorder, attributing it different characteristics. In 1911 Gilbert Ballet (1985) first described CHP, which has been subsequently considered by De Clérambault (1923), Ey (1934) and Pull (1987). These Authors underlined the central nature of the hallucinatory symptoms and suggested the nosographic autonomy of the syndrome, but each hypothesised different underlying pathogenetic mechanisms and disagreed about the prognosis.

The French concept of "Psychose Hallucinatoire Chronique" is characterised by late-onset psychosis, predominantly in females, with rich and frequent hallucinations, but almost no dissociative features or negative symptoms.

We propose the definition of "Hallucinatory Disorder" (HD) in order to underline the differences between the clinical picture we observed and the psychopathological profile of Chronic Hallucinatory Psychosis proposed by the French Authors.

Auditory verbal hallucinations are the prevalent psychopathological phenomena in HD, appearing in the absence of other types of hallucinations and of thought or behavioural disorganisation.

Chapter 13- Hallucinations are perceptions in the absence of an external stimulus and are accompanied by a compelling sense of their reality. They can occur in healthy individuals but they are a diagnostic feature of several illness. The differential diagnosis includes psychiatric diseases (e.g., schizophrenia, bipolar disorder), neurologic diseases (e.g., Alzheimer disease, Parkinson's disease, Lewy Body disease), Charles Bonnet syndrome. Hallucinations may also be prominent in delirium, drug-intoxication states and drug-withdrawal states (particularly alcohol withdrawal) and may also occur as an adverse effect of medication. Hallucinations may also occur in the hypnagogic (before sleep) and hypnopompic periods (after sleep). We present an overview of current understanding of neurobiologic / pathophysiologic mechanisms for these symptoms in healthy people and in mentioned diseases.

Hallucinations are defined as false sensory perceptions that arise in the absence of an external stimulus of the relevant sensory organ and are accompanied by a compelling sense of their reality [1].

Chapter 14- Hallucinations are very dramatic behavior that today is considered to be a distinguishing characteristic of a group of serious mental disorders, as is the case of schizophrenia. Despite the seemingly bizarre nature of this type of behavior, it should not be misconstrued that hallucinations hold no functionality for the person experiencing them or that they cannot be understood through different psychological or social mechanisms (Layng & Andronis, 1984).

To study this behavior, is it not only worthwhile to analyze people that suffer from schizophrenia, it is also useful to involve people with other disorders who experience voices (such as mood, dissociative and personality disorders, and posttraumatic stress) (Altman, Collins & Mundy, 1997; Dhossche, Ferdinand, van der Ende, Hostra & Verhulst, 2002; Romme & Escher, 1989; Ohayon, 2000; Tien, 1991), or even individuals within the normal population that may have similar experiences (Baker & Morrison, 1998; Cangas, Langer & Moriana, in press; Morrison & Wells, 2003; Serper, Dill, Chang, Kot & Elliot, 2005).

In: Hallucinations: Types, Stages and Treatments
Editor: Meredith S. Payne, pp. 1-32
ISBN: 978-1-61728-275-1
© 2011 Nova Science Publishers, Inc.

Chapter 1

About the Origin of Hallucinations: From a Phenomenological, Cognitive and Neurophysiological Point of View

Viola Oertel-Knoechel[*]
Laboratory for Neurophysiology and Neuroimaging, Dept. of Psychiatry,
Goethe-University, Frankfurt, Germany

Abstract

The main interest of this chapter is the investigation of the underpinnings of hallucinations, including phenomenological descriptions (Bentall, 1990; Oertel et al., 2009), cognitive models (Frith, 1992) and neurophysiological evidence (e.g., Dierks et al., 1999; Oertel et al., 2007; Sireteanu et al., 2008). The term *hallucination* was introduced in the psychiatric literature by Esquirol (1832), who first distinguished it from other disorders of perception. Hallucinations can occur in all sensory modalities, under several conditions (e.g., sensory deprivation) and pathological processes (e.g., epilepsy, Manford & Andermann, 1998; schizophrenia, Hahlweg, 1998), but can even occur in normal individuals in non-psychiatric environments (Johns & van Os, 2001).

A certain vividness of mental imagery is generally regarded as contributing to, if not the cause of, hallucinations. We investigated the occurrence and form of appearance of hallucinations (Aggerneas, 1972) and phenomenological issues and found no evidence for a linear relationship between vividness of mental imagery and predisposition to hallucinate (Oertel et al., 2009). Studies of cognitive biases, however, showed that hallucinating individuals failed to distinguish between internal and external phenomena (Bentall et al., 1991; Van de Ven & Merckelbach, 2003).

Important findings come from functional magnetic resonance imaging *(*fMRI) studies (Dierks et al., 1999; Lennox et al., 2000; Linden et al., 2002; Shergill et al., 2004; Van de Ven et al., 2005). They detected neurological evidence for a similar processing of

---

[*] Corresponding author: Viola Oertel-Knoechel, Laboratory for Neurophysiology and Neuroimaging, Dept. of Psychiatry, Heinrich-Hoffmann-Str. 10, Goethe-University, 60528 Frankfurt; E-Mail: Viola.Oertel@kgu.de; Phone: ++49 69 6301 83780; Fax: ++49 69 6301 3833.

auditory verbal hallucinations and real auditory perception in the brain. Studies regarding the visual modality of hallucinations found associations in the visual association cortex (Silbersweig et al., 1995; Oertel et al., 2007; Sireteanu et al., 2008), but not in the primary visual area, and an association between the locations of activity within specialized cortex and the contents of visual hallucinations (ffytche et al., 1998; Oertel et al., 2007). Surprisingly, memory-related areas were found involved during schizophrenia-induced hallucinations (Oertel et al., 2007), but not when they were artificially induced, e.g., by blindfolding (Sireteanu et al., 2008).

In general, attempts to define the distinctive features of hallucinations have drawn attention to the variety of hallucinatory phenomena and the difficulty in distinguishing between these phenomena and other normal or abnormal mental states. It is proposed that individual differences in psychopathology, as well as neuropsychological and psychosocial functioning may provide further means to understand the complex and highly dynamic aspects of hallucinations specifically and schizophrenia in general.

1. Introduction

In this chapter the consideration of the phenomenological (e.g., Bentall, 1990; Oertel et al., 2009), cognitive (e.g., Frith, 1992; Frenkel et al., 1995) and neural (e.g., Dierks et al., 1999; Oertel et al., 2007; Sireteanu et al., 2008) underpinnings of the phenomenon hallucinations is framed as a multivariate problem. Many studies have focused on the perceptual aspects of hallucinations, although, besides the individual's phenomenology and its correlation to several cognitive parameters, neural substrates and underlying processing mechanisms of the brain are known to be responsible for the outcome of hallucinations. This chapter follows a new line by describing anatomical and functional brain imaging findings together with behavioural data in order to connect different models into a multivariate psychopathological model of hallucinations.

Hallucinations are among the most severe and puzzling forms of psychopathology. The term hallucination (from the Latin *alucinari* = "to wander in mind") was introduced in the psychiatric literature by Esquirol (1832), who first distinguished it from other disorders of perception. In the DSM-IV (American Psychiatric Association [APA], 1994), hallucinations are defined as "sensory perceptions that have the compelling sense of reality of a true perception but that occurs without external stimulation of the relevant sensory organ". Hallucinations also serve the psychology of perception as the classic example of sensory experience in the absence of adequate external stimuli. They differ from mental imagery by the lack of control over the sensations (David, 1994; Hahlweg, 1998). However, their form of appearance and content are comparable to perception.

Slade and Bentall (1988) agree with this definition by defining hallucinations as "any perception-like experience which occurs in the absence of an appropriate stimulus, which has the full force or impact of the corresponding actual (real) perception and is not amenable to direct and voluntary control by the affected person". The current opinion is that hallucinations result from a perceptual error based on internal processes, with no evident relationship between perception and an external stimulus.

The phenomenology of hallucinations covers elementary acoustic, optic, olfactory, gustatory or tactile perceptions, as well as complex experiences based on different sensory information. Sireteanu et al. (2008) reported a case of a subject, who had simple and elementary visual hallucinations during 3 weeks of prolonged blindfolding. The hallucinations of the subject occurred when the subject was in a quiet state, and were mostly experienced as moving in depth. The hallucinations consisted of flashes, coloured and moving patterns, and intensely acoustic and haptic perception. Sireteanu et al. (2008) described that the subject reported the sensation of being in a "dome". In this dome, sound signals and visual images seemed to occur that were beyond the subject's control. The subject reported that the images were strikingly vivid and constantly in motion with brilliant colours at the beginning of the blindfolding. During progression of the blindfolding the images seemed to become more rare and gradually lost colour. At all times, the subject of the study by Sireteanu et al. (2008) was aware that the hallucinated images had no real content. According to the descriptions, the "inner images" (the subject preferred not to refer to these images as hallucinations) were floating in the three-dimensional space in front of the inner eye and had a virtual appearance.

Further description of the content and form of appearance is coming from a case report (Oertel et al., 2007), where a schizophrenic patient reported having visual hallucinations of common objects, faces and bodies of people in his surroundings, sitting or standing in a landscape. The patient was convinced that the people he perceived were actually in the room but that no other person could perceive them. The hallucinations varied in size and colour but not in content, and the images seemed well defined (Oertel et al., 2007).

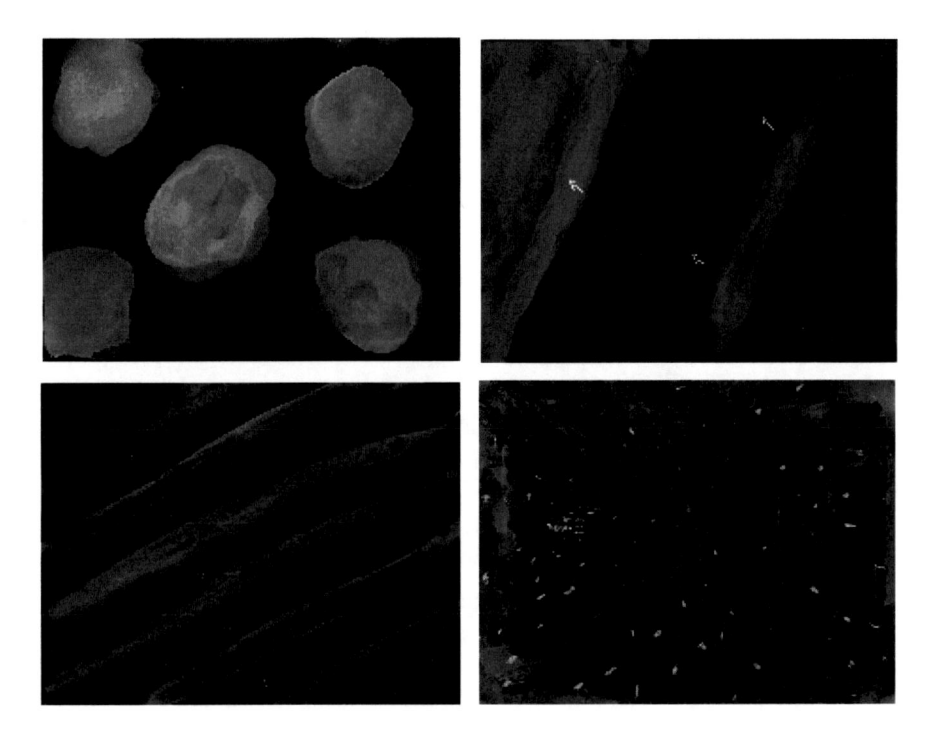

Figure 1. Examples of the perceived images, as drawn retrospectively by the subject. The upper row shows examples of elementary visual hallucinations; the lower row shows examples of less frequently experienced visual hallucinations. (Copyright© 2007: Marietta Schwarz; published with permission of the subject [Sireteanu et al., 2008; modified])

Of special interest are auditory verbal hallucinations, the perception of voices in the absence of corresponding agents in the external world. Hallucinations in other sensory modalities may also appear, but are much less prevalent. They are most common in the auditory modality (70%; Stephane et al., 2001; Verdoux and van Os, 2002), followed by the olfactory and visual (up to 32%; Bracha et al., 1989) and tactile (4%; Bracha et al., 1989) domains. Furthermore, auditory hallucinations are of special interest because they constitute an important clinical phenomenon, e.g. affecting about 60% of the patients with schizophrenia (Sartorius et al., 1978; Hahlweg, 1998). In many cases the voices cause considerable distress and anxiety because they produce derogatory comments and / or command the patients to engage in shameful, dangerous or otherwise undesirable behaviour.

In the clinical psychiatric routine, problems in investigating hallucinations occur through the fact that the persons experiencing them are, due to the underlying psychotic illness, not able to describe the form of appearance in a satisfactory way. Therefore, Oertel (2008) developed, based on the "Aggernaes criteria" (Aggernaes, 1972), a semi-structured interview to assess the psychopathology (contents, phenomenology, duration, severity and occurrence) of hallucinations in more details. This interview is meant to assess individuals who experience auditory hallucinations. The interview is divided into three categories, and the scores of the three categories will then be summed up as a total score for hallucinations. The questions along the following categories:

- 1st Category (form of appearance): clear as voices, gender, feed-back, recognizing of the voices, names, special knowledge, prognosing of the future, appearance in dreams, heard from other persons, seen as real.
- 2st Category (content): voices express emotions, voices include doubts, self protection, command voices, the appearance of hallucinations is typical/non-typical of the individual, physical manifestations, appearance in multiple sensory systems/modalities, extend in time/space, explanation of the voices regarding religion, voices are seen as real, because they appear repeatedly.
- 3st Category (Aggerneas criteria [Aggerneas, 1972]): sensation vs. ideation, relevance for the behaviour, publicness, objectivity, existence, non-voluntary, independence.

In general, there are different kinds of conditions and pathological processes usually connected with hallucinations. Hallucinations are most common in patients with schizophrenia (appear mainly in the auditory modality) and affective psychosis (Hahlweg, 1998), but also a minority of otherwise normal individuals report hallucinatory experiences (Barrett & Etheridge, 1992; Johns & van Os, 2001). In addition, hallucinatory experiences in the normal population can occur under conditions of sensory deprivation, emotional stress, religious exaltation, or great fatigue (Ohayon et al., 2000). Additionally, disturbance of sensory systems (Charles Bonnet syndrome), physiological disorders (sensory deprivation or fever) and migraine are known to be connected to hallucinatory experiences, either. Hallucinations were also reported during withdrawal from various drugs and alcohol and under the influence of hallucinogenic drugs such as LSD, mescaline and psilocybin. Some descriptions of acoustic hallucinations in dementia (Wilson et al., 2000) and epilepsy (Winawer et al., 2000; Manford & Andermann, 1998) can also be found in the literature. Bentall (1990) and Slade and Bentall (1988) suggested that hallucinations have a common origin in psychiatric patients and normal people.

Table 1. Summarized theories of origin and occurrence of hallucinations

THEORY	MAIN ARGUMENT	AUTHOR
PERCEPTUAL ABNORMALITIES		
"Perceptual error"	→ Appear in all sensory modality (mainly auditory) → Affect schizophrenic patients and others patients and healthy normals under special conditions	Barrett & Etheridge, 1992
Lack of control	Lack of control over the sensations	Mintz & Alpert, 1972; Slade, 1972
Continuum hypothesis	→ Perception → Mental imagery → Hallucinations	Bentall, 1990
Vividness of mental imagery	Relation between vivid mental images and proneness to hallucinations	Mintz & Alpert, 1972; Slade, 1972; Barrett & Etheridge, 1992
COGNITIVE THEORIES		
Cognitive deficit	Attribution bias Reality monitoring bias	Bentall, 1990; David, 1994 Brebion et al., 1997; Böcker et al., 2000; Aleman et al., 2003
Theory of mind	Self-monitoring-bias, disturbance of wilful movement	Frith, 1992
Capacity problem	of the information processing system	Kosslyn, 1994
Megacognitive processes	Attribution style, locus of control	Lyon et al., 1994; Frenkel et al., 1995; Fear et al., 1996
NEUROIMAGING STUDIES		
fMRI Similar processing	→ auditory hallucinations / real auditory perception (Heschl' gyrus, Broca' s area, Wernicke' s area)	Dierks et al. 1999; Lennox et al., 2000; Linden et al., 2002
fMRI "Cognitive Dissymmetry"	→ Disconnectivity between main brain areas (frontal, parietal, temporal) in SZ patients → Increased thalamo-cortical connectivity → Aberrant connectivity between limbic and sensory areas	Van de Ven et al., 2005 Schlösser et al., 2005 Kubicki et al., 2003
PET/fMRI Specialisation	Visual / auditory modality → visual association cortex during visual hallucinations Visual → specialized cortex / contents of hallucinations	Silbersweig et al., 1995 Kubicki et al., 2003
fMRI Arousal overload	Dopaminergic hyperactivity → damage to cholinergic projections to visual cortex	ffytche, 2005
DTI	Reduced anisotropy changes in the white matter Connection deficit between Broca's and Wernicke' area	Hubl et al., 2004, Agartz et al., 2001; Kubicki et al., 2003 Hubl et al., 2004

The quantity of the occurrence of hallucinations is a focus of research, too. Studies investigating the distribution of hallucinations in the general population yielded consistent findings showing that a considerable proportion of individuals experience hallucinations at some time in their lives (Johns & van Os, 2001). Bentall and Slade (1988) assumed that hallucinations in general have a lifetime prevalence of over 65 %. However, Tien (1991) reported a lifetime prevalence of hallucinations (not related to drugs or medical problems) of 10% for men and 15% for women. Interestingly, they reported that the overall rates were similar for visual, auditory, and tactile hallucinations.

Beside the description of the content, form of appearance and frequency of hallucinations, the question which processes are underlying the phenomenon "hallucinations" is of main interest. There exist different ways to explain hallucinations, including phenomenological descriptions, cognitive models and neurophysiological evidence. Table 1 summarizes the theories of origin and occurrence of hallucinations.

Psychological and neurobiological data suggest that hallucinations arise from a combination of both monitoring and perceptual abnormalities (Mintz & Alpert, 1972; Horowitz, 1975; Cahill & Frith, 1996; Brebion et al., 1997; Dierks et al., 1999; Behrendt, 2003). Attempts to define the distinctive features of hallucinations have drawn attention to the variety of hallucinatory phenomena and the difficulty in distinguishing between these phenomena and other normal or abnormal mental states. In sum, the present chapter deals with possible markers and an explanation for the occurrence of hallucinations in different kinds of conditions and pathological processes and their neural substrates and underlying processing mechanisms in the brain.

2. The Origin of Hallucinations: From Perception to Hallucination

2.1. The Role of Mental Imagery for the Occurrence of Hallucinations

To begin with phenomenological descriptions a number of authors have suggested that there exists a continuum from normal perceptual experiences over mental imagery to abnormal mental experiences, like hallucinations, and that hallucinations exist on a continuum ranging from relatively benign forms to pathological manifestations in schizophrenia (e.g. Bentall, 1990; Slade & Bentall, 1988).

A normal perception arises from an interaction between afferent signals and prior knowledge. Mental imagery is a perceptual experience ("seeing with the mind's eye"), that generates and manipulates mental representations in the absence of an adequate physical stimulus (Finke, 1989). It is associated with core psychological mechanisms such as perception and memory and may facilitate cognitive processes (Kosslyn, 1994). Normal mental imagery may be an example of a perception that is entirely dependent on prior knowledge. Such images are not hallucinations since we are aware that their origin is in our heads and not in the outside world. Thus, mental imagery is often believed to play a role in memory (Paivio, 1985) and motivation (McMahon, 1973). It is also commonly believed to be centrally involved in visuo-spatial reasoning and inventive or creative thought.

Vividness of mental imagery denotes the degree of perceptual detail that is experienced when mentally imagining sounds or speech, visual scenes or objects, touch, smells or tastes. Imagery vividness can be measured using a self-report questionnaire (e.g., Betts' Questionnaire of Mental Imagery; Sheehan, 1967), which probes the subjective vividness of imagery experience across different sensory dimensions. It has been proposed that increased mental imagery vividness may be associated with hallucinations, although the literature is inconsistent with respect to the role of mental imagery in hallucinations. Both constitute perceptual experiences which can occur in the absence of external stimuli, but, in contrast to hallucinations, mental images can be controlled and even stopped by the affected person (Kosslyn, 1994). Apart from that, the difference between hallucinations and mental images lies primarily in the intensity and the degree of reality similarity of the perceptual experience. Hallucinations evidently being a type of "mental image", the research tried to decode the complex "mental imagery" in order to assign hallucinations a place in the complex.

Kosslyn (1994) proposed that "imagery is a particular type of cognitive process or underlying representation that is involved in specific cognitive functions". These representations or processes are generally understood in the manner that their presence or activity can be consciously experienced as imagery in the original sense. Apart from that, it is supposed that the internal representation coincides with a certain brain state, which generates the conscious experience on the basis of stored information, not on the basis of actual sensory input. Therefore, there is an underlying brain state for imagery. If a person has the experience of *seeing with the mind's eye*, his brain state is attendant (Kosslyn, 1989).

Assuredly, imagery and perception are closely related. The purpose of imagery is to perceive optical characteristics of imaged objects. This supposes access to memory where information is stored. In addition, people are able to use imagery abilities to forecast the consequences of movements (Shepard & Metzler, 1971) and to achieve abstract learning and thinking. Sometimes the models of images are utilized to support higher-level reasoning. Through the storage of images or objects, events and faces, the matter is better preserved and can be retrieved more easily.

An interesting phenomenon is that imagery seems to use mechanisms specialized for processing in a specific sensory modality (Kosslyn, 1989). Some findings predicate that imagery selectively interferes with like-modality perception (Kosslyn, 1989). According to Formisano et al. (2002), visual perception is affected more when a visual image is received as combined with an auditory image. Investigating this interference, e.g. Goebel et al. (1998) stated that imagery uses central perceptual mechanisms. In addition, Sireteanu et al. (2008) provide detailed subjective descriptions and graphical illustrations of the progression of the experienced inner images during a longer period of visual deprivation. Throughout the deprivation period, the images did not depict specific objects or scenes, thus suggesting that they might be associated with activity in early processing stages of the central visual pathway.

The cognitive processes required to generate mental images and to analyze them are subserved by a distributed network of brain regions. Different authors examined the underlying neuronal processes of imagery and spatial analysis in several sensory modalities. The neurophysiological studies focused on a potential left hemispheric lateralisation during mental imagery tasks (Sato et al., 2004; Mazard et al., 2005), category-selective attention (Gardini et al., 2005; McGuire et al., 1996; Cohen et al., 1996; Silbersweig & Stern, 1998; Shergill et al., 2004), the potential involvement of primary / secondary brain regions

(Bunzeck et al., 2005; Ducreux et al., 2002) and the question of whether perception and imagery share similar brain areas (Slotnick et al, 2005; Jeannerod, 1994; Klein et al., 2004).

Furthermore, results from brain-damaged patients support the hypothesis that visual mental imagery and visual perception share many mechanisms. Nevertheless, both functions are not performed through identical processes (Trojano & Grossi, 1994). Perception does not require activation of information in the memory when the stimulus is not present. In contrast to perception, imagery does not require low-level processing (Kosslyn et al., 1994).

The current status of knowledge is puzzling. Some steps involved in mental imagery seem to share the same brain areas as during perceptual processes, while others seem to be more related to hallucination experiences. These results would prove the continuum-hypothesis of perception, mental imagery and hallucinations (Bentall, 1990). The next subchapter gives a survey of the current status of psychiatric literature regarding potential correlates of hallucinations and mental imagery, followed by a discussion of the current knowledge.

2.2. Findings of the Relationship between Mental Imagery and Hallucinations: From Normal Individuals to Schizophrenia

The study of imagery and its potential relation to hallucinations has not been confined to patients with a clinical diagnosis of schizophrenia. As a number of non-clinical populations report hallucinatory experiences as well (Barrett & Etheridge, 1992; Poulton et al., 2000), some authors (Mintz & Alpert, 1972; Slade, 1972) claimed that individuals who hallucinate are characterized by having very vivid images and a weak ability for distinguishing real perception from imagery. They showed higher mental imagery in hallucinating individuals and suggested that there is a capacity problem of the information processing and integrating system. In addition, Morrison et al. (2002a, b) developed a semi-structured interview to regard the connection between mental images and psychotic symptoms. 74.3 % of the subjects stated their psychotic symptoms to be dependent on their imagery ability. According to Mintz and Alpert (1972) and Slade (1972), an increase in mental imagery vividness would lead to an overload of information, which leads to an excessive demand on the information processing system. Here, a higher vividness of mental imagery is suggested to be responsible for the genesis of hallucinatory experiences.

However, several studies relying on various experimental paradigms support the understanding that vivid imagery per se does not account for reports of hallucinatory experiences (Aleman et al., 1999). In 1999, they investigated the relation between subjective and objective indices of vividness of imagery and disposition towards hallucinations in 74 college students. After assigning subjects to a high- and a low-hallucination group on the basis of scores on the *Launay Slade Hallucination Scale* (LSHS; Launay & Slade, 1981), two measurements of the vividness of mental imagery were carried out. The subjective measure was based on two subscales (visual, auditory) of the *Betts Vividness Upon Imagery* Scale (QMI; Sheehan, 1967). The objective task concerned the difference between a perceptual and an imagery condition of judgement of visual similarity of named objects. Subjects reporting hallucinatory experiences tended to show higher imagery vividness rating on the QMI than non-hallucinating subjects. It is important to note that this result could not be reconfirmed in an experimental imagery task.

More recent studies on the incidence of hallucinations in non-clinical populations have been carried out by Barrett (1993), and Barrett and Etheridge (1992). They revealed that people with hallucinations had a more vivid imagery, but no weaker control of images in comparison with people who did not experience hallucinations.

Van de Ven and Merckelbach (2003) examined a sample of undergraduate students with a task called *fantasy proneness task* and related it to measurements of vivid images and hallucinatory experiences. In the fantasy proneness task, subjects were asked to listen to "white noise" and instructed to press a button when they believed hearing a recording of Bing Crosby´s White Christmas Song without his record actually being presented. They found that participants who reported hallucinatory experiences during the White Christmas task scored higher on mental imagery and fantasy proneness compared with those who did not report such experiences. Self-reported imagery ability and fantasy proneness were strongly related. Furthermore, they found that increased reported hallucinatory experience was explained better by non-specific response bias than by increased imagery vividness (Merckelbach & Van de Ven, 2001; Van de Ven & Merckelbach, 2003).

This finding suggests that the role of mental imagery in non-clinical hallucinations is indirect, and may be associated with hallucinations via other traits or cognitive systems. Occasional reports of increased imagery vividness in relation to hallucinations (Mintz & Alpert, 1972; Morrison et al., 2002a, b) were not supported by other studies (Brett & Starker, 1977; Starker & Jolin, 1982). Several studies have suggested that vivid imagery per se does not account for reports of hallucinatory experiences (Aleman et al., 1999).

In contrast to categorical models of hallucinations that posit a qualitative difference between normal and psychotic experiences, some authors suggested that differences may be quantitative rather than qualitative (Hahlweg, 1998; Van Os, 2003) and that hallucinatory experiences are found on a continuum of clinical and non-clinical psychosis. The wider context for this hypothesis is provided by the identification of schizophrenia-like traits in the normal population, a condition that is often referred to as "schizotypy" (Claridge & Broks, 1984; Raine, 1991). Schizotypy is thus defined and identified by personality features that correspond to attenuated forms of psychotic symptoms typical of schizophrenia (Meehl, 1962, 1990). They may include perceptual aberration, magical thinking, delusional beliefs, a disposition to experience hallucinations, cognitive impairments and attentional dysfunction, and also symptoms corresponding to the negative symptoms of schizophrenia (Meehl, 1990; Lenzenweger, 1994; Van Kampen, 2006). The role of mental imagery for hallucinations in schizotypy has not been widely studied, and it seems that the association between imagery vividness and hallucinations is unclear at best (Van de Ven & Merckelbach, 2003).

Oertel et al. (2009) investigated the relationship between vividness of mental imagery and its possible relationship with the predisposition towards hallucinations across the putative psychosis continuum that includes high schizotypy participants and genetically vulnerable but unaffected participants (first-degree relatives). Vividness of mental imagery was assessed using the QMI (Sheehan, 1967), of which the items are statements regarding the imagery ability in seven different sensory modalities, the predisposition towards hallucinations was assessed using a self-administered questionnaire (RHS; Revised Hallucination Scale; Morrison et al., 2002a, b), which asks about 20 descriptions of psychotic experiences. The RHS is based on a widely used questionnaire to assess hallucination predisposition in nonclinical populations (Bentall & Slade, 1985). Some of the items are related to daydreams (Example item: "In my daydreams I can hear the sound of a tune as clearly as if I were actually listening to it"; Morrison et al., 2002a, b) while others refer to psychotic experiences (Example item: "I can hear the sound of my thoughts as clearly as spoken voices"; Morrison et al., 2002a, b). A high score on the RHS indicates an increased predisposition towards hallucinations.

Overall, the study by Oertel et al. (2009) suggested higher mental imagery vividness (QMI [Sheehan, 1967]) in first-degree relatives, high-schizotypy controls and patients, than in low-schizotypy controls. However, vividness of mental imagery was independent from predisposition towards hallucinations and cognitive test performance scores in all subject groups (view figure 2 for results of the RHS scores in Oertel et al. [2009]).

In conclusion, Oertel et al. (2009) suggested that, in contrast to previous studies (Barrett, 1993; Morrison et al., 2002a), imagery proneness exists independently of the actual presence of hallucinations. These results replicate previous studies (Brett & Starker, 1977; Starker & Jolin, 1982; Sack et al., 2005), and further support the hypothesis of an independence of the vividness of mental imagery and hallucination experiences.

Other studies investigating a possible connection between hallucinations and mental imagery in schizophrenic patients in contrast to healthy controls showed no overall consistence regarding the question of a proneness towards vivid mental imagery directly connected to hallucinations in this patient group. Some authors (Mintz & Alpert, 1972; Böcker et al., 2000) tested the hypothesis that hallucinations in schizophrenia are characterized by a tendency to perception-like internally generated experiences and a weak ability to distinguish real perception from imagery (*reality discrimination failure*). Thirteen hallucinating, nineteen non-hallucinating SZ patients and fourteen controls were tested with multiple tests of perception and vividness of mental imagery in the auditory and visual modalities by Böcker et al. (2000). They implicated that the hallucinating patients showed a higher level of vividness of mental imagery, especially in the auditory modality, in comparison with healthy participants. However, they found no group differences of perceptual acuity.

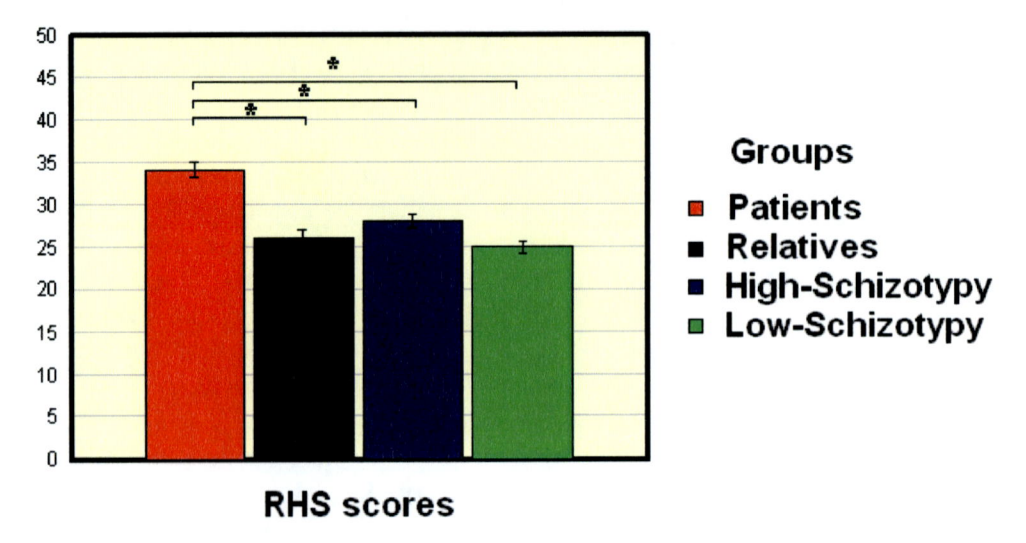

Figure 2. Results of the RHS scores in 4 different subject groups (Schizophrenia patients, first-degree relatives, high-schizotypy controls, low-schizotypy controls); modified version of the figure by Oertel et al. (2009)

It is important to note that Aleman et al. (2003), Chandiramani and Varma (1987) and Brebion et al. (1997) could not find any difference in the imagery ability between non-hallucinating, hallucinating schizophrenic patients and healthy control subjects. They suggested that there is no stable disposition towards abnormal mental imagery associated with hallucinations. This finding is consistent with Sack et al. (2005), who showed an independence of vividness of mental imagery and the predisposition towards hallucinations. Furthermore, Bentall and Slade (1985) used a signal detection task and suggested that, if hallucinatory experiences were related to vivid mental imagery, participants reporting such experiences would perform poorly on signal-detection tasks due to a decrease of sensitivity for their scores on an instrument measuring the predisposition towards hallucinating (Launay & Slade, 1981). The authors replicated other findings that imagery is *not* more vivid in hallucinatory SZ patients.

2.3. Mental Imagery and Hallucinations: Summary

The theories about mental imagery and a possible failure or increase in imagery abilities in hallucinating individuals are used as a way to find explanations for the rise of hallucinations. In sum, the involvement of mental imagery in hallucinations has proven to be a controversial issue. The difference between mental imagery and hallucinations is defined by the affected person itself, convinced that the phenomenon is occurring outside, in the real world. This lack of control contributes to the pathophysiology of the symptom. Hallucinations and mental imagery seem to have no clear boundary between them and maybe the difference lies mainly in the intensity and degree of reality similarity. Therefore, several authors propose a high connectivity between the vividness of mental imagery and the predisposition towards hallucinations (e.g. Mintz and Albert, 1972; Slade, 1972), while others could not find any connection between the two phenomena (Brett & Starker, 1977; Starker & Jolin, 1982; Sack et al, 2005; Oertel et al., 2009).

The inconsistent results regarding the connectivity between mental imagery and hallucinations could be due to the fact that most of the authors used self-administered questionnaires. Thus, the selection of the participants is not sufficient. So, some studies examined hallucinating vs. non-hallucinating individuals, while others compared hallucinating patients with normal controls etc.

Per se, it is not yet clear, which status vividness of mental imagery has in SZ patients. If vividness of mental imagery is not a cause of or connected with hallucinations, the question is to what kind of function mental imagery is related in such individuals. Mental imagery may not be directly related to hallucinations, but may be a general characteristic of pathological phenomena and disturbances, like schizophrenia (Sack et al., 2005). However, the hypothesis that an increased vividness of mental imagery is directly related to an increased tendency towards hallucinations, can be refuted.

3. The Origin of Hallucinations: From a Metacognitive and Cognitive Perspective

The cognitive theories are related to the knowledge of a deficit in the neurotransmitter-system of schizophrenic patients, the psychiatric patient group with the highest quantity of hallucinations. There is the assumption that the dopamine system is responsible for distinguishing important from non-important information. If there is an arousal overload, the system fails and leads to non-sensible associations (hallucinations). In this category of theories, hallucinations seem to occur because of an overload of information (drugs, neurotransmitter disturbance, epilepsy). What we know from schizophrenic patients is that they seem to suffer from a connectivity damage, which makes them unable to integrate incoming information into a whole (Uhlhaas et al., 2006). According to these underlying biological deficits, specific cognitive deficits have recently been linked to psychotic phenomena, including hallucinations and disorganized speech. The content of hallucinations is based on memory contents, and an overload or redundancy of sensory information leads to a lack of control over the memory-related information.

The *theory of mind* (Frith, 1992) sees a disturbance of the attribution of mind phenomena to exterior sources, followed by a disturbance of the attribution of mind phenomena to interior sources (*self monitoring*) and by a disturbance of wilful movement (*agency*), which could be responsible for the pathophysiology of hallucinations. Overall, hallucinating individuals may suffer from a cognitive deficit that prevents several memory contents to be formed into a whole.

The most common opinion is that hallucinations are caused by a damage that makes hallucinating individuals view internally generated information as coming from an external source. This deficit can be described as a loss of control by the mind which is known as *reality monitoring or attributing bias* (Bentall, 1990; David, 1994; Slade, 1994). The ability to distinguish between internal and external phenomena may be affected (Bentall et al., 1991). Neuroimaging studies showed increased activity of language production, motor and perception areas during the occurrence of positive symptoms (Dierks et al., 1999; Lennox et al., 2000; Van de Ven et al., 2005), which provides some support for the notion of vividly perceived inner processes misattributed to an external agent. This bias can be seen as a lack of control over the thoughts and the mind.

Specifically, some theoretical models posit that the occurrence of delusions and paranoid ideation are related to both bottom up deficits of source monitoring (i.e. deficient awareness of one's own actions and thoughts) (Frenkel et al., 1995) and metacognitive processes such as externalising locus of control and attribution style (Fear et al., 1996; Lyon et al., 1994). Therefore psychological models of psychotic symptoms have focused on cognitive biases, including the propensity of people to assume either external or internal causes for their perceptions and actions, termed locus of control (Rotter, 1966). A possible association between the subjective cognitive dysfunction and the predisposition to hallucinations would support cognitive deficit models of psychotic symptoms.

3.1. Toward a Metacognitive Model of Hallucinations

Locus of control refers to the extent to which individuals believe that they can control events that affect them. One's "locus" can either be internal, meaning the person believes that they control their life, or external, meaning they believe that their environment, some higher power, or other people control their decisions and their life (Zimbardo, 1985). Lefcourt (1980) extended the concept of locus of control to be a general personal disposition, and Bandura (1982) suggested that control orientation is relevant for the individual perception of the effect of one's own behaviour on the personal environment.

Studies investigating cognitive deficits and metacognitive biases and their potential relationship to psychotic symptoms, especially hallucinations and delusions, have often been done. For example, Baker and Morrison (1998) and Stirling et al. (1998) examined attributional bias and metacognitive beliefs in patients experiencing auditory hallucinations, and indicated that hallucinating patients misattributed internal events to an external source. Stirling et al. (1998) further investigated the self-monitoring hypothesis of hallucinations. They showed that patients with a history of hallucinations had greater difficulty than healthy controls with self-monitoring tests. The results were independent of neuropsychological or general cognitive function. These results offer considerable support to cognitive bias models of auditory hallucinations and delusions (Bentall & Slade, 1985; Stirling et al., 1998). Bentall (1989) found that psychotic patients, as compared with healthy controls, made more external attributions for negative events, and internal attributions for positive events.

Furthermore, links between locus of control and psychotic symptoms have been proposed by several investigators (Frenkel et al., 1995; Cromwell et al., 1961; Harrow & Ferrante, 1969; Cash & Stack, 1973; Varkey & Sathyavathi, 1984; Friedman et al., 1985-86). Ball et al. (2008) investigated the behaviour in depressive patients and found that these patients made more internal attributions for negative events in acute episodes. This effect disappeared after remission, which supports the view that these biases are not results of enduring cognitive deficits. Lasar (1997) found a constant external control orientation in SZ patients, which correlated with hallucinations. Furthermore, it has been proposed (Bentall & Fernyhough, 2008) that delusions and hallucinations, impressions without real stimulus, share similar mechanisms.

Oertel-Knöchel et al. (submitted) investigated the locus of control and its possible association to both hallucinations and delusions with individuals from the schizophrenia spectrum (schizophrenic patients, relatives and high schizotypy controls), because of the increasing evidence that at least hallucinations are quantitative phenomena (Van Os, 2003; Oertel et al., 2009). They investigated the control orientation (Rotter, 1966), using the German version of the Competence and Control Beliefs Scale (CCBS; German version: Krampen, 1991), the subjective cognitive dysfunction with the Eppendorf Schizophrenia Inventory (ESI; Mass, 2000) and the predisposition toward hallucinations (Revised Hallucination Scale [RHS], Morrison et al., 2002a, b), all with self-reported scales. The Competence and Control Beliefs Scale (CCBS; Krampen, 1991) is a 32-item self-report measure that was designed to evaluate the behaviour regarding the control and power orientation (locus of control; Rotter, 1966).

The study by Oertel-Knöchel et al. (submitted) showed that the control orientation and cognitive dysfunctions shared a common factor which predicts hallucinations measured with the PANSS (positive and negative symptom scale; Kay et al., 1987). They concluded that there is a general subjective cognitive dysfunction in the sense of dysfunctional thinking rather impairments in specific domains in hallucinating individuals.

3.2. Cognitive Theories: Summary

The study by Oertel-Knöchel et al. (submitted) showed that the control orientation seemed to be independent from subjective cognitive-perceptual deficits and the predisposition towards hallucinations. Moreover, the lack of a direct association with hallucinations suggests that a direct impact of the control orientation on the reality monitoring system, as supposed by Horowitz (1975), Cahill and Frith (1996) and others, is doubtful. One possible model to explain the lack of correlation between control orientation and hallucinations is that external locus of control is a trait marker of the schizophrenia spectrum but that other factors-like auditory uncertainty and deviant perception-have to be present in addition for hallucinations to arise. The tested model by Oertel-Knöchel et al. (submitted) indicates that subjective cognitive dysfunction and the external control orientation jointly explain some of the variance of hallucination scores.

The current knowledge provides evidence that hallucinations arise from a deficit in processing and integrating information, which is not per se related to imagery abilities. Hallucinations have been suggested to result from an increased influence of top-down sensory expectations on conscious perception. This would imply a new way of explaining hallucinations.

4. The Origin of Hallucinations: Neurophysiological Evidence

Beside phenomenological and cognitive approaches to hallucinations, neuroimaging studies concentrated on certain brain abnormalities and cognitive deficits which are associated with hallucinations (Whalley, 2005). The main multivariate approach for the analysis of functional imaging data sets of hallucinating individuals is the localisation of deficits in the auditory perception and processing brain areas. Analysis tools with methods for measuring functional and anatomical connectivity (e.g. diffusion tensor imaging) and behavioural data sets were combined in order to better understand the role functional and anatomical connections between sensory cortex and higher-order areas play in hallucinations.

Important findings of underlying processes during hallucinations come from fMRI-studies (Dierks et al., 1999; Lennox et al., 2000; Linden et al., 2002; Weiss & Heckers, 1999; Shergill et al., 2004; Van de Ven et al., 2005), who reported the auditory cortex, the limbic system and language areas, both motor and sensory, to be active during auditory hallucinations. In addition, during auditory hallucinations of patients with schizophrenia, they identified several brain areas involved in speech processing (Broca's area), for the encoding of speech (Wernicke's area), and for the processing of auditory stimuli (primary and higher level auditory areas) as active. This neurological pattern showed evidence for a similar processing of auditory verbal hallucinations and real auditory perception in the brain. Other studies (e.g. Van de Ven et al., 2005) found disconnectivity between main brain areas (frontal, parietal and temporal) during functional tasks in schizophrenic patients. Schlösser et al. (2005) analysed a group of schizophrenic patients and identified a disturbance of fronto-striato-thalamo-cortical circuits, especially an increased thalamo-cortical connectivity (cortical dissymmetry). Furthermore, Hoffmann et al. (1999) stimulated temporal brain regions of a small patient group in a repetitive magnetic-stimulation study and could influence the frequency and gravity of hallucinations.

Moreover, a number of structural imaging studies revealed decreased amounts of gray matter of individuals experiencing hallucinations in the left primary auditory cortex and superior temporal gyrus, which are important for complex analyses of auditory signals (e.g., language, object identity). Findings in a work by Oertel-Knöchel et al. (submitted) showed that a decrease of lateralisation of language areas is correlated with the severity of symptoms. Moreover, several studies reported that reductions in left HG volume correlated with hallucinations and delusions (Levitan et al., 1999; Sumich et al., 2005). Kircher et al. (2004) found that altered interaction between regions within the superior temporal gyrus and across hemispheres was in part responsible for language-mediated cognitive and psychopathological symptoms in schizophrenia. These structural changes are correlated with the presence and severity of auditory hallucinations. Other brain areas are known to be involved in hallucination processing as well. Anatomical changes may underlie the further detected functional connectivity abnormalities and contribute to the experience of positive symptoms like hallucinations. However, the exact relation between structure and hallucinations remains to be elucidated.

Furthermore, DTI (diffusion tensor imaging; Basser et al., 1994) that investigated auditory hallucinations showed controversial issues. Agartz et al. (2001) and Kubicki et al. (2003) showed a reduced anisotropy (anisotropy means the directionality of the water diffusion; the amount of anisotropy correlates with the directionality and the coherence of the fibre tracts in schizophrenic patients), whereas others (Lim & Helpern, 2002) could not find any difference in the anisotropy of patients compared with controls. Hubl et al. (2004) showed that there are changes in the white matter of the brain, in those parts which are known to be involved in auditory processing. These changes in the white matter could lead to abnormal activation of external stimuli. Hubl et al. (2004) suggested that these results contribute to the assumption that patients with schizophrenia are not able to distinguish between self-generated thoughts and external stimulation. At this point it may be possible to connect cognitive models of hallucinations with neurophysiological findings.

The study of several markers and their potential relation to hallucinations was not confined to patients with a clinical diagnosis of a psychiatric illness, because a substantial minority of non-clinical population report hallucinatory experiences as well (Poulton, 2000). While traditional models posit a qualitative difference between normal and psychotic experience, van Os (2003) suggested that the differences may be quantitative rather than qualitative. Such a concept of a "continuum" of hallucinations may challenge the view of hallucinations as a homogeneous disease entity.

However, beside the investigation of auditory hallucinations, several studies of visual hallucinations were done, although, in general, they have rarely been investigated so far. Most studies of visual hallucinations are reports of only a few, sometimes only one cases, so that the methodological issue has to be seen as critical. Inspite of that, we will describe two cases of visual hallucinations in this chapter-one schizophrenic patient, one blindfolded subject - in order to provide information about activation patterns during visual hallucinations and to compare them with those of auditory hallucinations. The activity pattern during visual stimulation and visual hallucination was compared in order to identify identical and different brain areas involved in the processing of the brain.

4.1. Functional Imaging of Visual Hallucinations

The neuronal mechanisms underlying visual hallucinations are still under debate. Visual hallucinations can be defined as involuntary images in the absence of sensory input. Visual hallucinations per se can be classified into simple and complex hallucinations. Simple hallucinations mostly consist of dots, lines, shapes and moving patterns. Complex hallucinations include the appearance of other people, animals and more rarely objects like cars or tables (Collerton et al., 2005). Merabet et al. (2004) reported both simple and complex visual hallucinations in ten out of thirteen subjects after 1-2 days of visual deprivation. Manford & Andermann (1998) classified the different types of complex hallucinations and suggested that "perturbations of a distributed matrix may explain the production of similar, complex mental phenomena by relatively blunt insults at disparate sites" (Manford & Andermann, 1998).

Many authors suggest that visual imagery and perception share similar sources (Farah, 1988; Kosslyn et al., 1997) and activations in the visual cortex have been reported during mental imagery (Kosslyn et al. 1997; Goebel et al., 1998). Oertel et al. (2007) suggested that the network of cortical areas involved in the voluntary generation of mental images is different from that related to the spontaneously occurring visual hallucinations. However, the relationship between visual hallucinations and mental imagery has not been investigated so far. Both phenomena share a neural substrate in early cortical areas on the ventral visual pathway, in some cases including area V1 (e.g. Meng et al., 2005; Komatsu, 2006; Muckli et al., 2005). Schultz and Melzack (1991) proposed that a lack of sensory input causes the release of stored images by disinhibition. In addition, Manford & Andermann (1998) suggested that defective visual input might result in hallucinations through an abnormal cortical release phenomenon.

ffytche and Howard (1999) classified the visual hallucinations and illusions secondary to degenerative eye diseases and observed remarkabe stereotyped experiences. ffytche and Howard (1999) suggested that visual loss can lead to both positive and negative perceptual disorders. Burke (2002) suggested that sensory deprivation might lead to an increase in the excitability of deafferented neurones in the visual cortex, which in turn result in an increased spontaneous activity. Collerton et al. (2005) developed the so-called Perception and Attention Deficit model (PAD) and assumed that impaired attentional binding and deficits in visual object perception cause the occurrence of complex visual hallucinations. They further suggested that these deficits may be based on disturbances in a lateral frontal cortex– ventral visual stream system.

In general, visual perception without adequate visual stimulation can occur in everyday life: visual phantoms were described for the normally occurring phenomenon of filling-in. And illusory perception of apparently moving stimuli is perceived along the illusory movement trace, in the absence of an actual stimulus. For example, flashes of light, called phosphenes, can be induced by mechanical, electrical or magnetic stimulation of the retina or the brain. The appearance of phosphenes depends on the stimulated location (Marg & Rudiak, 1994; Kammer, 1999); although they might appear in different colours, they are usually amorphous, but can develop into geometric patterns. Patients suffering from chronic migraineous headaches described migraine fortification spectra and scotomata. The percepts occurring during a migraine aura are usually black and white. They have specific geometric appearances, called 'fortification spectra', and they show a specific evolution in time, suggesting that they might be related to biochemical changes which invade portions of the topographically organized visual cortical areas (Lauritzen, 1994; Goadsby & Silberstein 1997; Spierings, 2004). Subjects with neurodevelopmental disorders like strabismic and anisometropic amblyopia (Barrett et al., 2003; Bäumer & Sireteanu, 2006; Sireteanu et al., 2007a; Sireteanu et al., 2007b) experience non-veridical visual percepts, consisting of idiosyncratic, moving and coloured distortions of the viewed images. They may be related to the prolonged disuse of the cortical structures connected to this eye.

The most prominent examples of non-veridical visual percepts are the visual hallucinations. Visual hallucinations in general can occur in a wide range of neurological and psychiatric diseases such as schizophrenia, narcolepsy, dementia with Lewy bodies, and can also be induced by hallucinogenic drugs or by pharmacological treatment (Slade & Bentall, 1988; Ohayon, 2000). In Charles Bonnet syndrome, which affects mostly healthy elderly persons, visual hallucinations are associated with blindness and social isolation (Schultz & Melzack, 1991). Visual hallucinations have also been reported during prolonged blindfolding in healthy subjects (Merabet et al., 2004; Sireteanu et al., 2008).

Neurophysiological studies regarding the visual modality of the hallucinations are rarely done. A positron emissions tomography study (Silbersweig et al, 1995) of a schizophrenic patient, with both visual and auditory hallucinations, found activation in the visual association cortex, but not in the primary visual area. An association between the location of activity within specialized cortex and the contents of visual hallucinations has been observed for patients with Charles Bonnet syndrome (Ffytche et al., 1998). Trojano et al. (2004) found - during the appearance of visual hallucinations - a prominent prefrontal activity, which reflects the active ideation. Possible pathophysiological mechanisms include dopaminergic hyperactivity in the mesolimbic pathway, which might also explain the common phenomenon of L-dopa-induced hallucinations in Parkinson's disease, damage to cholinergic projections to visual cortex (ffytche, 2005) and aberrant connectivity between limbic and sensory areas (Kubicki et al., 2003).

We will describe two interesting case reports of individuals experiencing visual hallucinations in more detail: a blindfolded subject and a schizophrenic patient. Both were the first fMRI studies to reveal the direct neural correlates in their fields. The visual percept experienced during blindfolding differs in several respects from the clinically experienced visual hallucinations. Patients with schizophrenia or under pharmacological influence usually do not distinguish between real images and those experienced during a hallucinatory episode; this is not the case with individuals under sensory deprivation. Therefore, terms like 'pseudohallucinations' or 'entoptic phenomena' (Tyler, 1978) might be more appropriate to describe their perceptual experience. However, since the subjective percepts occurring during prolonged blindfolding were already referred to as 'hallucinations' in the literature (Merabet et al. 2004; Sireteanu et al., 2008), we opted to use this term throughout this chapter.

4.1.1. Functional imaging of visual hallucinations in a patient with schizophrenia

Oertel et al. (2007) investigated a 27-year-old, right-handed male outpatient with paranoid schizophrenia (295.30 according to DSM-IV criteria; American Psychiatric Association, 1994). Their study provides evidence for the involvement of visual, attention (superior parietal lobule, precuneus) and memory-related (posterior cingulate, hippocampus) areas in the generation or experience of visual hallucinations in schizophrenia. Sensory cortex activity might underlie the vividness and subjective reality of hallucinations (Dierks et al., 1999). However, in contrast to the primary auditory cortex activation found by Dierks et al. (1999) for auditory hallucinations, they did not observe activation in primary visual areas.

Higher visual areas were activated in both hemispheres in Oertel et al.'s study (2007; view figure 3). The activation of higher visual areas during the patient's hallucinations of objects, faces and bodies corresponded to that commonly reported for visual stimulation with comparable material (view figure 4 for examples). They used retinotopic polar mapping, MT-mapping and a category localiser in order to identify primary and higher visual areas.

A previous positron emission tomography study (Silbersweig et al., 1995) of a schizophrenia patient, with both visual and auditory hallucinations, also found activation in visual association cortex. However, this study discovers category-selective higher visual areas and thus did not address the issue of content-specificity. The findings of Oertel et al. (2007) also conform to studies of visual hallucinations in Parkinson's disease (Oishi et al., 2005) and Charles Bonnet syndrome (ffytche et al., 1998). Oishi et al. (2005) used single photon emission tomography (SPECT) and found a hyperperfusion in the right superior and middle temporal gyri, which they related to the role of these regions in visual object recognition.

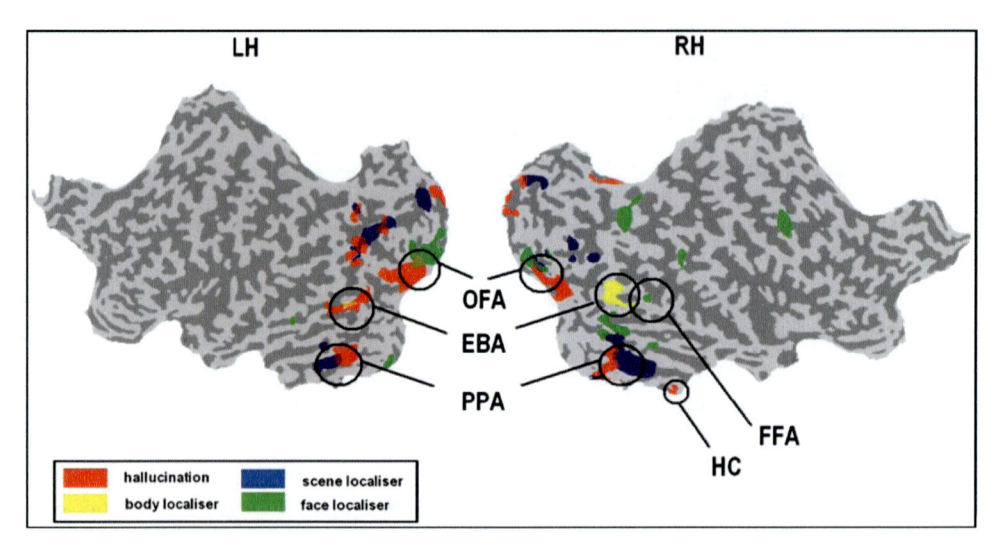

Figure 3. Cortical activation maps (displayed on a flatmap of the patient's anatomy) of a schizophrenia patient during a hallucination button press condition and a localiser condition. From left to right: (LH) flatmap of the patient's left hemisphere with the frontal pole pointing to the left, (RH) flatmap of the patient's right hemisphere with the frontal pole pointing to the right. Colour code (RGB system): red=hallucination button press, yellow=body localiser condition, blue=scene localiser condition, green=face localiser condition. OFA=occipital face area, FFA=fusiform face area, PPA=parahippocampal place area, EBA=extrastriate body area, HC=hippocampus. Note that some activated clusters were not captured by the flatmap (Oertel et al., 2007)

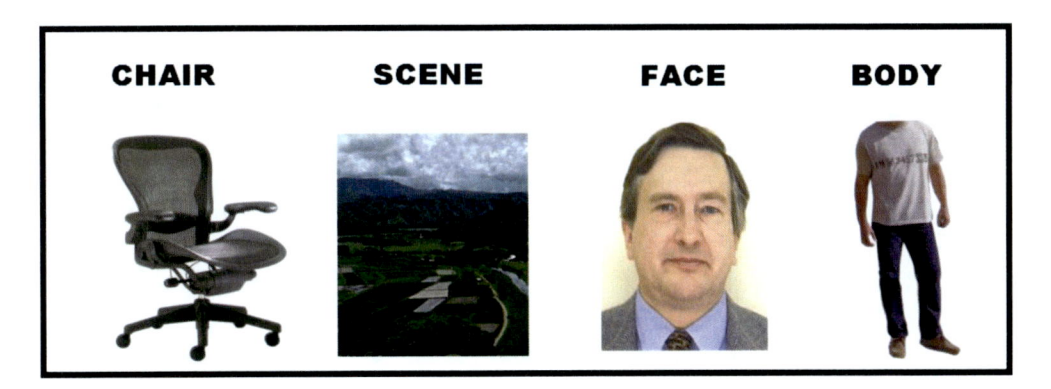

Figure 4. Examples of possible localiser for different visual areas

However, other studies did not report activity of memory-related areas, which suggests that the neural mechanisms underlying hallucinations in schizophrenia are at least partly distinct from those operational in cortical deafferentation (e.g. ffytche et al., 1998). The activation pattern during hallucinations was different from that commonly found in studies of visual imagery, where prominent prefrontal activity reflects active ideation (Trojano et al., 2004). In contrast to imagery, hallucinations are not under the subject's control, which might explain the absence of prefrontal activity in the study by Oertel et al. (2007).

4.1.2. Functional neuroimaging of visual hallucinations during prolonged blindfolding

Sireteanu et al. (2008) investigated the visual percepts and the associated brain activity in a 37-year-old healthy female subject who developed visual hallucinations during three weeks of blindfolding, and then compared this activity with the cortical activity associated with mental imagery of the same patterns. They found neural activity related to hallucinations in extrastriate occipital, posterior parietal, and several prefrontal regions. In contrast, mental imagery of the same percepts led to activation in prefrontal, but not in posterior, parietal, and occipital regions.

These results suggest that deprivation-induced hallucinations result from increased excitability of extrastriate visual areas, while mentally induced imagery involves active read-out under the volitional control of prefrontal structures. The ventral pathway is known to be responsible for processing of visual features like depth, colour, and motion. Sensory cortex activity might underlie the vividness and subjective reality of hallucinations (Dierks et al., 1999). Muckli et al. (2006) found that extrastriate areas on the ventral visual pathway (V2 and VP) show occasional hyperactivation in adult amblyopia. Interestingly, the same areas are the first to become active at the onset of a scintillating migraineous aura (Hadjikhani et al. 2001). These areas are especially sensitive to luminance and motion contrast (Tootell et al., 1997) and show increased activity in connection to illusory contours (Mendola et al., 1999). Extrastriate areas on the ventral visual pathway might prove to be especially prone to respond with aberrant neuronal firing to sensory or metabolic imbalance.

Apart from Dierks et al. (1999), who found primary cortex activation for auditory hallucinations, but in accordance with ffytche et al, (1998) and Silbersweig et al. (1995) for visual hallucinations, Sireteanu et al. (2008) and Oertel et al. (2007) did not observe hallucination-related activation in the primary visual area (V1), but activation of secondary and higher visual areas of the ventral pathway during simple and complex visual hallucinations.

In contrast to Oertel et al. (2007), who reported hippocampal activity during the occurrence of visual hallucinations in schizophrenia, Sireteanu et al. (2008) and ffytche et al. (1998) did not observe hallucination-related activity in memory areas for a blindfolded and a Charles Bonnet syndrome subject. The neural mechanisms underlying visual hallucinations in schizophrenia may be distinct from those activated in cortical deafferentation.

The finding of superior parietal lobule activation during blindfolding-induced visual hallucinations could have been due to increased spatial attention for the hallucinated images, or to the activation of an eye-movement network - as the subject was likely to scan her percepts. During mental imagery, no evidence for superior parietal activation was found. The higher activations in prefrontal areas during mental imagery than those during hallucinations may reflect a stronger top-down control in voluntary generation of mental images (Trojano et al., 2004). In contrast, during hallucinations, visual images emerge spontaneously, without voluntary top-down control of prefrontal areas.

We have to consider that a possible origin of visual sensations occuring in the absence of light stimulation may be due to spontaneous fluctuations in the dark-adapted retinal cells. Under normal circumstances, most of the random fluctuations generated within the retinal circuits do not reach the level of conscious perception, because they are filtered out through a retinal negative feedback system. Lack of retinal inhibition might increase the probability of occurrence of phosphenes (Cervetto et al., 2007). ffytche and Howard (1999) suggested that a similar process might arise in the deafferented cortical cells during prolonged visual deprivation (ffytche & Howard, 1999). Boroojerdi et al. (2000) reported that enhanced excitability in the visual cortex was described already after 45 minutes of light deprivation in normal subjects. The transient increase in visual cortical excitability after blindfolding is followed by a sustained decrease in excitability that quickly returns to baseline levels after re-exposure to light (Pitskel et al., 2007).

The descriptions of the visual hallucinations experienced during prolonged blindfolding, as well as their cortical localisation, place them somewhere between the hallucinations described by sufferers of the Charles Bonnet syndrome, the spatial distortions experienced in the chronically suppressed eyes of amblyopic subjects, and the visual phantoms experienced by healthy subjects in the absence of sensory stimulation. Together, they might reflect the constructive nature of the human brain.

4.2. Summary of the Neurophysiological Findings

The last chapter summarized studies which identified neural correlates of dysfunctional sensory processing that contribute to the development of hallucinations. Especially functional magnetic resonance imaging (fMRI) is now being used routinely to measure variations in the level of brain activity, with a spatial resolution of several millimetres and a temporal resolution of several seconds. This technological advance is enabling a new area of research, namely of the relationship between brain and behaviour in humans. By combining introspective reports with this technique, new insights into the functioning of the mind are possible.

Important findings of underlying processes during hallucinations come from fMRI-studies (Dierks et al., 1999; Lennox et al., 2000; Linden et al., 2002; Weiss and Heckers, 1999; Shergill et al., 2004; Van de Ven et al., 2005), detecting activity of the auditory cortex, the limbic system and language areas, both motor and sensory, to be active during auditory hallucinations. These detected neurological patterns showed evidence for a similar processing of auditory verbal hallucinations and real auditory perception in the brain.

Although it is not possible to infer patterns of lateralisation of hallucination-related activity from a single case, the findings of Oertel et al. (2007) and Sireteanu et al. (2008) about bilateral activation of sensory cortex conforms to the recent finding that sensory cortex activity related to auditory hallucinations is bilateral at least in some patients (Van de Ven et al., 2005). Interesting findings from a case report (Oertel et al.'s study, 2007) suggest that both limbic areas involved in retrieval from long-term memory and category-specific visual areas contribute to the generation of visual hallucinations in schizophrenia. Possible pathophysiological mechanisms include dopaminergic hyperactivity in the mesolimbic pathway, which might also explain the common phenomenon of L-dopa-induced hallucinations in Parkinson's disease, damage to cholinergic projections to visual cortex (ffytche, 2005) and aberrant connectivity between limbic and sensory areas (Kubicki et al., 2003). Furthermore, the findings of Sireteanu et al. (2008) support the assumption that blindfolding enhances the excitability of the deafferented, unimodal visual areas on the ventral visual pathway, and of regions in the parietal and frontal cortex involved in the control of visual attention.

We believe that these case reports are of general interest in a field where studies in larger samples cannot be easily performed. We have been screening patients with hallucinations on fMRI for years now, and this was the first schizophrenia patient with visual hallucinations who could be scanned. This seems to be of interest to a general medical audience because hallucinations are not confined to neuropsychiatric disorders but also occur in a number of medical conditions, i.e. sensory deprivation (toxic or metabolic, for example).

Controversial findings, regarding associations of reduced anisotropy to auditory hallucinations, were made through DTI-studies (Agartz et al., 2001; Kubicki et al., 2003; Rotarska-Jagiela et al., in press). Anatomical changes in general may underlie these functional connectivity abnormalities and contribute to the experience of positive symptoms. For example, several studies reported that reductions in left HG volume correlated with hallucinations and delusions (Gaser et al., 2004; Levitan et al., 1999; Sumich et al., 2005).

The results of the imaging parts of this chapter suggest several lines of future directions in research. Why do not all hallucinating patients show primary (sensory) cortex activity? Is it possible that such activity is associated with the phenomenological content of the hallucinations? Several studies have shown that higher-order, but not primary cortices are active during auditory mental imagery in healthy controls and non-hallucinating patients. On a different level, it is not well understood in what sense functional and anatomical connections between sensory cortex and higher-order areas play a role in hallucinations. Combining analysis tools with methods for measuring functional and anatomical connectivity (e.g. DTI) will likely be the path to answering these questions. We would suggest that it is of crucial conceptual importance to study hallucinations with functional imaging in order to determine their relationship with non-psychotic hallucinations, and with hallucinations in other sensory modalities. This method also demonstrates the power of functional imaging as a "window into the patient's mind".

Conclusion

In sum, the contents of the present chapter allow a number of conclusions regarding dysfunctional processes causing hallucinations. Why do hallucinations occur? This is a question which can be approached from different points of view, and ultimately these approaches will have to be unified. At the moment, some evidence exists from phenomenological, cognitive and neurophysiological approaches, albeit without a clear connection between the different manners of data collection. The goal of this chapter was to combine different approaches of investigation into one model to explain hallucinations.

From a neurophysiological point of view, neuroimaging studies showed increased activity of language production, motor and perception areas during the occurrence of positive symptoms (Dierks et al., 1999; Lennox et al., 2000; van de Ven et al., 2005), which provides some support for the notion of vividly perceived inner processes misattributed to an external agent. Therefore, findings from self-administered questionnaires were shown together with objective measurements of potential neural deficits on functional and structural imaging data, regarding the visual and the auditory modality. We summarized investigations of phenomenological and cognitive correlates of hallucinations. Results from different clinical scales which assess attribution bias and the personality structure and their relation to hallucinations were also reported.

It is proposed that individual differences in psychopathology, as well as neuropsychological and psychosocial functioning may provide further means to understand the complex and highly dynamic aspects of hallucinations. Providing associations between different models explaining hallucinations allows new insights into the mental imagery debate and the dysfunctional connectivity pattern known to be responsible for symptoms like hallucinations. However, no evidence was found for a linear relationship between vividness of mental imagery and predisposition to hallucinate. The associated cognitive impairments may be the expression of a single pathological factor, which is phenotypically expressed largely via negative symptoms. But the question of whether enhanced imagery ability causes the occurrence of hallucinations ought to be closed. They are independent.

Moreover, psychological models of psychotic symptoms have focused on cognitive biases, including the propensity of people to assume external or internal causes for their perceptions and actions, termed locus of control (Rotter, 1966). We focused on a study by Oertel et al. (submitted), who investigated cognitive correlates, a deficit in attribution systems ("attribution bias") and dysfunctional processing and integration of information which were suggested to be responsible for the genesis of hallucinations. Results showed an independence of control orientation and dysfunctional status from each other, as well as from the degree of predisposition towards hallucinations. Instead, the external locus of control correlated to delusions. Possibly, an attribution towards external power can lead to the appearance of delusions.

However, at the beginning, we supposed an abnormal activation pattern of hallucinations in the brain. This hypothesis could be approved. Several studies show evidence for the involvement of primary (auditory modality; Dierks et al., 1999) and higher (visual modality; Oertel et al., 2007; Sireteanu et al., 2008) sensory areas, very similar to perception and imagery, during the experience of hallucinations. Furthermore, the brain activity during visual hallucinations (Oertel et al., 2007; Sireteanu et al., 2008) followed the boundaries of category-selective areas, but, in contrast to a finding of activated memory-related areas found in a schizophrenic patient experiencing visual hallucinations (Oertel et al., 2007), Sireteanu et al. (2008) did not observe memory-related areas during visual hallucinations induced by blindfolding. This suggests that the neural mechanisms underlying hallucinations in schizophrenia are at least partly distinct from those operational in cortical deafferentation. This result suggests that alterations in visual and attentional regions are related to the experience of visual hallucinations. Furthermore, visual hallucinations seem to be more vivid and more strongly related to activations in visual areas than mental imagery.

The psychological and neurophysiological models of hallucination can be integrated if we consider that patients experiencing hallucinations might ascribe internal monologues or dialogues to external sources. The activity of language areas during hallucinations would conform to such a model while the activity in auditory cortex might explain why auditory hallucinations are often so vivid and real for the persons suffering from them. Moreover, the activation of the limbic system (e.g. Dierks et al., 1999) might correspond to the emotional aspects of the content of the voices and the accompanying arousal. While the neurophysiological models of hallucination are thus already rather refined, the attempt at suppressing auditory cortex activity with repetitive transcranial magnetic stimulation in order to alleviate treatment-resistant acoustic hallucinations still needs further study.

Limitations of studies regarding hallucinations and their connection to psychological processes like perception, mental imagery and cognitive bias are given through the fact that none examines the relationship between subjective cognitive dysfunction scores and objective cognitive deficits. The controversial results could be due to the fact that most of the authors used self-administered questionnaires. There are currently no available means to study hallucinations separately from the subjectivity of the patients that experience them. In addition, locus of control and the subjective cognitive dysfunction were assessed solely through the use of self-reports and it is well known that such measures are prone to bias through factors such as mood, current mental state, belief systems and social desirability. Such measures also depend on memory and observation and therefore cannot assess cognitive or emotional processes which occur at a pre-conscious level or at a speed which is not amenable to inspection. An interesting point is the question of the existence of good and bad imagers, independent of individual psychopathology but dependent perhaps on age, handedness, social behaviour or attribution bias.

Treatment schemes that are based on the psychological theories are more varied and have shown more consistent and long lasting effects but also suffer from the difficulty in measuring hallucinations quantitatively. Future research with functional and structural imaging should go beyond correlating brain activity and symptoms and also address the functional and structural connectivity patterns in the brain that enable hallucinations. The knowledge of the metacognitive dispositions of hallucinations and their biological mechanisms is important for any therapeutic interventions that improve personal skills by finding a model of the phenomenon. Furthermore, a better understanding of individuals' control orientation may help develop psychological interventions aimed at symptom reduction and relapse prevention.

Psychotherapeutic interventions to change the cognitive bias, if possible, could be useful to advance the treatment of hallucinations. Through training programs, in which learners can change their thoughts and can perceive themselves as responsible for their fate, individuals may be able to learn to change their individual beliefs into a more realistic way of thinking.

Reorganisation of dysfunctional thinking, which is widely known in the therapy of depressive patients, could be employed in the treatment of dysfunctional biases in individuals experiencing hallucinations as well. Shifting the way hallucinating persons think about their ability to influence their own fate could have important implications for further treatment of psychotic symptoms (Warner, 2009).

The results of the imaging parts of this chapter suggest several lines of future directions in research. Several studies have shown that higher-order, but not primary cortices, are active during auditory mental imagery in healthy controls and non-hallucinating patients. On a different level, it is not well understood in what sense functional and anatomical connections between sensory cortex and higher-order areas play a role in hallucinations in schizophrenia. Combining analysis tools with methods for measuring functional and anatomical connectivity (e.g. DTI) will likely be the path to answering these questions.

In sum, we found evidence that, during the occurrence of hallucinations, there is an increased activity of language production, motor and perception areas. But we don't know if the changed brain activity pattern is the origin of hallucinations or an effect of other processes. At the moment, we cannot with certainty identify a direct link between the occurrence of hallucinations and cognitive processes, personal dispositions or imagery vividness.

Acknowledgments

V.O.-K. was supported by the Scholarship for Graduate Students of the Goethe-University, Frankfurt, Germany, and A.R.-J. by a doctoral studentship of the Josef Buchmann Foundation. We are grateful to Marietta Schwarz (email: mariettaschwarz@netcologne.de) for the friendly permission to publish her pictures. The descriptions of the inner images are based on her project notes.

References

Agartz, I., Andersson, J. L. & Skare, S. (2001). Abnormal brain white matter in schizophrenia: a diffusion tensor imaging study. *Neuroreport, 12*, 2251-2254.

Aggerneas, A. (1972). The experienced reality of hallucinations and other psychological phenomena. An empirical analysis. *Acta Psychiatrica Scandinavica, 48*, 220-238.

Aleman, A., Böcker, K. B. E. & de Haan, E. H .F. (1999). Disposition towards hallucinations and subjective versus objective vividness of imagery in normal subjects. *Personality and Individual Differences, 27*, 707–714.

Aleman, A., Böcker, K. B., Hijman, R., de Haan, E. H. & Kahn, R. S. (2003). Cognitive basis of hallucinations in schizophrenia: role of top-down information processing. *Schizophr Res. 15*, 64(2-3), 175-85.

American Psychiatric Association (APA) (1994). *Diagnostic and Statistical Manual of Mental Disorders,* 4th ed. (DSM-IV). Washington, DC: APA.

Baker, C. A. & Morrison, A. P. (1998). Cognitive processes in auditory hallucinations: attributional biases and metacognition. *Psychol Med., 28(5)*, 1199-208.

Ball, H. A., McGuffin, P. & Farmer, A. E. (2008). Attributional style and depression. *Br J Psychiatry, 192(4)*, 275-8.

Bandura, A. (1982). Self-efficacy mechanism in human agency. *American Psychologist, 37*, 122-147.

Barrett, T. R. (1993). Verbal hallucinations in normals: II. Self-reported imagery vividness. *Personality and Individual Differences, 15*, 61-67.

Barrett, T. R. & Etheridge, J. B. (1992). Verbal hallucinations in normals: I. People who hear "voices". *Applied Cognitive Psychology, 6*, 379-387.

Barrett, B., Pacey, I. E., Bradley, A., Thibos, L. & Morill, P. (2003). Nonveridical visual perception in human amblyopia *Investigative Ophthalmology & Visual Science, 44*, 1555-1567.

Basser, P. J., Mattiello, J. & LeBihan, D. (1994). MR diffusion tensor spectroscopy and imaging. *Biophys Journal, 66*, 259-267.

Bäumer, C. & Sireteanu, R. (2006). Temporal instability in the perception of strabismic amblyopia. *Strabismus, 14*, 59-64.

Behrendt, R. P. (2003). Hallucinations: Synchronisation of thalamocortical gamma oscillations underconstrained by sensory input. *Consciousness and Cognition, 12*, 413-451.

Bentall, R. P. & Slade, P. D. (1985). Reality testing and auditory hallucinations: a signal detection analysis. *British Journal of Clinical Psychology, 24*, 159-169.

Bentall, R. P., Claridge, G. & Slade, P. D. (1989). The multi dimensional nature of schizotypal traits: a factor analytic study with normal subjects. *British Journal of Clinical Psychology, 28*, 363-375.

Bentall, R. P. (1990). The illusion of reality: A review and integration of psychological research on hallucinations. *Psychological Bulletin, 17*, 82-95.

Bentall, R. P., Baker, G. A. & Havers, S. (1991). Reality monitoring and psychotic hallucinations: a brief report. *British Journal of Clinical Psychology, 30*, 213-222.

Bentall, R. P. & Fernyhough, C. (2008). Social predictors of psychotic experiences: specificity and psychological mechanisms. *Schizophr Bull., 34(6)*, 1012-20.

Böcker, K. B. E., Hijman, R., Kahn, R. S. & de Haan, E. H. F. (2000). Perception, mental imagery and reality discrimination in hallucinating and non-hallucinating schizophrenic patients. *British Journal of Clinical Psychology, 39*, 397-406.

Boroojerdi, B., Bushara, K. O., Corwell, B., Immish, I., Battaglia, F., Muellbacher, W. & Cohen, L. G. (2000). Enhanced excitability of the human visual cortex induced by short-term light deprivation. *Cerebral Cortex, 10*, 529-534.

Brebion, G., Smith, M. J., Gorman, J. M. & Amador, X. (1997). Discrimination accuracy and decision biases in different types of reality monitoring in schizophrenia. *Journal of Nervous and Mental Disease, 185(4)*, 247–253.

Brett, E. A. & Starker, S. (1977). Auditory imagery and hallucinations. *Journal of Nervous and Mental Disease, 164*, 394-400.

Bracha, H. S.,Wolkowitz, O. M., Lohr, J. B., Karson, C. N. & Bigelow, L. B. (1989). High prevalence of visual hallucinations in research subjects with chronic schizophrenia. *American Journal of Psychiatry, 146*, 526-528.

Bunzeck, N., Wuestenbergb, T., Lutzc, K., Heinzea, H. J. & Janckez, L. (2005). Scanning silence: *Mental imagery of complex sounds. Neuroimage, 9.*

Burke, W. (2002). The neural basis of Charles Bonnet-hallucinations: a hypothesis. Journal of Neurology, *Neurosurgery & Psychiatry*, *73*, 535-541.

Cahill, C. & Frith, C. D. (1996). A cognitive basis for the signs and symptoms of schizophrenia. In: Pantelis, C., Nelson, H.E. and Barnes, T.R.E. (eds.). Schizophrenia: A neuropsychological perspective, 373-396. London, U.K: Wiley.

Cash, T. F. & Stack, J. J. (1973). Locus of control among schizophrenic and other hospitalized psychiatric patients. *Genetic Psychology Monographs*, *87*, 105-122, 1973.

Cervetto, L., Demontis, G. C. & Gargini, C, (2007). Cellular mechanisms underlying the pharmacological induction of phosphenes. *British Journal of Pharmacology*, *150*, 383-390.

Chandiramani, K. & Varma, V. K. (1987). Imagery in schizophrenic patients compared with normal controls. *British Journal of Medical Psychology*, *60*, 335-341.

Claridge, G. & Broks, P. (1984). Schizotypy and hemisphere function: I. Theoretical consideration and the measurement of schizotypy. *Personality and Individual Differences*, *5*, 633-648.

Cohen, M. S., Kosslyn, M., Breiter, H. C., DiGirolamo, G. J., Thompson, W. L., Anderson, A. K., Bookheimer, S. Y., Rosen, B. R. & Belliveau, J. W. (1996). Changes in cortical activity during mental rotation. A mapping study using functional MRI. *Brain*, *119*, 89-100.

Collerton, D., Perry, E. & McKeith I. (2005). Why people see things that are not there: a novel Perception and Attention Deficit model for recurrent complex visual hallucinations. *Behavioural Brain Science*, *28*, 737-757.

Cromwell, R. L., Rosenthal, D., Shakow, E. & Zahn, T. P. (1961). Reaction time, locus of control, choice behavior, and description of parental behavior in schizophrenic and normal subjects. *Journal of Personality*, *29*, 363-379.

David, A. S. (1994). The neuropsychological origins of auditory hallucinations. In: David, A.S., Cutting, J.C. (Eds.), *The Neuropsychology of Schizophrenia*. LEA, 269-313.

Dierks, T., Linden, D. E. J., Jandl, M., Formisano, E. & Goebel, R. (1999). Activation of Heschl's gyrus during auditory hallucinations. *Neuron*, *22(3)*, 414-5.

Ducreux, D., Petit-Lacour, M. C., Benoudiba, F., Castelain, V. & Marsot-Dupuch, K. (2002). Diffusion-weighted imaging in a case of Wernicke encephalopathy. *J. Neuroradiol.*, *29*, 39-42.

Esquirol, J. E. D. (1832). Sur les illusions des sens chez alienes. On the sensory illusions of the insane. *Archives Generales de Medicine*, *2*, 5-23.

Farah, M. J. (1988). Is visual imagery really visual? Overlooked evidence from neurophysiology. *Psychological Review*, *95*, 307-317 21.

Fear, C., Sharp, H. & Healy, D. (1996). Cognitive processes in delusional disorders. *Br J Psychiatry*, *168(1)*, 61-7.

Formisano, E., Esposito, F., Kriegeskorte, N., Tedeschi, G., Di Salle, F. & Goebel, R. (2002). Spatial independent component analysis of functional magnetic resonance imaging time-series: characterization of the cortical components. *Neurocomputing*, *49*, 241-254.

Ffytche, D. H. & Howard, R. J. (1999). The perceptual consequences of visual loss: 'positive' pathologies of vision. *Brain*, *122*, 1247-1260.

Ffytche, D. H., Howards, R. J., Brammer, M. J., David, A., Woodruff, P. & Williams, S. (1998). The anatomy of conscious vision: an fMRI study of visual hallucinations. *Nature Neuroscience*, *1*, 738-742.

Ffytche, D. H. (2005). Visual hallucinations and the Charles Bonnet Syndrome. *Current Psychiatry Reports,* 7, 168-179.

Finke, R. A. (1989). *Principles of Mental Imagery.* MIT Press: Cambridge.

Frenkel, E., Kugelmass, S., Natham, M. & Ingraham, L. J. (1995). Locus of control and mental health in adolescence and adulthood: Israeli high-risk study. *Schizophrenia bulletin,* 21(2), 219-226.

Friedman, R., Goodrich, W. & Fullerton, C. S. (1985-86). Locus of control and severity of psychiatric illness in the residential treatment of adolescents. *Residential Group Care and Treatment,* 3(2), 3-13.

Frith, C. D. (1992*). The cognitive neuropsychology of schizophrenia.* Hillsdale: LEA publishers.

Gardini, S., De Beni, R., Cornoldi, C., Bromiley, A. & Venneri, A. (2005). Different neuronal pathways support the generation of general and specific mental images. *Neuroimage,* 27(3), 544-52.

Gaser, C., Nenadic, I., Volz, H. P., Büchel, C. & Sauer, H. (2004). Neuroanatomy of "hearing voices": a frontotemporal brain structural abnormality associated with auditory hallucinations in schizophrenia. *Cereb Cortex.,* 14(1), 91-6.

Goadsby, P. J. & Silberstein, S. D. eds. (1997). *Headache.* Boston, Butterworth: Heinemann.

Goebel, R., Khorram-Sefat, D., Muckli, L., Hacker, H. & Singer, W. (1998). The contstructive nature of vision: direct evidence from functional magnetic resonance imaging studies of apparent motion and motion imagery. *European Journal of Neuroscience,* 10, 1563-1573.

Hadjikhani, N., Sanchez del Rio, M., Wu, O., Schwartz, D., Bakker, D., Fischl, B., Kwong, K. K., Cutrer, F. M., Rosen, B. R., Tootell, R. B. H. & Sorensen, A. G. (2001). Mechanisms of migraine aura revealed by functional MRI in human visual cortex. Proceedings of the *National Academy of Sciences,* 98, 4687-4692.

Hahlweg, K. (1998). Störungstheorien und -modelle. In: Hahlweg, K., Dose, M. (Eds.), Schizophrenie. *Hogrefe, Göttingen,* 25-35.

Harrow, M. & Ferrante, A. (1969). Locus of control in psychiatric patients. *Journal of Consulting and Clinical Psychology,* 33, 582-589.

Hoffmann, R. E., Boutros, N. N., Berman, R. M., Roessler, E., Belger, A., Krystal, J. H. & Charney, D. S. (1999). Transcranial magnetic stimulation of left temporo-parietal cortex in three patients reporting hallucinated voices. *Biological psychiatry,* 46, 130-132.

Horowitz, M. (1975). Hallucinations: an information processing approach. In: R. K., Siegel, L. J. West, (Eds.), *Hallucinations: behaviour, Experience and Theory,* pp. 163–196. NY: Wiley.

Hubl, D., Koenig, T., Strik, W., Federspiel, A., Kreis, R., Boesch, C. & et al. (2004). Pathways that make voices: white matter changes in auditory hallucinations. *Arch Gen Psychiatry,* 61, 658-668.

Jeannerod, M. (1994). The representing brain: neuronal correlates of motor intention & imagery. *Behavioral and Brain Sciences,* 3, 320-328.

Johns, L. C. & van Os, J. (2001). The continuity of psychotic experiences in the general population. *Clinical Psychological Review,* 21(8), 1125–1141.

Kammer, T. (1999). Phosphenes and transient scotomas induced by magnetic stimulation of the occipital lobe: their topographic relationship. *Neuropsychologia,* 37, 191-198.

Kay, S. R., Fiszbein, A. & Opler, L. A. (1987). The Positive and Negative Syndrome Scale (PANSS) for schizophrenia. *Schizophrenia Bulletin, 13*, 261-276.

Kircher, T. T., Rapp, A., Grodd, W., Buchkremer, G., Weiskopf, N., Lutzenberger, W., Ackermann, H. & Mathiak, K. (2004). Mismatch negativity responses in schizophrenia: a combined fMRI and whole-head MEG study. *Am J Psychiatry, 161(2)*, 294-304.

Klein, I., Duboisa, J., Mangina, J. F., Kherifa, F., Flandina, G., Polinea, J. B., Denisb, M., Kosslyn, S. M. & Le Bihana, D. (2004). Retinotopic organization of visual mental images as revealed by functional magnetic resonance imaging. *Cognitive Brain Research, 22,* 26-31.

Komatsu, H. (2006). The neural mechanisms of perceptual filling-in. *Nature Reviews of Neuroscience, 7*, 220-231.

Kosslyn, S. M. (1989). *Readings from the Encyclopedia of Neuroscience: Learning and Memory*. Boston.

Kosslyn, S. M. (1994). *Image and brain: the resolution of the imagery debate*. MIT Press: Cambridge, MA.

Kosslyn, S. M., Thompson, W. L. & Alpert, N. M. (1997). Neural systems shared by visual imagery and visual perception: a positron emission tomography study. *Neuroimage, 6*, 320-334.

Krampen, G. (1991). *Fragebogen zu Kompentenz- und Kontrollüberzeugung* (FKK). Göttingen, Hogrefe.

Kubicki, M.,Westin, C. F., Nestorm, P. G.,Wible, C. G., Frumin, M., Maier, S. E., Kikinis, R., Jolesz, F. A., McCarley, R. W. & Shenton, M. E. (2003). Cingulate fasciculus integrity disruption in schizophrenia: a magnetic resonance diffusion tensor imaging study. *Biological Psychiatry, 54*, 1171-1180.

Lasar, M. (1997). Kognitive Handlungsbewertung bei akut erkrankten chronisch schizophrenen Patienten. *Psychologische Beiträge, 39*, 297-311.

Launay, G. & Slade, P. D. (1981). The measurement of hallucinatory predisposition in male and female prisoners. *Personality and Individual Differences, 2*, 221-234.

Lauritzen, M. (1994). Pathophysiology of the migraine aura: The spreading depression theory" *Brain, 117*, 199-210.

Lefcourt, H. M. (1980). Personality and locus of control. In Garber J. and Seligman MEP (Eds.), *Human helplessness*, 245-260. New York, Academic Press.

Lennox, B. R., Park, S. B., Medley, I., Morris, P. G. & Jones, P. B. (2000). The functional anatomy of auditory hallucinations in schizophrenia. *Psychiatry Research Neuroimaging, 100*, 13-20.

Lenzenweger, M. F. (1994). Psychometric high-risk paradigm, perceptual aberrations, and schizotypy: an update. *Schizophrenia Bulletin, 20(1)*, 121-135.

Levitan, C., Ward, P. B. & Catts, S. V. (1999). Superior temporal gyral volumes and laterality correlates of auditory hallucinations in schizophrenia. *Biol Psychiatry, 46(7)*, 955-62.

Lim, K. O. & Helpern, J. A. (2002). Neuropsychiatric applications of DTI-a review. *NMR Biomed, 15*, 587-593.

Linden, D. E. J. & Dierks, T. (2002). Functional imaging of auditory hallucinations in schizophrenia. *Nervenheilkunde, 21*, 331-335.

Lyon, H. M., Kaney, S. & Bentall, R. P. (1994). The defensive function of persecutory delusions. Evidence from attribution tasks. *Br J Psychiatry, 164(5)*, 637-46.

Manford, M. & Andermann, F. (1998). Complex visual hallucinations. Clinical and neurobiological insights. *Brain, 121,* 1819-1840.

Marg, E. & Rudiak, D. (1994). Phosphenes induced by magnetic stimulation over the occipital brain: descriptions and probable site of stimulation. *Optometry & Visual Science, 71,* 301-311.

Mass, R., Haasen, C. & Wolf, K. (2000). Das Eppendorfer Schizophrenie-Inventar (ESI). Entwicklung und Evaluation eines Fragebogens zur Erfassung charakteristischer Selbstwahrnehmungen kognitiver Dysfunktionen schizophren Erkrankter. *Der Nervenarzt, 71(11),* 885-892.

Mazard, A., Laou, L., Joliot, M. & Mellet, E. (2005). Neural impact of the semantic content of visual mental images and visual percepts. *Brain Res Cogn Brain Res., 24(3),* 423-35.

McGuire, P. K., Silbersweig, D. A., Murray, R. M., David, A. S., Frackowiak, R. S. & Frith, C. D. (1996). Functional anatomy of inner speech and auditory verbal imagery. *Psychological medicine, 26,* 29-38.

McMahon, C. E. (1973). Images and Motives as Motivators: A Historical Perspective. *American Journal of Psychology, 86,* 465-490.

Meehl, P. E. (1962). Schizotaxia, schizotypy, schizophrenia. *American Psychologist, 17,* 827-838.

Meehl, P. E. (1990). Toward an integrated theory of schizotaxia, schizotypy, and schizophrenia. *Journal of Personality Disorders, 4,* 1-99.

Mendola, J. D., Dale, A. M., Fischl, B., Liu, A. K. & Tootell, R. B. H. (1999). The representation of illusory and real contours in human cortical visual areas revealed by functional Magnetic Resonance Imaging. *The Journal of Neuroscience, 19,* 8560-8572.

Merabet, L. B., Maguire, D., Warde, A., Alterescu, K., Stickgold, R. & Pascual-Leone, A. (2004). Visual hallucinations during prolonged blindfolding in sighted subjects. *Journal of Neuroophthalmology, 24,* 109-113.

Merckelbach, H. & Van de Ven, V. (2001). Another White Christmas: fantasy proneness and reports of "hallucinatory experiences" in undergraduate students. *Journal of Behavioral Therapy Exp Psychiatry, 32(3),* 137–144.

Meng, M., Remus, D. A. & Tong, F. (2005). Filling-in of visual phantoms in the human brain. *Nature Neuroscience, 8,* 1248-1254.

Mintz, S. & Alpert, M. (1972). Imagery vividness, reality testing and schizophrenic hallucinations. *Journal of Abnormal Psychology, 79,* 310-316.

Morrison, A. P., Wells, A. & Nothard, S. (2002a). Cognitive and emotional predictors of predisposition to hallucinations in non-patients. *British Journal of Clinical Psychiatry, 41,* 259-270.

Morrison, A. P., Beck, A. T., Glentworth, D., Dunn, H. & Reid, G. (2002b). Imagery and psychotic symptoms: a preliminary investigation. *Behaviour Research and Therapy, 40,* 1053-1062.

Muckli, L., Kiess, S., Tonhausen, N., Singer, W., Goebel, R. & Sireteanu, R. (2006). Cerebral correlates of impaired grating perception in individual, psychophysically assessed human amblyopes. *Vision Research, 46,* 506-526.

Muckli, L., Kohler, A., Kriegeskorte, N. & Singer, W. (2005). Primary visual cortex activity along the apparent-motion trace reflects illusory perception. *Plos Biol, 3,* 265.

Oertel, V., Rotarska-Jagiela, A., van de Ven, V. G., Haenschel, C., Maurer, K. & Linden, D. E. J. (2007). Visual hallucinations in schizophrenia investigated with functional magnetic resonance imaging. *Psychiatry Research, 15*, 156(3), 269-273.

Oertel, V. (2008). *Studying the brain correlates of hallucinations*. Dissertation zur Erlangung des Doktorgrades Dr. phil.nat: Deutsches Hochschulsystem.

Oertel, V., Rotarska-Jagiela, A., Van de Ven, V., Haenschel, C., Grube, M., Stangier, U., Maurer, K. & Linden, D. E. J. (2009). Mental imagery vividness as a trait marker across the schizophrenia spectrum. *Psychiatry Research, 15*, 167(1-2), 1-11.

Oertel-Knöchel, V., Rotarska-Jagiela, A., Van de, Ven, V., Haenschel, C., Grube, M.,Knöchel, C., Stangier, U., Maurer, K. & Linden, D. E. J. (submitted). External control orientation in the schizophrenia spectrum. *British Journal of Clinical Psychology*, submitted.

Ohayon, M. M. (2000). Prevalence of hallucinations and their pathological associations in the general population. *Psychiatry Research, 97*, 153-164.

Oishi, N., Udaka, F., Kameyama, M., Sawamoto, N., Hashikawa, K. & Fukuyama, H. (2005). Regional cerebral blood flow in Parkinson disease with nonpsychotic visual hallucinations. *Neurology, 65*, 1708-1715.

Paivio, A. (1985). Cognitive and motivational functions of imagery in human performance. *Can J Appl Sport Sci., 10(4)*, 22S-28S.

Pitskel, N. B., Merabet, L. B., Ramos-Estebanez, C., Kauffman, T. & Pascual-Leone, A. (2007). Timedependent changes in cortical excitability after prolonged visual deprivation. *Neuroreport, 18*, 1703-1707.

Poulton, R., Caspi, A., Mofitt, T. E., Cannon, M., Murray, R. & Harrington, H. (2000). Children's self-reported psychotic symptoms and adult schizophreniform disorder. *Archives of General Psychiatry, 57*, 1053-1058.

Raine, A. (1991). The SPQ: A scale for the assessment of schizotypal personality based on DSM-III-R criteria. *Schizophrenia Bulletin, 17*, 556-564.

Rotarska-Jagiela, A., Oertel, V., DeMartino, F., van de Ven, V., Formisano, E., Roebroeck, A., Rami, A., Schoenmeyer, R., Haenschel, C., Hendler, T., Maurer, K. & Linden, D. E. J. (in press). *Anatomical Brain Connectivity and Positive Symptoms of Schizophrenia: a Diffusion Tensor Imaging Study*. Psychiatry Research Neuroimaging.

Rotter, J. B. (1966). Generalized expectancies for internal versus external control of reinforcement. *Psychological Monographs, 80(609)*, 203-218.

Sack, A. T., Van de Ven, V., Etschenberg, S., Schatz, D. & Linden, D. E. J. (2005). Enhanced vividness of mental imagery as a trait marker of schizophrenia? Schizophrenia *Bulletin, 31*, 1-8.

Sartorius, N., Jablensky, A. & Shapiro, R. (1978). Cross-cultural differences in the short-term prognosis of schizophrenic psychoses. *Schizophrenia Bulletin, 4(1)*, 102-113.

Sato, M., Baciu, M., Loevenbruck, H., Schwartz, J. L., Cathiard, M. A., Segebarth, C. & Abry, C. (2004). Multistable representation of speech forms: a functional MRI study of verbal transformations. *Neuroimage, 23(3)*, 1143-51.

Schlösser, R., Wagner, G., Kohler, S. & Sauer, H. (2005). Schizophrenia as a disconnection syndrome. Studies with functional magnetic resonance imaging and structural equation modelling. *Radiology, 45(2)*, 137-40.

Schultz, G. & Melzack, R. (1991). The Charles Bonnet syndrome: 'phantom visual images'. *Perception, 20*, 809-825.

Sheehan, P. W. (1967). Reliability of a short test of imagery. *Perceptual and Motor Skills*, 25, 744.

Shepard, R. N. & Metzler, J. (1971). Mental rotation of three-dimensional objects. *Science*, 171, 701-703.

Shergill, S. S., Brammer, M. J., Amaro, E., Williams, S. C., Murray, R. M. & McGuire, P. K. (2004). Temporal course of auditory hallucinations. *Br J Psychiatry*, 185, 516-7.

Silbersweig, D. A., Stern, E., Frith, C., Cahill, C., Holmes, A., Grootoonk, S. & et al. (1995) A functional neuroanatomy of hallucinations in schizophrenia. *Nature*, 378, 176-179.

Silbersweig, D. A. & Stern, E. (1998). Towards a functional neuroanatomy of conscious perception and its modulation by volution: implications of human auditory neuroimaging studies. *Phil. Trans. R. Soc.* London. B., 353, 1883-1888.

Sireteanu, R., Bäumer, C., Sârbu, C. & Iftime, A. (2007a). Spatial and temporal misperceptions in amblyopic vision. *Strabismus*, 15, 45-54.

Sireteanu, R., Bäumer, C., Sârbu, C., Tsujimura, S. & Muckli, L. (2007b). Basiert der verzerrte Seheindruck bei Amblyopie auf einer erhöhten Aktivierung in der primären Sehrinde? Spatial misperceptions in amblyopic vision: abnormal activation of the primary visual cortex? *Klinische Monatsblätter für Augenheilkunde*, 224, 1-7.

Sireteanu, R., Oertel, V., Mohr, H., Linden, D. & Singer W. (2008). Graphical illustration and functional neuroimaging of visual hallucinations during prolonged blindfolding: a comparison to visual imagery. *Perception*, 37(12), 1805-21.

Slade, P. D., Bentall, R. P. (1988). *Sensory Deception: A Scientific Analysis of Hallucination*. London, Croom Helm.

Slade, P. D. (1972). An investigation of psychological factors involved in the predisposition to auditory hallucinations. *Psychol Med.*, 6(1), 123-32.

Slotnick, S. D., Thompson, W. L. & Kosslyn, S. M. (2005). Visual mental imagery induces retinotopically organized activation of early visual areas. *Cerebral Cortex*, 15(10), 1570-83.

Spierings, E. L. H. (2004). The aura-headache connection in migraine. *Archives of Neurology* 61, 794-799.

Starker, S. & Jolin, A. (1982). Imagery and hallucinations in schizophrenic patients. *Journal of Nervous and Mental Diseases*, 170, 448-451. In: Thurstone, L.L. (1938). *Primary Mental Abilities*. Chicago: university of Chicago Press.

Stephane, M., Barton, S. & Boutros, N. N. (2001). Auditory verbal hallucinations and dysfunction of the neural substrates of speech. *Schizophrenia Research*, 50, 61-78.

Stirling, J. D., Hellewell, J. S. & Quraishi, N. (1998). Monitoring dysfunction and the schizophrenic symptoms of alien control. *Psychological Medicine*, 28(3), 675-83.

Sumich, A., Chitnis, X. A., Fannon, D. G., O'Ceallaigh, S., Doku, V. C., Faldrowicz, A. & Sharma, T. (2005). Unreality symptoms and volumetric measures of Heschl's gyrus and planum temporal in first-episode psychosis. *Biol Psychiatry*, 57(8), 947-50.

Tien, A. Y. (1991). Distributions of hallucinations in the population. *Social Psychiatry and Psychiatric Epidemiology*, 26, 287-292.

Tootell, R. P., Mendola, J. D., Hadjikhani, N. K., Ledden, P. J., Liu, A. K., Reppas, J. B., Sereno, M. I. & Dale, A. M. (1997). Functional analysis of V3A and related visual areas in human visual cortex. *The Journal of Neuroscience*, 17, 7060-7078.

Trojano, L. & Grossi, D. (1994). A Critical Review of Mental Imagery defects. *Brain and Cognition*, 24, 213-243.

Trojano, L., Linden, D. E. J., Formisanom, E., Goebel, R., Sack, A. T. & Di Salle, F. (2004). What clocks tell us about the neural correlates of spatial imagery. *European Journal of Cognitive Psychology, 16*, 653-672.

Tyler, C. W. (1978). Some new entoptic phenomena. *Vision Research, 18*, 1633-1639.

Uhlhaas, P. J., Phillips, W. A., Mitchell, G. & Silverstein, S.M. (2006). Perceptual grouping in disorganized schizophrenia. *Psychiatry Res., 7*, 145(2-3), 105-17.

Van de Ven, V. & Merckelbach, H. (2003). The role of schizotypy, mental imagery, and fantasy proneness in hallucinatory reports of undergraduate students. *Personality and Individual Differences, 35*, 889-896.

Van de Ven, V. G., Formisano, E., Röder, C. H., Prvulovic, D., Bittner, R. A., Dietz, M. G., Hubl, D., Dierks, T., Federspiel, A., Esposito, F., Di Salle, F., Jansma, B., Goebel, R. & Linden, D. E. J. (2005). The spatiotemporal pattern of auditory cortical responses during verbal hallucinations. *Neuroimage, 27*, 644-55.

Van Kampen, D. (2006). The Schizotypic Syndrome Questionnaire (SSQ): psychometrics, validation and norms. *Schizophrenia Research, 84 (2–3)*, 305-322.

Van Os, J. (2003). Is there a continuum of psychotic experiences in the general population? *Epidemiol Psychiatr Soc., 12(4)*, 242-52.

Varkey, L. & Sathyavathi, L. (1984). Locus of control and other personality variables in psychotics. *Psychological studies, 29*, 83-87.

Verdoux, H. & van Os, J. (2002). Psychotic symptoms in non-clinical populations and the continuum of psychosis. *Schizophrenia Research, 54*, (1–2), 59-65.

Warner, R. (2009). Recovery from schizophrenia and the recovery model. *Curr Opin Psychiatry, 22(4)*, 374-80.

Whalley, H. C., Simonotto, E., Marshall, I., Owens, D. G. C., Goddard, N. H., Johnstone, E. C. & Lawrie, S. M. (2005). Functional disconnectivity in subjects at high genetic risk of schizophrenia. *Brain, 128(9)*, 2097-2108.

Weiss, A. P. & Heckers, S. (1999). Neuroimaging of hallucinations: a review of the literature. *Psychiatry Research, 20*, 92(2-3), 61-74.

Wilson, R. S., Gilley, D. W., Bennett, D. A., Beckett, L. A. & Evans, D. A. (2000). Hallucinations, delusions, and cognitive decline in Alzheimer's disease. *J Neurol Neurosurg Psychiatry, 69(2)*, 172-7.

Winawer, M. R., Ottman, R., Hauser, W. A. & Pedley, T. A. (2000). Autosomal dominant partial epilepsy with auditory features: defining the phenotype. *Neurology, 13, 54(11)*, 2173-6.

Zimbardo, P. G. (1985). *Psychology and life 11th edition*. Glenview, III, Scott, Foresman.

Chapter 2

Auditory Verbal Hallucination in Schizophrenic Patients and the General Population: The Sense of Agency in Speech

Tomohisa Asai[*], *Eriko Sugimori and Yoshihiko Tanno*
Department of Cognitive and Behavioral Science, Graduate School of Arts and Sciences, University of Tokyo, 3-8-1 Komaba, Meguro-ku,
Tokyo 153-8902, Japan

Abstract

Recently, the boundaries between "normal" and "abnormal," even with regard to mental disorders, like schizophrenia even, have blurred. Thought auditory verbal hallucinations (AVH) are a cardinal feature of schizophrenia, recent studies have suggested that even healthy general population might experience the AVH (i.e., auditory verbal hallucination like experiences) (e.g., Barrett et al., 1992), indicating the continuum of schizophrenic symptoms. In this chapter, we reviewed the results of the studies about AVH both in schizophrenic patients, and the general population with AVH in terms of self-monitoring or sense of agency in speech, including our own studies. A perspective that situates schizophrenia on a continuum implies that this disorder constitutes a potential risk for everyone, and, thus,, helps toin promoteing understanding and correction ofing misunderstandings, whichthat contribute to prejudice within communities.

We first reviewed the phenomenology of AVH in the general population including quality and quantity, as compared with patients with AVH. According to these previous studies, we developed the auditory hallucination experience scale (AHES) for general population because a scale for directly measuring AVH was needed. What causes AVH,

---

[*] Corresponding author: Tel: +81-3-5454-6259, Fax: +81-3-5454-6979, as@beck.c.u-tokyo.ac.jp

even in the general population? Recent studies have suggested the relationship with to the sense of agency in speech.

The sense of agency is the feeling of causing our own actions, in this case, speech (Gallagher, 2000). One's own speech could seem to be AVH (McGuigan, 1966). The activation of Broca's area, which can produce, but cannot listen to speech, has been associated with AVH (McGuire et al., 1993). ThereforeThus, these people might produce speech, but not think that they actually spoke. As a result, they may hear their own voices as the voices of others. Indeed, schizophrenic patients with AVH tend to misattribute their own speech (self-speech recognition task: e.g., Johns et al., 1999; 2001). To measure the subjective aspect of the sense of agency, we developed a scale to measure the sense of agency in a general population.

The sense of agency approach to AVH could be a key not only to not only understanding schizophrenic cardinal symptom but also to understanding the sense of "self" in the healthy general population in the sense that, even the general population even could experience AVH. We Ffinally, we discussed on the neurocognitive model of the sense of agency in speech and its potential disturbance in people with AVH.

Introduction

According to the Diagnostic and Statistical Manual-Fourth Edition-Text Revision (DSM-IV-TR; American Psychiatric Association; APA, 2000), a hallucination is "a sensory perception that has the compelling sense of reality of a true perception, but occurs without external stimulation of the relevant sensory organ." An auditory hallucination is a false perception of sound, and it is the most common form of hallucination. Whileereas auditory hallucinations are one of the most characteristic symptoms, of schizophrenia, many epidemiological studies have suggested the possibility that some normal healthy people have similar experiences (Stevenson, 1983; Barrett & Etheridge, 1992; Sidgewick, Johnson, Myers, et al., 1894; Tien, 1991; Johns, 2005; Choong, Hunter, & Woodruff, 2007). In this chapter, we defined theis experience occurring in healthy people as an auditory hallucination-like experience, with the means of in order to differentiatinge this it from the sort of auditory hallucinations which that occur in schizophrenia.

To describe the phenomenology of auditory hallucination in patients with schizophrenia, Nayani and David (1996) administered a comprehensive semi-structured questionnaire to 100 psychotic patients, who had experienced auditory hallucinations. They concluded that, the essential characteristics of the form and content of auditory hallucinations in psychotic patients can be summarized as follows: they are repetitive, emotive utterances which are context dependent, spatio-temporally organized and appear to originate from stereotypical personifications. Auditory hallucinations seem to evolve by accretion and, increasingly, come, to invadinge the patient's private life. Many retain some degree of control of them, probably reducing their distress (Nayani & David, 1996). On the other hand, among normal and healthy individuals, those in their 20s are most likely to have experienced auditory hallucination-like experiences (Sidgewick, et al., 1894) and 37-39% of undergraduates report auditory hallucination-like experiences (Barrett, et al., 1992). Although certain qualitative differences distinguish between the auditory hallucinations experienced in schizophrenia and the auditory hallucination-like experiences reported inby normal healthy people (or for example, in the psychiatric population, these tend to be frequent, intrusive, and distressing. In contrast, in the nonclinical population, these are often predominantly positive and nonthreatening: see for review, Choong, et al., 2007), previous research provides a foundation for conceptualizing a continuum of auditory hallucinations ranging from experiences of auditory hallucinations accompanying schizophrenia, to the experiences of auditory hallucination-like phenomena reported by normal healthy people. At present, many researchers assume a certain degree of continuity with regard to auditory hallucinations, and focus on analog studies involving individual differences among normal people (e.g., Claridge & Davis, 2003; Cella, Taylor, & Reed, 2007).

Analog studies are conducted because people with schizophrenia show differences from normal healthy controls with regard to almost all experimental tasks. It is difficult to determine whether these differences are derived from the mechanisms of schizophrenia (the first symptom) or from the reduction in cognitive functioning that which results from the onset of schizophrenia, hospital admission, or medication (the second symptom) (Vollema,1999). Analog research on schizophrenia involves the study of normal healthy people, who reporting an experience like such as the first symptom. This approach offers the advantage of potentially examining the pathological mechanisms while avoiding the aforementioned difficulties associated with the samples comprised of those diagnosed with schizophrenia.

Measuring the Auditory Hallucination-like Experiences in the General Population: AHES-40

Although the number of analog studies of schizophrenia is increasing (e.g., Claridge, 1997), a scale for to directly measuringe auditory hallucination-like experiences directly has not yet been developed. The Launay-Slade Hallucination Scale (LSHS; Launay & Slade, 1981) and its revised version (LSHS-R; Waters, Badcock, & Matbery, 2003) measure hallucination-like experiences, including auditory hallucinations, but do not focus on auditory hallucinations separately. In order toTo investigate auditory hallucinations directly, a scale is needed, as that measuringes auditory hallucination-like experiences separately from other hallucinations or hallucination-like experiences.

We drew from the LSHS (Launay & Slade, 1981), the Body Image Aberration Scale (BIAS; Chapman, Chapman, & Raulin, 1978), and the Perceptual Aberration Scale (PAS; Chapman, et al., 1978) and thereby developed the Auditory Hallucination-like Experience Scale (AHES 40), which consistings of 40 items whichand measures auditory hallucination-like experiences (Sugimori, Asai, and Tanno, 2009; Table 1). We showed that the AHES has high reliability and validity as a measure of auditory hallucination-like experiences. Onari (1998) investigated the relationship between auditory hallucination-like experiences and delusional ideation by using the AHES-40 and the Delusional Ideation Checklist (DICL; Tanno, Ishigaki, & Sugiura, 2000) and findingound a correlation between these measures. This finding is consistent with the status of both auditory hallucinations and delusions as positive symptoms of schizophrenia as well as with the high rate with which these phenomena are associated with complications of this disorder (Verdoux et al., 1998). These results suggest, that the AHES-40 has high reliability and validity as a measure of auditory hallucination-like experiences.

Asai, Sugimori, & Tanno (2008) used the AHES-40 as one questionnaire in a test battery and investigated the relationship between the results of the entire battery and an experimental self-monitoring task. These researchers found strong correlations between the AHES-40 and theose scales that are thought to be strongly related to schizophrenia and no correlation between the AHES-40 and the scales that which are viewed as not being directly related to schizophrenia. Adding to the criterion-related validity, a high correlation between the AHES-40 and the experimental self-monitoring task also emerged, which showsing that, as scores on the AHES-40 increased, performance on the experimental self-monitoring task declined. Asai et al. (2008) hypothesized that, hallucinations are based on disorders of speech self-monitoring (self-monitoring hypothesis; Frith, 1992), and their results suggest construct validity.

Developing the Shorten Version of AHES-40

Our purpose in this subsection was to develop the brief version (AHES-17) of the AHES-40 in order forto reducinge the burden on participants and to facilitatinge the measure's global use as a self-report screening instrument for auditory hallucination-like experiences. We investigated reliability (test–retest reliability and internal reliability), the factor structure of the AHES-17, and criterion-related validity (the relationship between the AHES and other scales), and we then constructed path models forto investigatinge the relationship between schizophrenia and auditory hallucinations.

Method

Participants

There were three groups. First, 145 undergraduates (115 men, 30 women; mean age 19.06, SD = 1.06) participated. Second, 145 undergraduates (90 men, 46 women; mean age 19.07, SD = 0.82) participated. Third, 172 undergraduates (52 men, 120 women; mean age 19.61, SD = 0.98) participated. In order to investigate test–retest reliability, undergraduates in group1 participated in the research twice. The period from the first and the second research was one month and 96 undergraduates (71 men, 25 women; mean age 19.02, SD = 1.10) participated in both first and second research, whom we used for for measure of the test–retest reliability. We conducted AHES-17, LSHS, STA, SPQ, STAI, and SDS for group 1, AHES-17, LSHS, O-Life, STAI, and SDS for group 2, and AHES-17, LSHS, STAI, and SDS for group 3 (described below).

Materials

We used the data collected by Sugimori et al. (2009), in with which 139 participants (45 men, 94 women; mean age 20.06, SD = 1.08) completed the AHES-40, a self-report 40-item questionnaire with responses based on a 5-point Likert scale (1–5) measuring the frequency of auditory hallucination-like experiences. In Sugimori, et al., (2009), skewness was 0.00, identical to that of a normal distribution (skewness of a normal distribution is 0). However, kurtosis was 2.15, which is smaller than that of a normal distribution (which is 3). Therefore, we first reduced the number of items by eliminating items whose mean scores minus 1 Standard Deviation (SD) were below 1 or whose mean scores plus 1 SD were above 5 to makeso that the distribution would more closely resemble that of a normal distribution. As a result, we reduced the number of items from 40 to 35. Secondly, we conducted a factor analysis of the 35 items using the maximum likelihood method with promax rotation for latent roots. Factor analysis revealed theat the AHES to consists of four factors: 1. Auditory hallucinations caused by internal speech or thinking, 2. Delusions or thought insertion related to auditory hallucinations, 3. Auditory hallucinations related to music, and 4. Auditory hallucination related to the voices of others. We eliminated the items with factor loadings below 0.5. As a result, 17 items remained. ThusAs such, we identified the remaining items as the AHES-17.

We used six scales to investigate criterion-related validity. Four scales are thought to be directly related to auditory hallucination-like experiences. The LSHS (Launay & Slade, 1981; Bentall, Claridge, & Slade, 1989) is a 12-item self-report questionnaire measuring hallucination-like experiences. The STA (Claridge & Broks, 1984; Cyhlarova & Claridge, 2005) is 37-item self-report questionnaire based on the diagnostic criteria for Schizotypal Personality Disorder included in the Diagnostic and Statistical Manual, Third Edition (DSM-III; APA, 1980). This instrument measures schizotypal traits, especially perceptual aberrations that which are analogous to positive symptoms, and including auditory hallucinations. The O-LIFE (Mason, Claridge, & Jackson, 1995) is a 104-item, true/false self-report questionnaire measuring comprehensive schizotypal personality traits, according to four subscales: Unusual Experiences (UnEx), Introvertive Anhedonia (InAn), Cognitive Disorganization (CoDi), and Impulsive Nonconformity (ImNo). The Schizotypal Personality Questionnaire-Brief (SPQB; Raine & Benishay, 1995), is a 22-item, true/false self-report questionnaire, with items selected from the SPQ, a 74-item self-report scale modeled on The Diagnostic and Statistical Manual, Third Edition, Revised (DSM-III-R; APA, 1987) criteria for schizotypal personality disorder. The latter has a three-factor structure similar to that of schizophrenia, with Cognitive (Positive), Interpersonal (Negative), and Disorganization (Disorganized Schizotpy) as factors (Gruzelier, 1996; Fossati et al., 2003). The SPQB has the same three-factor structure as the SPQ. The State–Trait Anxiety Inventory-Trait version (STAI-T; Spielberger, Gorsuch, & Lushene, 1970) is a well known 20-item self-report questionnaire, with responses based on a 4-point Likert scale, which measuresing anxiety traits. The Self-rating Depression Scale (Zung, 1965) is a well known 20-item self-report questionnaire, which measuresing depressive tendencies, with the responses based on a 4-point Likert scale.

Procedure

We conducted the research in a group format. In both the first and second sessions, the AHES-17 was distributed to participants. The first and the second investigations were separated by 1 month. Alpha coefficients for the scales were calculated in order to investigate internal reliability, and correlations between scores from the first and the second sessions were calculated to investigate test–retest reliability.

We conducted the research in a group format. Participants in Group 1 were given a booklet containing the AHES, the LSHS, and the STAI during the second research meeting to examine the test–retest validity. Participants in Group 2 were given a booklet containing the

AHES, the LSHS, the O-Life, the SDS, and the STAI. On a different day, participants in Group 3 were given a booklet containing the AHES, the LSHS, the SPQB, the SDS, and the STAI.

Table 1. AHES-40 Items

	For each of the following questions, please circle 5 if you very often have this experience, 4 if you sometimes have this experience, 3 if you cannot say either way, 2 if you do not have this experience very often, and 1 if you do not have this experience at all.
1.	When you had some sort of problem, you used concrete and clear words to express vague thoughts and feelings.
2.	When you were in a difficult situation, you tried to reassure yourself using clear phrases such as "get a grip" or "calm down" or "I have to. . .".
3.	You contemplated something while having a conversation in your head with another person.
4.	To gather your thoughts, you had a conversation in your head with an imaginary person.
5.	You muttered to yourself, when you were thinking about something.
6.	You laughed to yourself, when you were thinking about something.
7.	Your thoughts were so strong, it was as if you had said them aloud.
8.	You felt that there was a "voice of conscience" inside of you.
9.	You felt that there was a "voice calling you towards bad things" inside of you.
10.	You had random thoughts that which would not go away even though you wanted them to.
11.	You had thoughts about criticizing someone or breaking something, and these thoughts did not go away or you could not forget them.
12.	You had a thought that you might have forgotten to do something (for example, you forgot to lock the house, turn off the stove, or sign your name).
13.	You had a thought that you or your family were in danger, and this thought would not go away.
14.	You thought you could hear in your head the television commercial in your head for the product you bought at the store.
15.	You are confident about your memory of music and melodies, and you thought that you wouldn't forget a melody, once you heard it.
16.	You were bothered when things said by people close to you lingered in your ear.
17.	You clearly remembered talking with people and you felt as if you could even hear their voices.
18.	You clearly heard a melody in your head.
19.	You clearly heard music from a television commercial in your head.
20.	You clearly heard sounds in your imagination.
21.	You heard music in your head and, it was hard to erase it from your mind.
22.	Your ears became very sensitive and little sounds seemed irritating to you.
23.	Your own voice felt distant and foreign.
24.	The voices of people talking near you seemed far away.
25.	You heard sounds that did not actually exist (such as car or the cries of animals).
26.	Your ears played tricks on you (you thought you heard something even ifthough you didn't actually hear anything).
27.	What you thought was a person's voice was actually a different sound.

28.	You turned around in a crowd because you thought you heard someone call your name.
29.	When you were alone, you felt like that someone called your name.
30.	You heard a person's voice, but no one was there.
31.	You saw people laughing, and felt they were laughing about you.
32.	You heard people talking, and it sounded like they were gossiping and saying bad things about you.
33.	You felt thatlike sounds or voices around you had something to do with you.
34.	When you were on the verge of falling asleep or when you woke up, you heard a voice calling your name or someone talking.
35.	When you were on the verge of falling asleep or when you woke up, you had a vision of a person or an event from that day.
36.	When you were on the verge of falling asleep or when you woke up, you had a temporary feeling of paralysis and you couldn't move.
37.	Even though you were awake, you felt thatlike you were in a dream and you hallucinated or had strange experiences.
38.	You felt thatlike you heard a voice from God, or a friendly spirit.
39.	You felt thatlike you heard a voice from the devil, or a bad spirit.
40.	When you drank alcohol or the morning after drinking, you felt like you were in a dream, and you had hallucinations.

Results and Discussion

This study used the Pearson product–moment correlation coefficient, r, as a measure of effect size to enable comparisons involving each r (Cohen, 1988). First, the use of an interval of 1 month to measure test–retest reliability for the scales was shown to be reasonable (r = 0.78, p < .0001); the internal reliability was also shown to be reasonable (α = 0.84).

We decided to use two factors to examine the screeplot and conducted a factor analysis of the 17 items of AHES-17 using the maximum likelihood method with promax rotation for latent roots (Table 2).

The first factor included auditory hallucinations as caused by internal speech or thinking (Factor 1 from the factor analysis of the original AHES), auditory hallucinations related to music (Factor 3 of AHES), and auditory hallucinations related to the voices of others (Factor 4 of AHES); the alpha coefficient was 0.82. The second factor included delusions or thought insertion as related to auditory hallucinations (Factor 2 of AHES); the alpha coefficient was 0.87. We referred to the first factor as Voice and music, because it included auditory hallucinations related to one's own voice, the voices of others, and music. We found a strong correlation between the first and second factors (r = 0.54). The second factor was referred to as Paranoid ideation because it involved auditory hallucinations as related to paranoid ideation. This finding is consistent with the status of both hallucinations and delusions as positive symptoms of schizophrenia as well as with the high rate of complications associated with this disorder (Verdoux, et al., 1998).

Table 3 shows the correlations between the AHES-17 and the LSHS (hallucination-like experiences), the STA (positive symptoms of schizotypy), the SPQB (schizotypal personality disorder), the O-Life (schizotypal personality traits), the STAI (anxiety), and the SDS (depression). As we predicted, the strongest correlation emerged between the AHES and the

LSHS (r = 0.76). Correlations between the AHES and the STA, the Unusual Experiences (UnEx) scale of the O-Life, and the Cognitive–Perceptual Deficits scale of the SPQB were also high (r = 0.44, r = 0.50, r = 0.50, respectively). These three scales measure positive symptoms of schizophrenia, including auditory hallucinations. Furthermore, we also found high correlations between scores on the AHES and scores for the Cognitive Disorganization (CoDi) and Impulsive Nonconformity (ImNo) factors of the O-Life (r = 0.47, r = 0.44, respectively). The Unusual Experiences (UnEx) and CoDi factors of the O-Life often show strong correlations (e.g., Asai, & Tanno, 2009; Kecskemeti, & Loas, 2001). Asai, Sugimori, and Tanno (in press) suggested that positive and negative factors might be foundational and might cause disorganized schizotypy. The fourth factor, ImNo, focuses on the affective dimension in psychiatric disorders (Claridge & Davis 2003) and which is more strongly related to bipolar disorder and borderline personality disorder than to schizophrenia (Mason, Claridge, & Williams, 1997). That is, Impulsive Nonconformity might not be a central characteristic of schizotypal personality.

Table 2. AHES-17 Items and Factor Loadings

		1	2
4	Your thoughts were so strong, it feltwas as if you had said them aloud.	**0.58**	-0.10
13	When you were alone, you felt like someone called your name.	**0.55**	0.10
5	You felt there was a "voice of conscience" inside you.	**0.54**	0.02
14	You heard a person's voice, but no one was there.	**0.53**	0.16
6	You felt there was a "voice calling you towards bad things" inside you.	**0.52**	0.03
8	You clearly heard clearly a melody in your head.	**0.51**	-0.05
11	What you thought was a person's voice was actually a different sound.	**0.50**	0.11
9	You clearly heard music from a television commercial in your head.	**0.49**	-0.03
12	You turned around in a crowd because you thought you heard someone calling your name.	**0.48**	0.15
10	You heard music in your head, and it was hard to erase it from your mind.	**0.47**	0.00
1	You contemplated something while having a conversation in your head with another person.	**0.41**	-0.03
7	You are confident about your memory of music and melodies, and you thought that you wouldn't forget a melody once you heard it.	**0.41**	-0.12
2	To gather your thoughts, you had a conversation in your head with an imaginary person.	**0.40**	0.01
3	You muttered to yourself when you were thinking about something.	**0.30**	0.13
16	You heard people talking which, and it sounded to you like they were gossiping and saying bad things about you.	-0.11	**0.99**
15	You saw people laughing and felt they were laughing about you.	-0.10	**0.95**
17	You felt thatlike sounds or voices around you had something to do with you.	0.20	**0.59**
	Correlation between factors		
	Factor 1	-	
	Factor 2	0.54	-

Table 3. Pearson Correlations for Scores on the AHES-17 and Other Scales

		1	2	3	4	5	6	7	8	9	10	11	12	13
AHES	1.Total	—												
	2.Voi and Mu	0.97**	—											
	3.Para	0.69**	0.49**	—										
4.LSHS		0.75**	0.73**	0.50**	—									
SPQB	5.Cog	0.46**	0.42**	0.36**	0.45**	—								
	6.Int	0.17**	0.10	0.30**	0.18**	0.32**	—							
	7.Dis	0.31**	0.27**	0.28**	0.30**	0.37**	0.30**	—						
8.STA		0.47**	0.40**	0.41**	0.44**	0.52**	0.40**	0.49**	—					
O-Life	9.UnEx	0.50**	0.50**	0.38**	0.52**					—				
	10.InAn	0.47**	0.39**	0.55**	0.38**					0.52**	—			
	11.CoDi	0.25*	0.25*	0.20	0.26*					0.08	0.31**	—		
	12.ImNo	0.44**	0.37**	0.50**	0.48**					0.51**	0.41**	0.12	—	
13.STAI		0.35**	0.25**	0.50**	0.34**	0.33**	0.41**	0.37**	0.45**	0.39**	0.72**	0.28**	0.35**	—
14.SDS		0.36**	0.28**	0.44**	0.37**	0.35**	0.36**	0.39**	0.53**	0.35**	0.61**	0.36**	0.38**	0.78**

* p < .05, ** p < .01

Voi and Mu = Voice and music, Para = Paranoid ideation.
Cog = Cognitive, Int = Interpersonal, Dis = Disorganization.
UnEx = Unusual Experiences, InAn = Introvertive Anhedonia, CoDi = Cognitive Disorganization, ImNo = Impulsive Nonconformity.

We used the data from the SPQB to investigate the relationship between schizotypy and the AHES-17 asbecause the sample size was sufficient for the path analysis. The results of correlation analyses involving the subscales of AHES-17 and those of the SPQB (Table 2) showed that the Interpersonal subscale was highly related to Paranoid ideation (r = 0.30) but not to Voice and music (r = 0.10), whereas correlations between Paranoid ideation and Cognitive and Disorganization, and those between Voice and music and Cognitive and Disorganization were equally high. Based on these results, we constructed path models and examined these relationships using SPSS 17.0 and Amos 17.0 for the statistical analysis. When we investigated whether Voice and music explained Paranoid ideation or, alternatively, whether Paranoid ideation explained Voice and music (the difference being the direction of the arrow), the former showed better fitness than did the latter. However, the correlation between Paranoid ideation and Disorganization was not significant (r = 0.08; Figure 1); we therefore omitted the arrow from Paranoid ideation and Disorganization, and reexamined these relationships (Figure 2).

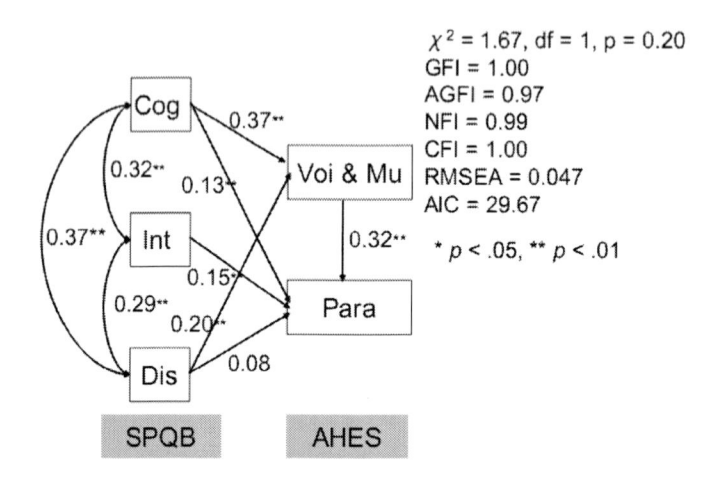

Figure 1. The path model from SPQB to AHES

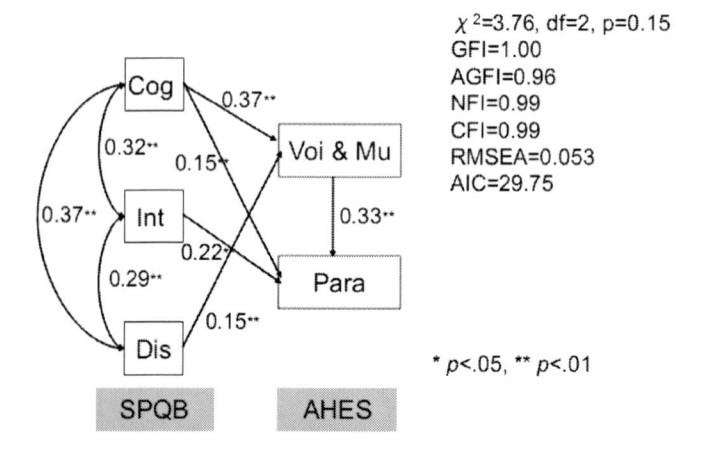

Figure 2. The path model from SPQB to AHES

These data reveal two new findings. First, Voice and music explained the Paranoid ideation and not vice versa, and Interpersonal explained Paranoid ideation. MacBeth, Schwannauer, and Gumley (2008) showed that, higher levels of interpersonal problems were associated with higher paranoia scores. It might be suggested that complications associated with auditory hallucinations related to voice and music, as well as negative symptoms of schizophrenia, may cause auditory hallucinations related to paranoid ideation. Second, Disorganization explained Voice and music but Disorganization did not directly explain Paranoid ideation, although previous studies showed a relationship between positive symptoms, including auditory hallucination-like experiences, and schizotypal personality (e.g., Asai, & Tanno, 2007; Kecskemeti, & Loas, 2001), or between delusional ideation and schizotypal personality disorder (Bockian, 2006). It may be that schizotypal personality disorder is directly related to auditory hallucination-like experiences, involving voices and music and indirectly related to other positive symptoms through such experiences such as auditory hallucination-like experiences related to voice and music.

Our purpose in this study was to develop a brief measure of auditory hallucination-like experiences (AHES-17). Test–retest reliability and internal reliability were adequate. Factor analyses revealed that the AHES-17 consists of two factors: Voice and music, and Paranoid ideation. The investigation of criterion-related validity showed that the AHES was highly correlated with scales measuring positive symptoms of schizophrenia, including auditory hallucinations. Furthermore, we examined the path model of the AHES and the SPQB based on the results obtained investigating criterion-related validity. The results of this analysis suggested the possibility, that auditory hallucinations are not initially related to paranoia, but emerge as a complication of the auditory hallucinations and negative symptoms associated with schizophrenia and thereafter manifest as paranoid auditory hallucinations. Based on these results, we conclude that the AHES-17 is suitable for use as a scale measuring auditory hallucination-like experiences and should prove helpful, to research into auditory hallucination-like experiences.

Auditory Verbal Hallucination and the Sense of Agency

What couldmay cause the auditory verbal hallucinations in the patients with schizophrenia or the auditory hallucination-like experiences in the general population? Many people with schizophrenia describe a sense of passivity to their experiences, in that their actions, thoughts, or emotions are experienced as something created for them by some external agent rather than through just by their own will. These positive symptoms of schizophrenia are included among Schneider's first-rank symptoms for the diagnosis of schizophrenia (Mellors, 1970; Schneider, 1959). Phenomena such as delusions of control, auditory hallucinations, and thought insertion canmay all be caused by an abnormal sense of agency (Frith et al., 2000a; Gallagher, 2004; Lindner, Their, Kircher, Haarmeier & Leube, 2005). For example, one's own speech could seem to be an auditory hallucinations (McGuigan, 1966). The activation of Broca's area,, which couldan produce but cannot listen to speech, has been associated with auditory hallucinations (McGuire, Shah & Murray, 1993).

ThereforeThus, these people mayight produce speech but may not think that they actually spoke. Then aAs a result,, they may hear their own voices as the voices of others.

The abnormal sense of agency in schizophrenia has been shown empirically. Some studies reported, that when required to make judgments about the origin of hand actions or movements based upupon biased feedback (self-action recognition task), people with schizophrenia or schizotypal personality were more likely than normal controls to misattribute their own actions (Asai & Tanno, 2007; 2008; Daprati et al., 1997; Franck et al., 2001), which might be interpreted as a delusions of control. As well, Sschizophrenic patients with auditory hallucinations tend to misattribute their own speech as well (self-speech recognition task: e.g., Johns et al., 1999; 2001). With the objective ofTo measuringe the subjective aspect of the sense of agency, we developed a scale to measure the sense of agency in a general population (Asai, Takano, Sugimori & Tanno, 2009). In the following subsection, we introduced that scale, asbecause it was developed in Japanese.

Developing the Sense of Agency Scale

Cognitive neuropsychological studies based on theories of the social brain or social cognition have recently reported, on how our brain recognizes the "self." Gallagher (2000) suggested that self-consciousness can be divided into two components: the narrative self, aswhich is related to our identity, and the minimal self. The latter can also be divided into two parts: the sense of agency, or the sense that "I am the one who generates the action," and the sense of ownership, or the sense that "This acting hand is my own hand." This sense of self has been the focus of research in many fields bBecause thea sense of agency is reliantsts upon the experience of one's own actions., this sense of self has been the focus of research in many fields.

The sense of agency refers to the experience of attributing one's own action or its neurological correlate to the self. Because this sense generally occurs implicitly and automatically in general, humans do n noot consciously experience thisa sense of agency when in the process ofwhen acting. ThisIt is, however, observable in the psychopathology of schizophrenia, which canmight involve a disordered sense of self.

Schizophrenia, which is characterized by delusions or hallucinations, has a lifetime incidence of about 1% (Kendler et al., 1996). McGuigan (1966) conducted the pioneering study that first suggestinged the relationship between symptoms of passivity and an abnormal sense of agency in schizophrenia. In that study, auditory hallucinations (in most cases, experienced as emanating from someone else; Nayani & David, 1996) were considered to possibly represent as one's own speech. On the basis of these studies, Frith hypothesized that schizophrenic patients mayight lack a sense of agency over their own speech and might consequently interpret their own speech as emanating from someone else (Frith, 1987, 1992).

The sense of agency has been examined empirically, including throughby research in the domain of brain science. Measures of this phenomenon thatthat eliminated participants' subjective experiences would enable the objective comparisons. On the other hand, however, we assume that data on the participants' subjective feelings should be integrated with the results of the objective measures used in experiments. In any event, the only evidence concerning sense of agency has derived from clinical observations focused on such questions such as "Do schizophrenic patients really not experience a sense of agency when they act?" A questionnaire methodology might could represent an effective approach, towards understanding of subjective feelings. Using this technique,, we could can compare the subjective sense of agency of patients in terms of both quantity and quality. To A scale measuring the sense of agency is necessary to examinee this phenomenon and identify peoplethose with impairments in this domain, a scale is necessary, with the objective of measuring the sense of agency.

Method

Development of the scale

After reviewing existing schizotypal personality scales (STA, Claridge & Broks, 1984; O-LIFE, Mason et al., 1995; SPQ, Raine, 1991), we selected 31 items related to the sense of agency as defined in the present study (i.e., the sense of attributing of one's own actions to one's self). These items seemed to be potentially characterized by a three-factor structure: mentality or perception, physicality or action, and interpersonal relationships or sociability. The first factor included seven items (e.g., "I sometimes hear voices or sounds when I am thinking."). The second factor included eight items (e.g., "I sometimes feel as if my own body doesn't really exist."). The third factor included six items (e.g., "I sometimes feel that the casual comments or sounds made by others are really related to me.").

Drawing on the extant literature, we added 19 original items. we We added six items (e.g., "I sometimes cannot distinguish what I am thinking from what is real." (Ditman & Kuperberg, 2005)) to the first factor. We added eight items (e.g., "I sometimes feel that I don't have control of my own body" (Lenzenweger & Maher, 2002)) to the second factor. We added five items (e.g., "I sometimes feel like my behavior has some effect on society.") to the third factor.

High scores on these 40 items used in my study indicate an abnormal or unstable sense of agency. Participants were asked, "How much do the following items apply to you in your daily life?" and were instructed to respond on a scale ranging from 1 to 4, where 1 indicated "never," 2 indicated "not much," 3 indicated "a little," and 4 indicated "very much."

Participants and procedure

The sample was comprised of university students (N = 242; males: 178, females: 65; average age: 18.9 years, SD = 1.03) who had participated in three previous longitudinal studies (of two, two, and five weeks), as described below.

I obtained valid data from 210 respondents to the first survey mentioned above (males: 156, females: 54), which included the STA, the Self-monitoring Scale (SMS; Snyder & Gangestad, 1986), and the Rosenberg Self-esteem Scale (RSES; Rosenberg, 1965). The STA was developed to address schizotypal passive experiences. Because passivity experiences caused by an abnormal sense of agency seem to be included among these passive experiences, we predicted a relationship between this measure and the sense-of-agency scale, demonstrating convergent validity. The SMS was developed with the objective to address self-monitoring traits, which relate to selecting actions within a social context. Because the concept of self-monitoring resembles the sense of agency, we predicted that a relationship would emerge between these constructs. The RSES was developed with the objective to assess self-esteem in terms of ability and sense of personal worth. We predicted that a relationship between this construct and social factors would emerge, within my scale.

I obtained valid questionnaires from 184 respondents in the second survey (males: 125, females: 59), which included the State–Trait Anxiety Inventory (STAI-T; Spielberger et al., 1970), the State–Trait Anger Expression Inventory (STAXI-T; Spielberger, 1988), the Paranoia Checklist (PC; Freeman et al., 2005), and the Liebowitz Social Anxiety Scale (LSAS; Liebowitz, 1987). The STAI-T and STAXI-T were developed with the objective to measure trait anxiety and trait anger, respectively. We predicted that the validity of these constructs would be independent of the Sense of Agency scale because these traits might not be related to sense of agency (e.g., Asai et al., 2008). The PC was developed to measure persecutory delusions in the general population. This trait is included in schizophrenic experiences, but might not be related to sense of agency (Frith et al., 2000), and we predicted that it would be independent of the sense of agency. The LSAS was developed to measure tendencies to avoid social situations. We predicted a relationship between this phenomenon and the social factor, within the sense-of-agency scale.

I received 157 valid questionnaires in the third survey (males: 108, females: 49), which included the newly developed Sense of Agency Scale temporary (SOASt), and the Self-rating Depression Scale (SDS; Zung, 1965). The SDS was developed with the objective to measure depression in the general population. We predicted no relationship to occur between these measures because depression might not be conceptually related to sense of agency.

I obtained 132 valid questionnaires in the fourth survey (males: 93, females: 39), which included the SOASt to confirm its reliability.

Results

On the basis of the results obtained by the SOASt in the third survey, we eliminated 18 items because their distributions were skewed (i.e., ceiling or floor effects: their average scores ±1 SD were beyond the score sphere). We conducted factor analysis with maximum likelihood estimation and promax rotation on the 22 remaining items because we assumed that the three potential factors were related to one another. We fixed the number of factors at three, and this three-factor structure showed the best fit to the data (eigenvalues were 7.19, 2.29, 1.50, 1.29, and 0.83…). Furthermore, wWe eliminated the five items with factor loadings under 4.0, and we reversed the score for item 17 because its factor loading value was negative. As a result, the final Sense of Agency Scale (SOAS) included 17 items reflecting three factors (Table 4).

Because the first factor included the item like "I sometimes turn around, feeling as if someone called my name in a crowd," we interpreted this factor as measuring the sense of agency experienced during the stage in which information is received (input level), and we labeled this "the misattribution of the agent in mental activity" ("mental"). Because the second factor included items such as "I sometimes don't have control of my own body," this factor was interpreted as measuring the sense of agency during the stage involving somatic output (output level), and we named this factor "the uncontrollability of one's own body in physical activity" ("physical"). Because the third factor included items such as "I sometimes stick to my opinion, not compromising with others," this factor was interpreted as measuring sense of agency, with respect to social activities, and we named this "self-assertiveness in social activities" ("social").

Table 4. The factorial structure in SOAS

	Item	1	2	3	commonality
1	I sometimes turn around feeling as if someone called my name in a crowd	**.67**	-.15	.04	.473
2	I am sometimes told that I speak loud	**.53**	-.29	.27	.437
3	I sometimes feel that the casual voice or sounds made by others is related to me	**.47**	.19	.03	.257
4	What I thought I had actually seen was in fact mistaken at times	**.47**	.31	-.01	.317
5	I sometimes find that what I thought was my idea was actually that of others	**.47**	.15	-.13	.260
6	I sometimes cannot distinguish what I actually said from what I intended to say	**.45**	.02	-.11	.215
7	I sometimes mistake things or shadows for a person	**.44**	-.02	.02	.194
8	I sometimes feel that I can never understand what others are thinking	-.17	**.62**	.14	.432
9	However As hard I try to concentrate, unrelated matters sometimes still enter my thoughts	.14	**.49**	.04	.261
10	I am sometimes asked to repeat myself as I speak in a low voice	-.04	**.47**	-.30	.312
11	I sometimes feel I cannot move my body as I want	.14	**.47**	.11	.252
12	I sometimes smile over my memories	.02	**.46**	.01	.212
13	I sometimes forget what I had wanted to say	.36	**.42**	-.08	.312
14	I sometimes stick to my opinion, not compromising with others	-.08	.13	**.72**	.541
15	I sometimes push things forward with my own initiative	.04	-.02	**.60**	.362
16	I sometimes feel that my behavior has some effect on society	.14	.20	**.49**	.299
17	I feel more comfortable to follow a leader than to open up a new field by myself	.17	.06	**-.52**	.302
	Correlations among factors after rotation				
	Factor 1	-			
	Factor 2	.45	-		
	Factor 3	.27	-.18		

Confirmation of Reliability

I examined the reliability of the SOAS. The test–retest results showed that the r values both for total scores and for each factor were about 0.70 (total score, r(107) = .73; first factor, r(107) = .68; second factor, r(107) = .68; third factor, r(107) = .72; p < 0.0001). We also examined internal coherence and α values were .77, .72, .68, and .68 for the total score and for the first through third factors, respectively. Thus, weWe thus confirmed that the stability and coherence of the SOAS were sufficient to warrant its use.

Confirmation of Validity

I first examined sex differences, and fiounding no significant differences for the SOAS total score, for each factor of the SOAS, and for the other questionnaires. We also conducted correlation analyses to confirm the validity of the SOAS (Table 5). The results showed that all combinations of each factor in the SOAS were significant. The STA, which was used to confirm convergent validity, was significantly correlated with the SOAS total score and with each of its factors. However, the STA was a source of some items for the SOASt and was significantly correlated with the other five scales used in this study. For this reason, we conducted partial correlation analysis, controlling for the STA to examine the relationship with the SOAS (Table 6).

When we focused on the SOAS total score, the simple correlation analysis revealed significant correlations with the PC, STA (moderate), STAI-T, STAXI-T, and SDS (marginal). When we conducted the partial correlation analysis controlling for STA scores, however, these significant correlations disappeared. A significant negative correlation between the SOAS and the SMS was observed, indicating that individuals with an unstable sense of agency might lack an appropriate sense of control over their own actions in social situations. Furthermore, the partial correlation analysis revealed that the SOAS was distinguishable from other scales, including the SDS, STAI-T, STAXI-T (emotional aspects), LSAS, and RSES (social aspects). On the other hand, the PC included schizotypal personality traits, but no significant correlation with the SOAS emerged because the PC seems to be conceptually unrelated to the SOAS. In summary, in the simple correlation analysis, the SOAS was correlated with the STA and PC more strongly than it was with the other scales; in the partial correlation analysis, the SOAS was significantly correlated with the SMS, which is conceptually similar to the SOAS. These findings suggested the validity of the entire SOAS.

The first factor, "the misattribution of the agent in mental activity," was not significantly correlated with other variables according to the results of the partial correlation analysis, indicating that this factor might relate to the characteristics as associated with schizotpy (STA), with the exception of paranoia (PC), and couldmight be distinguishable from emotional or social traits. The second factor, "the uncontrollability of one's own body in physical activity," was negatively correlated with scores on the SMS and positively correlated with scores on the STAI-T and SDS, indicating that, those with an unstable sense of agency in physical activities might lack the experience of being able to control their own actions in social situations and tend incline toward depression and anxiety. This "physical" factor was distinguishable from social traits, including those as addressed by the LSAS and RSES, and was not always unique to schizotypy. The third factor, "self-assertiveness in social activities," was positively correlated with scores on the SMS and RSES and negatively correlated with those on of the STAI-T, LSAS, and SDS, indicating that individuals who were assertive or had an unstable sense of agency in social activities might have appropriate self-control in social situations, higher self-esteem, resistance to depression and anxiety, and indifference to social situations.

Table 5. Correlation matrix among questionnaires

		N	Mean	SD	1	2	3	4	5	6	7	8	9	10	11
1	SOAS	157	40.2	7.65	-										
2	Factor 1	157	14.9	4.07	.82**	-									
3	Factor 2	157	16.1	3.68	.77**	.42**	-								
4	Factor 3	157	9.20	2.73	.56**	.23**	.17*	-							
5	SMS	209	37.8	8.02	-.01	.03	-.24**	.26**	-						
6	STAI-T	184	48.6	10.9	.24**	.23**	.38**	-.17	.28**	-					
7	SDS	157	44.4	8.44	.16*	.22**	.28**	-.25**	-.14	.72**	-				
8	STAXI-T	184	48.6	10.9	.29**	.25**	.21**	.14	.28**	.41**	.25**	-			
9	RSES	209	32.0	8.42	.02	.03	-.14	.18	.17*	-.22**	-.32**	.08	-		
10	LSAS	181	47.3	14.2	.00	.08	.18*	-.35**	-.25**	.33**	.32**	-.01	-.07	-	
11	STA	210	10.5	6.33	.54**	.48**	.40**	.27**	.26**	.46**	.35**	.46**	-.06	.09	-
12	PC	183	34.4	12.0	.45**	.43**	.31**	.19**	.16*	.46**	.34**	.45**	-.15	.11	.62**

* *p*<.05, ** *p*<.01

Table 6. Partial correlation matrix between SOAS and other questionnaires controlling STA as covariance

SOAS	1	2	3	4	5	6	7
Factor 1	-.16	.00	-.02	-.03	.09	-.03	.14
Factor 2	-.42*	.32**	.22*	.06	-.12	.17	.12
Factor 3	.21*	-.34**	-.41**	.05	.21*	-.39**	.07
Total	-.22*	.02	-.07	.03	.08	-.10	.17

* p<.05, ** p<.01
Note. 1=SMS, 2=STAI-T, 3=SDS, 4=STAXI-T, 5=RSES, 6=LSAS, 7=PC

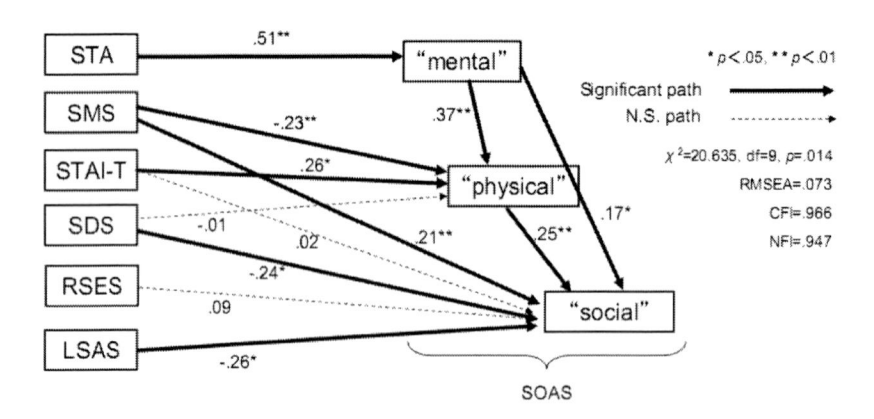

Figure 3. Hierarchic structure in SOAS

This "social" factor might could include emotional and social aspects, and it might not always be unique to schizotypy, as noted with regard to the second factor. These relationships might could be interpreted as appropriate and as demonstrative ofng valid correlations in general.

Thus, the three factors in the SOAS were related to emotional or social traits, and these relationships were independent of schizotypal personality traits, thereby suggesting a hierarchical structure for the SOAS. The mental factor is reflective ofs the ability to distinguish between self and other, irrespective of emotional and social traits. The physical factor is related to emotional traits, and the social factor mayight constitute a general personality trait whichthat includes both emotional and social features. Can we assume a directional path originating in self–other misattribution and moving through a sense of being unable to control one's own body to an assertive attitude in social situations? We conducted path analysis, to examine the potential hierarchical structure of the SOAS.

On the basis of the significant correlations presented in Table 6, we assumed the aforementioned path and hierarchical structure (Figure 3). We conducted path analysis using Amos 16.0J, and each relevant measure indicated that this model showed good fit to the data (Schermelleh-Engel et al., 2003). The relationship between the SOAS and other scales was replicated in this analysis, and a hierarchical structure among the three factors in the SOAS was suggested. That beingis, the mental factor, which is unique to schizotypal personality, could could explain the physical and social factors as well as other emotional and social traits, and the physical factor also explaininged the social factor. This relationship suggests a hierarchical structure, in the sense of agency in which each factor might may have a different relationship to other emotional or social personality traits.

Discussion

In the present study, we developed the Sense of Agency Scale (SOAS) in order to measure the sense of beingthat "I am the one who generates the action." The results of statistical analyses showed that, the 17-item SOAS had a three-factor structure, which was consistent with the hypothesized three factors (mental, physical, and social), although some items were included in unexpected factors. Simple correlation analysis revealed that, each factor was related to schizotypal personality; when this effect was controlled, the SOAS total score was related to self-monitoring traits (SMS), including mental, physical, and social features (i.e., extroversion and the sense of control over one's own actions). Because the SOAS and SMS include shared traits, their relationship seems to be valid.

The mental factor in the sense of agency, which might be unique to schizophrenia or schizotypal personality, is characterized by the misattribution of what is seen or heard. The relationship between schizophrenia and misattribution in source memory (Ditman & Kuperberg, 2005) or between schizophrenia and misattribution in regard to one's own action or speech (Daprati et al., 1997; Franck et al., 2001; Cahill et al., 1996) might be related to this mental factor. The physical factor in the sense of agency is characterized by the sense of a lack of control over one's own body or experiencing one's self as acting automatically. This factor is not always unique to schizophrenia and is related to emotional traits, including depression and anxiety. For example, people with depression have reported feeling a lack of control over their actions (Thomas et al., 2008). On the other hand, the relationship between schizophrenia or schizotypal personality and feeling a lack of control over one's own movements (Blyler et al, 1997; Lenzenweger & Maher, 2002) might may be associated with this physical factor. The social factor in the sense of agency is characterized by self-assertiveness or over-estimation of self. Although the attribution of external events to the self (Haggard et al, 2003) has been suggested in schizophrenia, this factor couldmight be seen as a general personality trait, such as "openness," in the five-factor model of personality (O'Connor, 2002). The sense of agency might be related to a type of personality found in the general population, gGiven that schizotypal personality canmight be observed as a personality type within the general population (Rawlings & Feeman, 1997) and that the sense of agency constitutes the nature of main component of self-consciousness., the sense of agency might be related to a type of personality found in the general population.

These results suggest the validity of the SOAS as well as an acceptable level of reliability. Although the number of items (17 items in the present form) might be suitable for an experimental procedure, it would be useful to increase the number of items to achieve a number such as in the STAXI (Spielberger, 1999). The test–retest reliability was also acceptable. This suggests some ambiguity with regard to the the effect of external stress on the sense of agency. Auditory hallucinations, which might could be caused by an abnormal sense of agency, seem to be associated with reports that the patients hear others' voices immediately after emotional reactions, including sadness or fear (Nayani & David, 1996), which indicatesing that thethese stressful events mayight have lead to thisan unstable sense of agency. Further studies should examine whether or not the sense of agency might be related to traits or states.

Positive correlations were observed among all factors. On the surface, the mental and physical factors measured by the SOAS appearseem to represent negative aspects, but the social factor in this scale might not be problematic. Indeed, the social factor couldmight be related to resistance to negative emotions, including depression and anxiety. However, the positive correlation between the social and physical factors indicates that the feeling ofa lack of control over physical activities mayight lead to assertiveness in social situations. Asai et al. (2008) suggested a relationship between schizotypal personality and an underestimation of one's own movements (i.e., overreaching). Overreaching (self-assertiveness or lack of humility) canmight be observed in movements as well as in social activities.

The present study suggests an internal hierarchical structure, for the sense of agency, as beingwhich is a component of self-consciousness. Because self-consciousness might could be characterized by a hierarchic structure, it is reasonable that the sense of agency would also be characterized by a hierarchical rather than a one-dimensional structure. TAlthough the statistical analyses suggested that misattributions of agency could lead to failure in accounting for one's own actions and that this could lead to assertiveness in social situations, causal relationships among these variables should be examined in detail.

Speech predictive pathway

Speech executive pathway

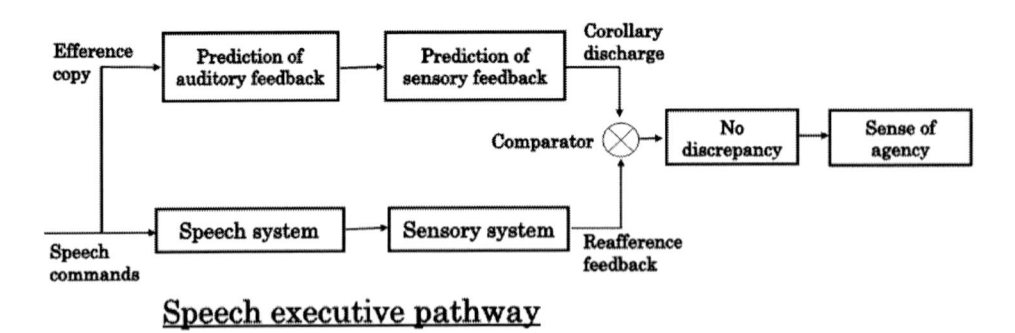

Figure 4. Neurocognitive model of the speech control and the sense of agency

In summary, we developed the Sense of Agency Scale. First, an unstable sense of agency is not always unique to schizophrenia or schizotypal personality. Second, an unstable sense of agency can be divided into three factors. Third, each factor in this case has a relationship to emotional or social traits and the three are characterized by a hierarchical structure. Because the social factor includes only a few items, we should carefully consider whether to use the total SOAS score or the score for each factor when employing this scale. In addition, this measure should be standardized with a very large sample.

Neurocognitive Model for the Sense of Agency and the Auditory Verbal Hallucination

The forward model, which is part of the computational model of motor control (Wolpert, Ghahramani & Jordan, 1995), explainings the neuropsychological mechanism of the sense of agency (Frith et al., 2000b; Wolpert, 1997). This model includes two information-processing pathways, the action-predictive and the executive pathway; the former deals with action planning, and the latter with action execution (Asai, Sugimori & Tanno, 2008; Miall & Wolpert, 1996; Schmidt, 1988). This model can be applied in several ways, including in the differentiation of self-produced sensations from externally generated sensations (Miall & Wolpert, 1996). Prediction of the actual outcome of motor commands can be compared with the desired outcome (forward dynamic model). When a movement is made, an efferent copy of the motor command is used to make a prediction of the sensory consequences of the movement (forward output model). This sensory prediction can then be compared with the actual sensory feedback from the movement. As the discrepancy between the predicted and actual sensations increases, likewiseso does the likelihood that the sensation is externally produced (Sato & Yasuda, 2005). In this way, the forward model can differentiate self-produced sensations from externally generated sensations and can thereby generate a sense of agency (Blakemore & Frith, 2003; Blakemore, Wolpert & Frith, 2002; Frith et al., 2000b; Wolpert, 1997; Wolpert et al., 1995). According to a review by Miall & Wolpert (1996), the circuit linking the ventral premotor cortex (F5), the PF part of the posterior parietal cortex (PPC), and the superior temporal sulcus (STS) may act as a forward model, along with the cerebellum, to predict movement outcome. Furthermore, the extrastriate body area (EBA), as which might supporting the disentangling of one's own behavior from that of another (David et al., 2007), may act as comparator to generate a sense of agency.

Frith et al. (2000a; 2000b) and Blakemore et al. (2002) suggested that, the abnormal sense of agency experienced by people with schizophrenia might be caused by an abnormal prediction system in their motor control or forward model. In this model, people with schizophrenia are aware that an action matches an intention, but do not experiencehave no awareness of initiating the action or of its predicted consequence. That is, the action executive pathway or actual sensory feedback may still produce a sense of self-ownership ("I am moving"), but the sense of agency is compromised ("I am not causing the movement") even if the actual movement matches the intended movement (Gallagher, 2000). Indeed, Carnahan, Aguilar, Malla, and Norman (1997) showed that people with schizophrenia demonstrated abnormal movement planning, which is associated with action prediction, although they had normal movement execution. How does the level of the abnormal prediction pathway in the forward model lead to an abnormal sense of agency? Frith (2005) suggested at least three possibilities: the abnormal forward dynamic model, the forward output model, and the comparator. EThe evidence that schizophrenic patients conform to the abnormal forward output model has increased. It has been claimed that schizophrenia may be a disorder of the corollary discharge systems (Blakemore, Rees, & Frith, 1998; Feinberg & Guazzelli, 1999; Shergill, Samson, Bays, Frith & Wolpert, 2005), which that are emphasized in the forward output model. Furthermore, some studies have suggested that people with schizophrenia exhibit an abnormal forward dynamic model, as being which predictive ofs the next state of our body when given motor commands. Frith and Done (1988) showed that schizophrenics are unable to rapidly correct their arm movements. The forward dynamic model makes this 'online' correction of movement possible (Miall & Wolpert, 1996). Asai et al. (2008) suggested that people with high scores on measures of schizotypy might exhibit an abnormal action prediction. Their predictive control of arm movements underperformed that of the low schizotypal people.

Although an abnormal sense of agency in schizophrenics was first suggested by studies of auditory hallucinations (e.g., McGuigan, 1966), the model of the sense of agency in speech has been suggested only recently, throughby the application ofying the model in action (Figure 4). Seal, Alemam, & McGuire (2004) and Jones & Fernyhough (2007) proposed a model for the sense of agency over speech that is congruent with the forward model of motor control in order to resolve the mechanism of auditory hallucination. Both models share the idea that the motor command for speech is accompanied by a parallel efferent copy of this motor command. The comparator integrates the latter with information about the current state of the system in order to predict the outcome of actually speaking as planned. These researchers suggest that if the actual sensory feedback matches the prediction, thate speech is regarded as emanating from the self. WThat is, when the speech has been predicted that is, a sense of agency over speech is the results. In line with the studies that suggesting the presence in schizophrenia of an abnormal action prediction system according to the forward model (e.g., Blakemore et al., 1998), some studies have suggested a schizophrenic abnormal speech prediction system (Ford & Mathalon, 2004, 2005; Ford et al., 2001). For example, Ford and Mathalon (2004) suggested the electrophysiological evidence of corollary discharge dysfunction in schizophrenia, showing that a corollary discharge from frontal areas where thoughts are generated failed to alert the auditory cortex that those discharges are were self-generated, leading to the misattribution of inner speech to external sources and producing the experience of auditory hallucinations. On the other hand, although few behavior studies have been conducted along these lines, the speech tracking tasks in schizophrenia (Hoffman et al., 1999; Lee et al., 2004) might may be related to this problem. Schizophrenic people have difficulty tracking auditory sentences.

Conclusion

In this chapter, we presented the scales for the auditory hallucination experiences and the abnormal sense of agency in the general population. These phenomena couldmight be linked with to the neurocognitive model for motor control including speech production. To focus on the subjective experiences including passivity phenomena, the questionnaire approach might may also be useful as well as behavioral experiments or brain imaging. A multi-level approach would be needed in the future.

References

American Psychiatric Association. (1980). *Diagnostic and statistical manual of mental disorders* (3rd ed.). Washington, DC: American Psychiatric Association.
American Psychiatric Association. (1987). *Diagnostic and statistical manual of mental disorders* (3rd ed.- Text Revision). Washington, DC: American Psychiatric Association.
American Psychiatric Association. (2000*). Diagnostic and statistical manual of mental disorders* (4th ed.- Text Revision) Washington, DC: American Psychiatric Association.
Asai, T. & Tanno, Y. (2007). The relationship between the sense of self-agency and schizotypal personality traits. *Journal of Motor Behavior*, *39*, 162-168.
Asai, T. & Tanno, Y. (2008). Highly schizotypal students have a weaker sense of self-agency. *Psychiatry and Clinical Neurosciences*, *62*, 115-119.
Asai, T., Bando, N., Sugimori E. & Tanno Y. (in press). The hierarchic structure in schizotypy and the five-factor model of personality, *Psychiatry Research*.
Asai, T., Sugimori, E. & Tanno, Y. (2008). Schizotypal personality traits and prediction of one's own movements in motor control: What causes an abnormal sense of agency? *Consciousness and Cognition*, *17*, 1131-1142.
Asai, T. & Tanno, Y. (2009). Schizotypy and handedness in Japanese participants revisited. *Laterality*, *14*, 86-94.

Asai, T., Takano, K., Sugimori, E. & Tanno, Y. (2009). Development of the sense of agency scale and its factor structure. *The Japanese Journal of Psychology*, *80*, 414-421. (in Japanese).

Barret, T. R. & Etheridge, J. B. (1992). Verbal hallucinations in normals, I : People who hear 'Voices'. *Applied Cognitive Psychology*, *6*, 379-387.

Barret, T. R. & Etheridge, J. B. (1992). Verbal hallucinations in normals: People who hear 'voices.' *Applied Cognitive Psychology*, *6*, 379-387.

Bentall, R. P., Claridge, G. S. & Slade, P. D. (1989). The dimensional nature of schizotypal traits: A factor analytic study with normal subjects. *British Journal of Clinical Psychology*, *28*, 363-375.

Blakemore, S. J. & Frith, C. (2003). Self-awareness and action. *Current Opinion in Neurobiology*, *13*, 219-224.

Blakemore, S. J., Rees, G. & Frith, C. (1998). How do we predict the consequences of our actions? A functional imaging study. *Neuropsychologia*, *36*, 521-529.

Blakemore, S. J., Wolpert, D. M. & Frith, C. D. (2002). Abnormalities in the awareness of action. *Trends in Cognitive Sciences*, *6*, 237-242.

Blyler, C. R., Maher, B. A., Manschreck, T. C. & Fenton, W. S. (1997). Line drawing as a possible measure of lateralized motor performance in schizophrenia. *Schizophrenia Research*, *26*, 15-23.

Bockian, N. R. (2006). Depression in schizotypal personality disorder. In: Bockian, N. R. (Ed.), *Personality-guided therapy for depression* (91-108). Washington, DC: American Psychological Association.

Cahill, C., Silbersweig, D. & Frith, C. D. (1996). Psychotic experiences induced in deluded patients using distorted auditory feedback. *Cognitive Neuropsychiatry*, *1*, 201-211.

Carnahan, H., Aguilar, O., Malla, A. & Norman, R. (1997). An investigation into movement planning and execution deficits in individuals with schizophrenia. *Schizophrenia Research*, *28*, 213-221.

Cella, M., Taylor, K. & Reed, P. (2007). Violation of expectancies produces more false positive reports in word detection tasks in people scoring high on the unusual experiences scale. *Personality and Individual Differences*, *43*, 59-70.

Chapman, L. J., Chapman, J. P. & Raulin, M. L. (1978). Body-image aberration in schizophrenia. *Journal of Abnormal Psychology*, *87*, 399-407.

Choong, C., Hunter, M. D. & Woodruff, P. W. R. (2007). Auditory hallucinations in those populations that do not suffer from schizophrenia. *Current Psychiatry Reports*, *9*, 206-212.

Claridge, G. (Eds.). (1997). *Schizotypy: Implication for illness and health*. Oxford, UK: Oxford University Press.

Claridge, G. & Broks, P. (1984). Schizotypy and hemisphere function: Theoretical considerations and the measurement of schizotypy. *Personality and Individual Differences*, *5*, 643-670.

Claridge, G. & Davis, C. (2003). *Personality and psychological disorders*. London: Arnold.

Cohen, J. (1988). *Statistical power analysis for the behavioral sciences* (2nd ed.). Hillsdale, NJ: Lawrence Erlbaum.

Cyhlarova, E. & Claridge, G. (2005). Development of a version of the Schizotypy Traits Questionnaire (STA) for screening children. *Schizophrenia Research*, *80*, 253-261.

Daprati, E., Franck, N., Georgieff, N., Proust, J., Pacherie, E., Dalery, J. & Jeannerod, M. (1997). Looking for the agent: An investigation into consciousness of action and self-consciousness in schizophrenic patients. *Cognition, 65*, 71-86.

David, N., Cohen, M. X., Newen, A., Bewernick, B. H., Shah, N. J., Fink, G. R. & Vogeley, K. (2007). The extrastriate cortex distinguishes between the consequences of one's own and others' behavior. *Neuroimage, 36*, 1004-1014.

Ditman, T. & Kuperberg, G. R. (2005). A source-monitoring account of auditory verbal hallucinations in patients with schizophrenia. *Harvard Review of Psychiatry., 13*, 280-299.

Feinberg, I. & Guazzelli, M. (1999). Schizophrenia - a disorder of the corollary discharge systems that integrate the motor systems of thought with the sensory systems of consciousness. *The Royal College of Psychiatrists, 174*, 196-204.

Ford, J. M. & Mathalon, D. H. (2004). Electrophysiological evidence of corollary discharge dysfunction in schizophrenia during talking and thinking. *Journal of Psychiatric Research, 38*, 37-46.

Ford, J. M. & Mathalon, D. H. (2005). Corollary discharge dysfunction in schizophrenia: Can it explain auditory hallucination? *International Journal of Psychophysiology, 58*, 179-189.

Ford, J. M., Mathalon, D. H., Heinks, T., Kalba, S., Faustman, W. O. & Roth, W. T. (2001). Neurophysiological evidence of corollary discharge dysfunction in schizophrenia. *American Journal of Psychiatry, 158*, 2069-2071.

Fossati, A., Raine, A., Carretta, I., Leonardi, B, & Maffei, C. (2003). The three-factor model of schizotypal personality: Invariance across age and gender. *Personality and Individual Differences, 35*, 1007-1019.

Franck, N., Farrer, C., Georgieff, N., Marie-Cardine, M., Dalery, J., d'Amato, T. & Jeannerod, M. (2001). Defective recognition of one's own actions in patients with schizophrenia. *American Journal of Psychiatry, 158*, 454-459.

Freeman, D., Garety, P. A., Bebbington, P. E., Smith, B., Rollinson, R., Fowler, D., Kuipers, E., Ray, K. & Dunn, G. (2005). Psychological investigation of the structure of paranoia in a non-clinical population. *British Journal of Psychiatry, 186*, 427-435.

Frith, C. (2005). The neural basis of hallucinations and delusions. *Comptes Rendus Biologies, 328*, 169-175.

Frith, C. D. (1987) The positive and negative symptoms of schizophrenia reflect impairments in the perception and initiation of action. *Psychological Medicine, 17*, 631-48.

Frith, C. D. (1992). *The cognitive neuropsychology of schizophrenia*. Mahwah, NJ: Erlbaum.

Frith, C. D. & Done, D. J. (1988). Experiences of alien control in schizophrenia reflect a disorder in the central monitoring of action. *Psychological Medicine, 19*, 359-363.

Frith, C. D., Blakemore, S. J. & Wolpert, D. M. (2000a). Explaining the symptoms of schizophrenia: Abnormalities in the awareness of action. *Brain Research Reviews, 31*, 357-363.

Frith, C. D., Blakemore, S. J. & Wolpert, D. M. (2000b). Abnormalities in the awareness and control of action. *Philosophical Transactions of the Royal Society of London: Biological Sciences, 355*, 1771-1788.

Gallagher, S. (2000). Philosophical conceptions of the self: Implications for cognitive science. *Trends in Cognitive Science, 4*, 14-21.

Gallagher, S. (2004). Neurocognitive models of schizophrenia: a neurophenomenological critique. *Psychopathology, 37*, 8-19.

Gruzelier, J. (1996). The factorial structure of schizotypy: Part I affinities with syndromes of schizophrenia. *Schizophrenia Bulletin, 22(4)*, 611-620.

Haggard, P., Martin, F., Taylor-Clarke, M., Jeannerod, M. & Franck, N. (2003). Awareness of action in schizophrenia. *Neuroreport, 14*, 1081-1085.

Hoffman, R. E., Rapaport, J., Mazure, C. M. & Quinian, D. M. (1999). Selective speech perception alterations in schizophrenic patients reporting hallucinated "voices." *American Journal of Psychiatry, 156*, 393-399.

Johns, L. C. (2005). Hallucinations in the general population. *Current Psychiatry Reports, 7*, 162-167.

Johns, L. C. & McGuire, P. K. (1999). Verbal self-monitoring and auditory hallucinations in schizophrenia. *Lancet, 353*, 469-470.

Johns, L. C., Rossell, S., Frith, C., Ahmad, F., Hemsley, D., Kuipers, E. & McGuire, P. K. (2001). Verbal self-monitoring and auditory verbal hallucinations in patients with schizophrenia. *Psychological Medicine, 31*, 705-715.

Jones, S. R. & Fernyhough, C. (2007). Thought as action: Inner speech, self-monitoring, and auditory verbal hallucinations. *Consciousness and Cognition, 16*, 391-399.

Kecskemeti, S. & Loas, G. (2001). Relationship between hallucinations and disorganization in schizophrenic patients. *Psychological Reports, 89*, 106.

Kendler, K. S., Gallagher, T. J., Abelson, J. M. & Kessler, R. C. (1996). Lifetime prevalence, demographic risk factors, and diagnostic validity of nonaffective psychosis as assessed in a US community sample. The National Comorbidity Survey. *Archives of General Psychiatry, 53*, 1022-1031.

Larøi, F., Van der Linden, M. & Marczewski, P. (2004). The effects of emotional salience, cognitive effort, and metacognitive beliefs on a reality monitoring task in hallucination-prone subjects. *British Journal of Clinical Psychology, 43*, 221-233.

Launay, G. & Slade, P. (1981). The measurement of hallucinatory predisposition in male and female prisoners. *Personality and Individual Differences, 2*, 221-234.

Lee, S. H., Chung, Y. C., Yang, J. C., Kim, Y. K. & Suh, K. Y. (2004). Abnormal speech perception in schizophrenia with auditory hallucinations. *Acta Neuropsychiatrica, 16*, 154-159.

Lenzenweger, M. F. & Maher, B. A. (2002). Psychometric schizotypy and motor performance. *Journal of Abnormal Psychology, 111*, 546–555.

Liebowitz, M. R. (1987). Social phobia. *Modern Problems of Pharmacopsychiatry, 22*, 141-173.

Lindner, A., Their, P., Kircher, T. T. J., Haarmeier, T. & Leube, D. T. (2005). Disorders of agency in schizophrenia correlate with an inability to compensate for the sensory consequences of actions. *Current Biology, 15*, 1119-1124.

MacBeth, A., Schwannauer, M. & Gumley, A. (2008). The association between attachment style, social mentalities, and paranoid ideation: An analogue study. *Psychology and Psychotherapy: Theory, Research and Practice, 81*, 79-83.

Mason, O., Claridge, G. & Jackson, M. (1995). New scale for the assessment of schizotypy. *Personality and Individual Differences, 18*, 7-13.

Mason, O., Claridge, G. & Williams, L. (1997). Questionnaire measurement. In Claridge, G. (Ed.), *Schizotypy: Implication for illness and health* (19-37). Oxford: Oxford University Press.

McGuigan, F. J. (1966). Covert oral behaviour and auditory hallucinations. *Psychiatry, 158*, 307-316.

McGuire, P. K., Shah, G. M. & Murray, R. M. (1993). Increased blood flow in Broca's area during auditory hallucinations in schizophrenia. *Lancet, 342*, 703-706.

Mellors, C. S. (1970). First rank symptoms of schizophrenia. *British Journal of Psychiatry, 117*, 15-23.

Miall, R. C. & Wolpert, D. M. (1996). Forward models for physiological motor control. *Neural Networks, 9*, 1265-1279.

Miyaji, Y. & Yama, H. (2002). Making Japanese lists which induce false memory at high probability for the DRM paradigm, *The Japanese journal of psychonomic science, 21*, 21-26.

Nayani, T. H. & David, A. S. (1996). The auditory hallucination: a phenomenological survey. *Psychological Medicine, 26*, 177-189.

O'Connor, B. P. (2002). A quantitative review of the comprehensiveness of the five-factor model in relation to popular personality inventories. *Assessment, 9*, 188-203.

Onari, Y. (1998). Psychological examination on the auditory hallucination experience. Graduation thesis, The University of Tokyo).

Osaka, N. (1998). Brain Model of Self-consciousness Based on Working Memory. *Japanese Psychological Review, 41*, 87-95. (in Japanese).

Raine, A. (1991). The SPQ: A scale for the assessment of schizotypal personality besed on DSM-III-R criteria. *Schizophrenia Bulletin, 17*, 555-564.

Raine, A. & Benishay, D. (1995). The SPQ-B: A brief screening instrument for schizotypal personality disorder. *Journal of Personality Disorder, 9*, 346-355.

Rankin, P. M. & O'Carroll, P. J. (1995). Reality discrimination, reality monitoring and disposition towards hallucination. *British Journal of Clinical Psychology, 34*, 517-528.

Rawlings, D. & Freeman, J. L. (1997). Measuring paranoia/ suspiciousness. In G. Claridge (Eds.). *Schizotypy: Implication for Illness and Health*. Oxford: Oxford University Press. 3-18.

Rosenberg, M. (1965). *Society and the adolescent self-image*. Prinston, NJ: Prinston Univ. Press.

Ross, S. R., Lutz, C. J. & Bailley, S. E. (2002). Positive and negative symptoms of schizotypy and the five-factor model: A domain and facet level analysis. *Journal of Personality Assessment, 79(1)*, 53-72.

Sato, A. & Yasuda, A. (2005). Illusion of self-agency: Discrepancy between the predicted and actual sensory consequences of actions modulates the sense of self-agency, but not the sense of self-ownership. *Cognition, 94*, 241-255

Schermelleh-Engel, K., Moosbrugger, H. & Muller, H. (2003). Evaluating the fit of structural equation models: Test of significance and descriptive goodness-of-fit measures. *Methods of Psychological Research, 8*, 23-74.

Schmidt, R. A. (1988). Motor Control and Learning: A Behavioral Emphasis. *Human Kinetics,* Champaign, IL.

Schneider, K. (1959). *Clinical psychopathology*. New York: Grune & Stratton.

Seal, M. L., Aleman, A. & McGuire, P. K. (2004). Compelling imagery, unanticipated speech and deceptive memory: Neurocognitive models of auditory verbal hallucinations in schizophrenia. *Cognitive Neuropsychiatry, 9*, 43-72.

Shergill, S., Samson, G., Bays, P., Frith C. & Wolpert, D. (2005). Evidence for sensory prediction deficits in schizophrenia. *American Journal of Psychiatry, 162*, 2384-2386.

Sidgewick, H., Johnson, A., Myers, F. W. H. et al. (1894). Report on the census of hallucinations. *Proceedings of the Society for Psychical Research, 34*, 25-394.

Snyder, M. & Gangestad, S. (1986). On the nature of self-monitoring: Matters of assessment, matters of validity. *Journal of Personality and Social Psychology, 51*, 125-39.

Spielberger, C. (1988). State-Trait Anger Expression Inventory, Research Edition. Professional Manual. Odessa, FL: *Psychological Assessment Resources*.

Spielberger, C. D. (1999). State-Trait Anger Expression Inventory-2: Professional Manual. Florida: *Psychological Assessment Resources*, Inc.

Spielberger, C. D., Gorsuch, R. L. & Lushene, R. E. (1970). In cursive: STAI. *Manual for the state-trait anxiety inventory*. Palo Alto, CA: Consulting Psychologist.

Stevenson, I. (1983). Do we need a new word to supplement 'hallucination'? *American Journal of Psychiatry, 140*, 1609-1611.

Sugimori, E., Asai, T. & Tanno, Y. (2009). Reliability and validity of the Auditory Hallucination-like Experience Scale. *The Japanese Journal of Psychology, 80*, 389-396. (in Japanese).

Tanno, Y., Ishigaki, T. & Sugiura, Y. (2000). Construction of scales to measure thematic tendencies of paranoid ideation. *The Japanese Journal of Psychology, 71*, 379-386.

Thomas, A. J., Gallagher, P., Robinson, L. J., Porter, R. J., Young, A. H., Ferrier, I. N. & O'Brien, J. T. (2008). A comparison of neurocognitive impairment in younger and older adults with major depression. *Psychological Medicine, 30*, 1-9.

Tien, A. Y. (1991). Distribution of hallucinations in the population. *Social Psychiatry and Psychiatric Epidemiology, 26*, 287-292.

Verdoux, H., Maurice-Tison, S., Gay, B., van Os, J., Salamon, R. & Bourgeois, M. L. (1998). A survey of delusional ideation in primary-care patients. *Psychological Medicine, 28*, 127-134.

Vollema, M. (1999). The current study: Context and outline. In Vollema, M. (Author & Ed.). *Schizotypy: toward the psychological heart of schizophrenia* (25-27). City, ST: Shaker Publishing.

Waters, F., Badcock, J. C. & Maybery, M. (2003). Revision of the factor structure of the Launay-Slade Hallucination Scale (LSHS-R). *Personality and Individual Differences, 35*, 1351-1357.

Wolpert, D. M. (1997). Computational approaches to motor control. *Trends in Cognitive Science, 1*, 209-216.

Wolpert, D. M., Ghahramani, Z. & Jordan, M. I. (1995). An internal model for sensorimotor integration. *Science, 269*, 1880-1882.

Zung, W. (1965). A self-rating depression scale. *Archives of General Psychiatry, 12*, 63-70.

Chapter 3

The Roles of Negative Affect in Auditory Hallucinations

Georgie Paulik and Johanna C. Badcock

Abstract

You hear a voice saying "Everyone is looking at you. You're making a fool of yourself *again*. You're pathetic". It's the voice of a young man, he sounds angry and he seems to be close by. You start to reply, then look around. No one is there.

Auditory hallucinations (AHs) are frequently pessimistic in content and intrusive in nature, and – not surprisingly – they are most often perceived by the individual as confronting and distressing. This potentially explains the high co-occurrence of AHs with depression, anger, fear, anxiety, low self-esteem, and suicide. However, in recent years it has become increasingly evident that negative affect plays more than one role in an hallucinatory event: it may be a trigger, a maintenance mechanism, a determinant of content, and an outcome. This chapter will start by briefly defining and describing the phenomenology of AHs in different populations, and then proceed to review the literature pertaining to each of the roles of negative affect in an hallucinatory event, and make recommendations for the treatment of AHs according to this multifaceted relationship.

Auditory Hallucinations

Auditory hallucinations (AHs) are broadly defined as auditory sensory experiences that occur in the absence of external stimuli that is perceived by the individual as a true perception (Gelder, Gath, & Mayou, 1993), that is of non-self origin (Nayani & David, 1996a), beyond the individual's control (Bentall, 1990), intrusive, unwanted, and interrupt ongoing reality (Slade & Bentall, 1988). AHs are traditionally associated with schizophrenia-spectrum disorders, in which they are highly prevalent, however they also occur in other mental-health disorders – especially mood and anxiety disorders – and in the general population. The phenomenology of hallucinatory experiences in these varied populations will be briefly reviewed in turn.

AHs are one of the most common symptoms experienced by individuals with schizophrenia, with approximately 74% of individuals with schizophrenia experiencing an AH at some stage during the course of their illness (Sartorius, Shapiro, & Jablensky, 1974). In schizophrenia, although non-verbal AHs are frequently experienced (i.e., music and environmental sounds), hearing "voices" is the most common form of AH, and are typically personal and negative in content, with individuals commonly reporting that their voices are commanding, critical and even abusive (Haddock, McCarron, Tarrier, & Faragher, 1999; Nayani & David, 1996a). Active voice hearers typically hear their voices between once a week to continuously, and may be perceived to originate from either outside or inside the head. In many cases the gender, identity (often a relative or friend) and even accent of hallucinated voices can be described (Haddock et al., 1999; Nayani & David, 1996a). The grammatical construction of voices also varies; second person (i.e. "you are a slob"), third person (i.e. "he's going to bed"), or purely descriptive non-personal comments (i.e. "the grass is green"), and sometimes - though less often - first person narration (i.e. "I am doing the dishes"). Most commonly voices are described as a similar loudness to one's own speaking voice and most likely to occur when alone (Haddock et al., 1999; Nayani & David, 1996a). The subjective experience of AHs in schizophrenia has been found to correlate with the neural regions involved in the motor mechanisms of speech comprehension (in particular the inferior frontal gyri), with contributions from neural regions involved in sensory salience-detection and self-monitoring (Raij et al., 2009). Research has also found an array of cognitive deficits associated with AHs in schizophrenia – including deficits in intentional inhibition (e.g., Paulik, Badcock, & Maybery, 2009; Waters, Badcock, Maybery, & Michie, 2003), context memory and source monitoring (e.g., Waters, Badcock, & Maybery, 2006), verbal source monitoring (e.g., Johns et al., 2001), and meta-cognitive beliefs (e.g., Morrison & Wells, 2003) – accounting for the multitude of explanatory models of AHs in the literature (for review see Seal, Aleman, McGuire, & Seal, 2004).

Although typically associated with schizophrenia, auditory hallucinations can also occur in mood disorders - during major depressive and manic episodes – and anxiety disorders, in particular posttraumatic-stress disorder (PTSD). For instance, research has shown that between 50% and 80% of individuals with bipolar disorder (during a manic episode), and between 10% and 30% of individuals with major depressive disorder, experience psychotic symptoms, including AHs (Carlson & Goodwin, 1973; Johnson, Horwath, & Weissman, 1991; Ohayon & Schatzberg, 2002), and that the presence of psychotic symptoms is related to the severity of the mania or depression (Abrams & Taylor, 1981; Ohayon & Schatzberg, 2002). A recent study of AHs in schizophrenia and 'psychotic depression' reported similar phenomenological qualities of this experience in each of these conditions. Moreover, anxiety was the strongest predictor of hallucination intensity irrespective of diagnosis, suggesting that anxiety may play a similar role in the production of AHs in schizophrenia and mood disorders (Delespaul, deVries, & van Os, 2002). (The role of anxiety will be reviewed and discussed in more detail in this chapter). The most consistently reported difference between the AHs experienced in schizophrenia and mood disorders is that a greater percentage of hallucinations are mood-congruent (Coryell & Tsuang, 1985; Coryell, Tsuang, & McDaniel, 1982; Fennig, Bromet, Karant, Ram, & Jandorf, 1996; Winokur, Scharfetter, & Angst, 1985). For instance, in depression hallucinated voices are typically negative in content, berating the voice hearer for his/her short comings, while in mania the voices are typically grandiose in content, commonly taking the identity of God or other influential/famous individuals (APA, 2000).

The predisposition to hallucinations and the occurrence of AHs in individuals with schizophrenia have also been linked to traumatic life experiences (e.g., Freeman & Fowler, 2009; Hardy et al., 2005; Morrison & Petersen, 2003; Read, van Os, Morrison & Ross, 2005). Consistent with this, PTSD is characterised by intrusive hallucinatory-like flashbacks of the trauma, and – although less common – full-blown hallucinatory experiences, with the content of most AHs related to the trauma (APA, 2000; Hamner, 1997; Hamner et al., 2000; Kastelan et al., 2007). It has been documented that as many as 40% of combat veterans with PTSD have co-morbid psychotic symptoms, and that the severity of PTSD and psychotic symptoms correlate (Hamner, 1997). It should be noted that AHs also occasionally occur in some other non-affect related disorders, such as dissociate identity disorder and Alzheimer's disease (Bassiony & Lyketsos, 2003; Ross, 2007).

AHs are not limited to clinical populations. There is strong evidence that a symptom continuum exists for AHs between individuals from the general population and individuals with full-blown psychosis (e.g., Choong, Hunter, & Woodruff, 2007; Paulik, Badcock, & Maybery, 2007; Shevlin, Murphy, Dorahy, & Adamson, 2007). Numerous large scale community projects have reported an annual prevalence rate for AHs of around 4%, and that between 10% and 25% of individuals in the general population report having experienced an hallucination (not including hallucinatory experiences during altered states of consciousness) at some stage during their lives, of whom less than half have received any psychological services or met criteria for the diagnosis of a mental illness (Johns, Nazroo, Bebbington, & Kuipers, 1998; Kendler, Gallagher, Abelson, & Kessler, 1996; Ohayon, 2000; Romme, Honig, Noorthoorn, & Escher, 1992; Sidgewick, et al., 1894; Tien, 1991). These prevalence rates are similar for children and adolescents (Altman, Collins, & Mundy, 1997; Escher, Delespaul, Romme, Buiks, & Van Os, 2003; McGee, Williams, & Poulton, 2000). The AHs experienced by non-clinical and clinical individuals share many phenomenological characteristics, such as type, form, pragmatics and perceived reality characteristic (Barrett & Caylor, 1998; Choong et al., 2007; Honig et al., 1998; Leudar, Thomas, McNally, & Glinski, 1997). Nevertheless, several differences have been documented, possibly contributing to, or predicting the need for care. Firstly, non-patient voice hearers report a lower frequency of AHs than patient voice hearers (Badcock, Chhabra, Maybery, & Paulik, 2008). Furthermore, by and large, studies have found that non-patient voice hearers report that their AHs are predominantly positive or neutral in content, that they have some control over the experience, and are less distressed and functionally impaired by the experience than patient voice hearers (Escher, Romme, Buiks, Delespaul, & van Os, 2002; Honig et al., 1998; Tien, 1991). Despite the reported differences in emotional content and affective responses to AHs by patient and non-patient voice hearers, high levels of anxiety and depression are reported in both hallucinating groups (Barrett & Etheridge, 1994; McGee et al., 2000; Ohayon, 2000; Paulik, Badcock, & Maybery, 2006), suggesting that affective disturbance may play a similar role in the onset and/or maintenance of AHs across the continuum.

Negative Affect

The term *affect* encompasses a wide range of emotion-related phenomena, with the preceding term *negative* describing emotion-related experiences that are generally perceived as being unpleasant. According to Gross (1998), affect is the 'superordinate category for valanced states, including emotions such as anger and sadness.., moods such as depression and euphoria, dispositional states such as liking and hating, and traits such as cheerfulness and irascibility' (p. 273). The following review will focus primarily on depression and anxiety, since these affective states have been linked most closely to the positive symptoms (including hallucinations, delusions and thought disorder) of schizophrenia.

Negative Affect and Schizophrenia

Given the intrusive nature of positive symptoms and the negative impact the disorder typically has on the individual's social and occupational life, it is not surprising that high rates of co-morbid depression and anxiety have been documented across the lifespan of the disorder. Some schizophrenia studies have shown as many as two thirds of individuals report being depressed and/or anxious (Huppert & Smith, 2001; Siris, 1995). Furthermore, the rate of suicide in schizophrenia is 10 times higher than in the general population, with 10% of sufferers taking their own lives (APA, 2000; Limosin, Loze, Philippe, Casadebaig, & Rouillon, 2007). Other studies have shown that depression and anxiety are characteristic of the prodromal phase of psychosis, evident even prior to symptom onset. Two large-scale prodromal studies reported that between 57% and 76% of individuals had depressive symptomatology, and between 62% and 86% of individuals had high levels of anxiety (Birchwood et al., 1989; Herz & Melville, 1980). Such findings suggest that negative affective disturbances may not only be a consequence of the frightening and disabling symptoms of schizophrenia but may be important causal factors. Furthermore, neuroimaging studies of individuals with schizophrenia have shown abnormal volumes in areas of the brain involved in the production and modulation of emotion and storing of emotion-cued memories: the amygdala, thalamus, hippocampus and insula (Aleman & Kahn, 2005; McCarley, Wible et al., 1999; Wright et al., 2000).

Until recently, the study of affective disturbance in schizophrenia has almost exclusively focused on negative (deficit) symptoms, since the most common negative symptoms, namely flat affect and anhedonia, respectively mimic the behavioural and subjective emotional experience of depression (Bentall, 2003). Researchers in the area have sought to determine whether these symptoms are independent of, or merely part of, the high co-morbidity of depression in schizophrenia. Refuting the speculated link between negative symptoms and negative affect, empirical studies have typically found that schizophrenia individuals with these negative symptoms do not differ from controls or schizophrenia individuals without negative symptoms on subjective ratings of the valence and arousal of their experiences of emotional stimuli (e.g., Berenbaum & Oltmanns, 1992; Burbridge & Barch, 2007; Myin-Germeys, Delespaul, & deVries, 2000). Despite this empirical focus, studies have consistently found depression and anxiety to be more closely related to positive symptoms – hallucinations and delusions in particular – than negative symptoms (e.g., Guillem,

Pampoulova, Stip, Lalonde, & Todorov, 2005; Norman & Malla, 1991; Norman, Malla, Cortese, & Diaz, 1998; Norman & Malla, 1994; Smith, Fowler et al., 2006; Tibbo, Swainson, Chue, & LeMelledo, 2003). The literature pertaining to affect and delusions will not be reviewed in this chapter, however in a recent literature review, Freedman and Garety (2003) concluded that the *content* of delusions 'are a direct representation of emotional concerns, and that emotion contributes to delusion formation and maintenance' (pg. 923). The following subsection of this chapter will review the literature which has examined the specific relationship(s) between negative affect and AHs.

Negative Affect and Auditory Hallucinations

Auditory hallucinations are predominantly ominous in content and intrusive in nature, and are most often perceived by the individual as confronting and distressing (Nayani & David, 1996a). Although this potentially explains the high co-occurrence of AHs with depression, anger, fear and anxiety (Alpert & Silvers, 1970; Carter, Mackinnon et al., 1996; Close & Garety, 1998; Delespaul et al., 2002; Gallagher, Dinan, Sheehy, & Baker, 1995; Hustig & Hafner, 1990; Johns et al., 2002; Walsh et al., 1999), in recent years it has become increasingly evident that negative affect plays more than one role in an hallucinatory event. Negative affect may not only be a bi-product of the experience, but also a trigger, a maintenance mechanism, a determinant of content. The literature pertaining to each of these roles will be reviewed.

The Role of Negative Affect in the Onset and Maintenance of Auditory Hallucinations

Depression and anxiety have not only been found to accompany the experience of AHs, but have also been found to precede the initial – and subsequent – onset of AHs, suggesting that emotional disturbance plays a direct *causal* role in the onset of AHs (e.g., Allen & Agus, 1968; Delespaul et al., 2002; Myin-Germeys, Delespaul, & van Os, 2005; Nayani & David, 1996a; Slade, 1976b). For instance, in a phenomenological survey of AH experiences in individuals with a psychotic disorder conducted by Nayani and David (1996a), 52% reported feelings of sadness and 45% reported having anxiety-related bodily sensations (i.e., churning or butterfly sensations in their stomach) prior to the onset of hallucinatory episodes. Overcoming the potential limitations of using a retrospective design, Delespaul and colleagues (2002) employed a time-sampling procedure and found that hallucinating individuals with schizophrenia or 'psychotic depression' reported a rise in anxiety levels immediately prior to the onset of a hallucinatory episode, with anxiety restoring to baseline levels shortly after the episode ceased. Interestingly, this study found that anxiety was the strongest predictor of hallucination severity – more so than depression-related mental states – irrespective of diagnosis. Another time-sampling study found that increases in psychosis intensity (including AHs) was associated with daily life stress in both schizophrenia participants and their first degree relatives, but not control participants (Myin-Germeys,

Delespaul et al., 2005), providing further evidence of an interplay between negative affect and the mechanisms or 'diathesis' underlying psychotic symptoms. In a much earlier study, Allen and Agus (1968) demonstrated in a series of case studies that AHs could be induced in individuals with schizophrenia by stimulating the somatic symptoms that often accompany anxiety and panic attacks. Clinical studies have also found that by effectively reducing anxiety and depression in patients with schizophrenia through cognitive-behavioural intervention or antidepressant medication, the severity of AHs is also reduced (e.g., Cornblatt, Lencz, & Obuchowski, 2002; Cornblatt et al., 2007; Kuipers et al., 1998; Slade, 1972, 1973). Taken together, the findings of these studies strongly implicate negative affect as being a contributing factor in the onset or triggering of AHs.

Studies examining the emergence of psychosis in at-risk and community samples have largely found that depression, anxiety, stress and trauma are amongst the strongest predictors of psychosis onset (e.g., Bebbington et al., 1993; Cunningham, Miller, Lawrie, & Johnstone, 2005; Goodwin, Fergusson, & Horwood, 2004; Jones, Rodgers, Murray, & Marmot, 1994; Svirskis et al., 2005; Tien & Eaton, 1992; Yung et al., 2003). It has also been found that the sub-clinical psychotic-experiences reported in youths identified as being at ultra-high-risk (UHR) for developing psychosis remit, and the likelihood of transition to psychosis is significantly reduced, with reduction/remission of mood symptoms (Yung et al., 2007) and the targeted treatment of mood symptoms with antidepressant medication (Cornblatt et al., 2007). Studies examining the temporal order of symptom emergence in the prodromal phase have reported that depressive symptoms precede all other schizophrenia-specific and non-specific symptoms, while anxiety symptoms do not appear until prior to positive symptom onset (Hafner et al., 2005). In line with this finding, the few studies that have examined the initial onset of hallucinations specifically, report that anxiety disorders and anxious mood are strong predictors of hallucination onset, more so than depression (e.g., Krabbendam et al., 2002; Nayani & David, 1996a; Tien & Eaton, 1992), while both anxiety and depression are related to the continuation of AHs (Escher et al., 2002). In a series of studies conducted by Krabbendam and colleagues, it was found that the presence of depressed mood was able to predict the onset of psychosis in individuals who *already* experience AHs in the general population, and furthermore that this relationship was partly mediated by negative and delusional appraisals of hallucinatory experiences (Krabbendam et al., 2005; Krabbendam & van Os, 2005). Taken together, these separate findings implicate the involvement of anxiety in the initial and subsequent onset of AHs, and the involvement of depression in the onset of psychosis more generally, with both likely to contribute to the maintenance of hallucinations by shaping cognitive appraisals of aberrant experiences (Freeman & Garety, 2003; Garety et al., 2001; Kuipers et al., 2006; Yung & McGorry, 1996).

Several socio-psychological and cognitive theories have been proposed to explain the involvement of negative affect in the onset and maintenance of AHs, which can be organised into two main categories: (1) direct theories, those that argue that affect may trigger the underlying mechanisms (or some of) involved in the development of AHs (rather than advocating that affect *is* the underlying mechanism), and (2) indirect theories, those that argue that hallucinations are a form of defence mechanism against negative emotion (Freeman & Garety, 2003). Indirect theories originate from psychoanalytic explanations of AHs (Freud, 1924; Gillibert, 1968), with modern indirect theoretical models postulating that intrusive cognitions that threaten the integrity of the individual (causing 'cognitive dissonance') are automatically rejected by the individual as belonging to – or a product of – one's own mind, and consequently are attributed to an external source (e.g., Baker & Morrison, 1998; Kapsambelis, 2005; Morrison, 2001; Morrison & Wells, 2003). Although Morrison and colleagues have found evidence that voice hearers have meta-cognitive beliefs regarding punishment, responsibility, uncontrollability, and the unacceptability of negative thoughts (Baker & Morrison, 1998; Morrison & Wells, 2003), there has been no documented evidence that meta-cognitive beliefs impact on an individuals' attribution of the source of an event to self or other.

Direct theories however, have received substantial empirical support in the literature (Freeman & Garety, 2003). These models typically propose some form of maintenance cycle, often in which negative affect either directly or indirectly influences or biases a person's interpretations/appraisals/beliefs about their AHs (i.e., beliefs regarding malevolence, omnipotence, and controllability of voices) which further exacerbates negative affect, and in turn triggers further AHs (e.g., Chadwick & Birchwood, 1994; Garety et al., 2001; Morrison, 1998; Morrison, 2001; Slade, 1976a). The processes themselves which lead to this faulty and distressing appraisal of a voice are processes empirically found to contribute to the maintenance of anxiety disorders/symptoms, such as avoidance and safety behaviours (Morrison, 1998; Northard, Morrison & Wells, 2008); cognitive biases, such as an externalising attribution bias, jumping to conclusions, catastrophizing, belief inflexibility, belief confirmation bias, and circular and emotional reasoning (e.g., Baker & Morrison, 1998; Beck & Rector, 2003; Bentall, Baker, & Havers, 1991; Morrison & Haddock, 1997; Morrison, Nothard, Bowe, & Wells, 2004); meta-cognitive beliefs regarding the uncontrollability of thoughts (Baker & Morrison, 1998; Morrison & Wells, 2003); self-focused attention (Ensum & Morrison, 2003); and thought suppression (Garcia-Montes, Perez-Alvarez, & Fidalgo, 2003; Perona-Garcelán et al., 2008). While these direct theoretical accounts adequately address how negative affect may contribute to the maintenance of AHs and further exacerbate affective distress, more research is needed to explain *how* – the precise mechanisms by which – emotions contribute to the onset of AHs (Bentall, 2003; Freeman & Garety, 2003).

Negative Affect and the Phenomenology of Auditory Hallucinations

It has been proposed that the mood state preceding an AH may have a direct influence on the phenomenological characteristics of the hallucinatory experience (Freeman & Garety, 2003; Nayani & David, 1996b). For instance, Garety et al. (2001) proposed that the emotions which trigger AHs and the emotions caused by AHs, feed back into the content of voices, such that the content of an AH is a reflection of the affective state. Several theoretical models of AHs attempt to explain this. Firstly, since inner-speech is mostly congruent with – or a reflection of – current emotional concerns, inner-speech models of AHs (which propose that AHs are misidentified fragments of inner-speech) predict that that the content of AHs should mostly be consistent with the individual's current mood state (Frith, 1992). Nayani and David's (1996b) model of AHs as misidentified memories resulting from contextual memory deficits, has also been used to explain the reciprocal nature of negative affect and AHs. They propose that because memories are organised in a semantic network, affect laden memories that are congruent with an individual's current mood state will be automatically activated and retrieved if the emotional intensity of the current mood is above the critical activation threshold. Accordingly, a mood such as anxiety or paranoia may result in the automatic retrieval of memories of threat or abuse. According to Nayani and David (1996b), a vicious cycle emerges making AHs increasingly more frequent and severe, since the re-pairing of the emotion with the memory reinforces the triggering emotion, the memory (or at least the misidentification of the memory as a 'voice'), and the memory-emotion link, making the memory more readily accessible.

Numerous studies have provided partial empirical support for Nayani and David's (1996b) conjecture that AHs are misidentified memories. For instance, Nayani and David's (1996a) survey study of 100 patient voice hearers found that 61% of voice hearers can identify their voices as people they know (and a further 15% report familiarity). Additionally, several studies have found that the content of AHs experienced by individuals who have experienced trauma are predominantly negative and paranoid, and are typically related to – or flash backs of – the traumatic event itself (Hardy et al., 2005; Honig et al., 1998; Read & Argyle, 1999). However, the empirical evidence supporting the specific link between mood state and AH content – shared by both Nayani and David's model and inner speech models – has been somewhat inconsistent. In support, several studies have reported significant correlations between depression/self-esteem and negative/distressing content of AHs in schizophrenia (e.g., Smith, Fowler et al., 2006). However, studies that have examined the prevalence of mood-congruent AHs in different clinical populations have reported that while most AHs experienced in mood disordered samples are mood-congruent, the AHs experienced in schizophrenia are both mood-congruent and mood-incongruent (e.g., Fennig et al., 1996; Winokur et al., 1985). However, a limitation of mood congruency studies is that 'mood' is typically determined by a single trait measure or by diagnostic label, rather than a measure of ones mood *state* at the time of the hallucinatory episode. Similar to Nayani and David's (1996b) conjecture, it has been proposed that the content of AHs reflect affect-triggered self-schemas (Freeman & Garety, 2003), and indeed several studies have found that the content of AHs reported by individuals with schizophrenia is closely tied to the individual's self-schema, self esteem and social status (e.g., Close & Garety, 1998; Hayward, 2003). However, these findings are not inconsistent with Nayani and David's proposal, since memories are thought to be linked to a person's self-schema, reciprocally activating one another.

The relationship between negative affect and the phenomenology of AHs is thought to be a reciprocal one, with several aspects of the AH experience contributing to one's affective response. It has long been assumed that the predominantly negative content of AHs is primarily responsible for the resulting distress. However, research findings suggest that the relationship between AH phenomenology and affective responding is more complex than this (Soppitt & Birchwood, 1997). Honig et al. (1998) compared the AHs of patient and non-patient voice hearers and reported that only patients found their voices distressing. The two AH features distinguishing these groups was the amount of negative content (patients reported predominantly negative content, while non-patients reported predominantly positive control) and perceived control over voices (patients reported little control, while non-patients felt they had some control), suggesting that content and control may influence affective responding. Similar findings have also been reported in samples of patient and non-patient adolescent voice hearers (Escher et al., 2002), and in a large scale community studies (Tien,

1991). Similarly, one study reported that 26% of schizophrenia participants rated their experience of AHs as enjoyable, and that these 'enjoyable' AHs were almost always positive or neutral in content and controllable (Sanjuan, Gonzalez, Aguilar, Leal, & van Os, 2004). It is possible however that perceived control over AHs is more integral to the affective response than content (Nayani & David, 1996a). Johns et al. (2002) compared the AHs experienced by individuals with tinnitus and schizophrenia, and found that the tinnitus participants predominantly experienced non-verbal AHs (music, singing, birds, etc) with positive or neutral content, while the schizophrenia participants mainly head voices with negative content. Despite these differences in form and content, both groups reported high levels of resulting distress, which was primarily attributed in both groups to the perceived uncontrollability of their AHs.

In addition to content and control, studies have also linked affective and behavioural responses to AHs to the individual's beliefs regarding the voice's omnipotence (all-powerfulness) and malevolence versus benevolence (evil versus good intent/purpose) (Birchwood & Chadwick, 1997; Chadwick & Birchwood, 1994; Morrison, Nothard, Bowe, & Wells, 2004; Soppitt & Birchwood, 1997). In Chadwick and Birshwood's (1994, Study 1) survey of patient voice hearers, they not only found that the perceived omnipotence and benevolence of the voice was related to the voice hearer's affective and behavioural response to it (namely higher perceived omnipotence and malevolence was related to higher resulting negative affective and compliance), but that the perceived identity of the voice was the greatest predictor of perceived omnipotence and malevolence/benevolence. This, in part, led to the modification of the original cognitive model of AHs, and the development of a complimentary theory, called the social rank theory. According to the social rank theory, 'the interpersonal relationship a voice-hearer has with his/her voice is partly shaped via recruitment of specialized social processing systems (social mentalities) that act as guides for social roles and scripts' (Birchwood et al., 2004, p. 1572), such that if the voice is perceived as being more powerful/knowledgeable than themselves the person is more likely to follow through with requests or else fear disobedience, while if the reverse is true the voice hearer may be able to chose to ignore the voice. According to the social rank theory, if the person hears the voice of someone they know or have known in the past, their relationship with the voice will mimic the power dynamic they have with that person in real life, such that a person who hears the voice of their fourth grade teacher may resume the social power/rank of a fourth grader and fear the voice and/or concede to its demands. In support of the social rank theories, empirical studies have provided evidence that the perceived social power/rank of the voice relative their own plays a large role in the affective and behavioural response to the voice (Birchwood et al., 2004; Birchwood, Iqbal, & Upthegrove, 2005; Birchwood, Meaden, Trower, Gilbert & Plaistow, 2000; Vaughan & Fowler, 2004). Using covariance structural equation modelling, Birchwood and colleagues (2004) compared three models which proposed different directions in the relationship between psychosis, depression and feelings of social subordination. The results supported their model that perceptions of their own social power/rank lead to the appraisal of voice power, distress and resulting depression, rather than depression influencing appraisals of voices. This further emphasises the importance of targeting perceived social power/rank and faulty appraisals of voices in the treatment of auditory hallucinations, in addition to treating negative affect, as discussed in the next section.

Clinical Implications

The overwhelming empirical evidence that negative affect plays a significant role in the onset and maintenance of AHs emphasises the importance of targeting affective disturbance in the treatment and prevention of AHs. The most effective treatments for depression are antidepressant medication, cognitive-behavioural therapy (CBT), and interpersonal psychotherapy (IPT), while for anxiety disorders the most effective treatment options are CBT, antidepressant medications and benzodiazepines (which act as relaxants). Indeed, as reviewed earlier, clinical research studies have found evidence that the successful treatment of mood or anxiety symptoms can lead to a reduction in the severity and frequency of AHs in individuals who hear voices. This is a particularly appealing approach for individuals who hear voices who do not meet criteria for psychosis and for young people at ultra-high risk for psychosis, since antipsychotic medications can have negative side effects and may be perceived to be stigmatising. Suicide rates in individuals with schizophrenia are alarmingly high, with one in 10 people with schizophrenia taking their life. It has recently been found that suicidal ideation in individuals with schizophrenia is not related to the severity of AHs, but rather the resulting distress and mood disturbance due to the experience (Fialko, 2006). This further emphasises the importance of treating negative affective disturbances in voice hearers.

CBT for AHs has been developed specifically to challenge the perceived malevolence and omnipotence of the voices, as well as the voice hearer's perceived lack of control (Chadwick, Birchwood & Trower, 1996). This approach has been developed in light of the findings that these three aspects of the experience are closely tied to a person's affective response to their voices. Numerous randomised clinical control trials of CBT for AHs have been conducted, most of which have reported a reduction in the conviction of the voices' omnipotence and malevolence and increased sense of control over – and their behavioural responses to – their voices, as well as reduced levels of negative affect and even reduced frequency/severity of AHs (e.g., Wiersma, Jenner, van de Willige, Spakman & Nienhuis, 2001). There is also preliminary evidence to suggest that beliefs relating to voices can be indirectly modified through mindfulness training, resulting in reduced affective responding to AHs (Taylor, Harper, & Chadwick, 2009).

Finally, since the content of AHs and peoples' affective and behavioural response to AHs has been closely tied to their perceived social rank, self-schema, and self esteem (e.g., Close & Garety, 1998; Hayward, 2003), working directly on modifying the power dynamic with the dominant voice(s) in therapy is likely to reduce the negative content and/or appraisal of AHs, and also lessen the negative affective response to the AHs. It may also prove beneficial to additionally treat individuals for poor self esteem and self-image, using approaches such as schema therapy and CBT (Byrne, Birchwood, Trower & Meaden, 2006), and increase their social skills/confidence and social network, through assertiveness and social skills training, mental health rehabilitation (etc). The effect of this may be to reduce the negative content and/or appraisal of AHs, in turn lessen associated distress, and even potentially reduce the frequency of AHs, since you are effectively eliminating/reducing one of the principal triggers – negative affect (Birchwood et al., 2004). The successful implementation of many of these suggested approaches has been documented in clinical case studies (e.g., Hayward, Overton,

Dorey, Denney, 2009), however larger controlled outcome studies are needed to establish efficacy.

In sum, these studies have exposed that the relationship between affect and AH phenomenology is both complex and reciprocal in nature. It is clear however that emotion is an important precursor to the onset on AH, yet the precise mechanisms by which emotions contribute to the production of AHs is still unknown (Bentall, 2003; Freeman & Garety, 2003). This is an especially important area of research, since treatment may be more effective and less costly if targeted to the specific route of action.

References

Abrams, R., & Taylor, M. A. (1981). Importance of schizophrenic symptoms in the diagnosis of mania. *American Journal of Psychiatry, 138*, 658-661.

Aleman, A., & Kahn, R. S. (2005). Strange feelings: Do amygdala abnormalities dysregulate the emotional brain in schizophrenia? *Progress in Neurobiology, 77*, 283-298.

Allen, T. E., & Agus, B. (1968). Hyperventilation leading to hallucinations. *American Journal of Psychiatry, 125*, 632-637.

Alpert, M., & Silvers, K. N. (1970). Perceptual characteristics distinguishing auditory hallucinations in schizophrenia and acute alcoholic psychoses. *American Journal of Psychiatry, 127*, 298-302.

Altman, H., Collins, M., & Mundy, P. (1997). Subclinical hallucinations and delusions in nonpsychotic adolescents. *Journal of Child Psychology and Psychiatry, 38*, 413-420.

APA. (2000). *Diagnostic and Statistical Manual of Mental Disorders (DSM-IV-TR)* (4th ed.). Washington DC: American Psychiatric Association.

Badcock, J. C., Chhabra, S., Maybery, M. T., & Paulik, G. (2008). Context binding and hallucination predisposition. *Personality and Individual Differences, 45*(8), 822-827.

Baker, C. A., & Morrison, A. P. (1998). Cognitive processes in auditory hallucinations: Attributional biases and metacognition. *Psychological Medicine, 28*, 1199-1208.

Barrett, T. R., & Caylor, M. R. (1998). Verbal hallucinations in normals, V: Perceived reality characteristics. *Personality and Individual Differences, 25*, 209-221.

Barrett, T. R., & Etheridge, J. B. (1994). Verbal hallucinations in normals: III. Dysfunctional personality correlates. *Personality and Individual Differences, 16*, 57-62.

Bassiony, M. M., & Lyketsos, C. G. (2003). Delusions and hallucinations in Alzheimer's disease: Review of the brain decade. *Psychosomatics, 44*, 388-401.

Bebbington, P., Wilkins, S., Jones, P., Foerster, A., Murray, R., Toone, B., et al. (1993). Life events and psychosis. Initial results from the Camberwell Collaborative Psychosis Study. *British Journal of Psychiatry, 162*, 72-79.

Beck, A. T., & Rector, N. A. (2003). A cognitive model of hallucinations. *Cognitive Therapy and Research, 27*, 19-52.

Bentall, R. P. (1990). The illusion of reality: A review and integration of psychological research on hallucinations. *Psychological Bulletin, 107*, 82-95.

Bentall, R. P. (2003). *Madness explained: Psychosis and human nature.* London: Penguin Books Ltd.

Bentall, R. P., Baker, G. A., & Havers, S. (1991). Reality monitoring and psychotic hallucinations. *British Journal of Clinical Psychology, 30*, 213-222.

Berenbaum, H., & Oltmanns, T. F. (1992). Emotional experience and expression in schizophrenia and depression. *Journal of Abnormal Psychology, 101*, 37-44.

Birchwood, M., & Chadwick, P. (1997). The omnipotence of voices: Testing the validity of a cognitive model. *Psychological Medicine, 27*, 1345-1353.

Birchwood, M., Gilbert, P., Gilbert, J., Trower, P., Meaden, A., Hay, J., et al. (2004). Interpersonal and role-related schema influence the relationship with the dominant 'voice' in schizophrenia: A comparison of three models. *Psychological Medicine, 34*, 1571-1580.

Birchwood, M., Iqbal, Z., & Upthegrove, R. (2005). Psychological pathways to depression in schizophrenia: Studies in acute psychosis, post psychotic depression and auditory hallucinations. *European Archives of Psychiatry and Clinical Neuroscience, 255*, 202-212.

Birchwood, M., Meaden, A., Trower, P., Gilbert, P., & Plaistow, J. (2000). The power and omnipotence of voices: Subordination and entrapment by voices and significant others. *Psychological Medicine, 30*(2), 337-344.

Birchwood, M., Smith, J., Macmillan, F., Hogg, B., Prasad, R., Harvey, C., et al. (1989). Predicting relapse in schizophrenia: The development and implementation of an early signs monitoring system using patients and families as observers. *Psychological Medicine, 19*, 649-656.

Burbridge, J. A., & Barch, D. M. (2007). Anhedonia and the experience of emotion in individuals with schizophrenia. *Journal of Abnormal Psychology, 116*, 30-42.

Byrne, S., Birchwood, M., Trower, P. E., & Meaden, A. (2006). *A casebook of cognitive behaviour therapy for command hallucinations: A social rank theory approach*: New York, NY, US: Routledge/Taylor & Francis Group.

Carlson, G. A., & Goodwin, F. K. (1973). The stages of mania. A longitudinal analysis of the manic episode. *Archives of General Psychiatry, 28*, 221-228.

Carter, D. M., Mackinnon, A., & Copolov, D. L. (1996). Patients' strategies for coping with auditory hallucinations. *Journal of Nervous and Mental Disease, 184*, 159-164.

Chadwick, P., & Birchwood, M. (1994). The omnipotence of voices: A cognitive approach to auditory hallucinations. *British Journal of Psychiatry, 164*, 190-201.

Chadwick, P. D., Birchwood, M. J., & Trower, P. (1996). *Cognitive therapy for delusions, hallucinations and paranoia*. Chichester: Wiley.

Choong, C., Hunter, M. D., & Woodruff, P. W. (2007). Auditory hallucinations in those populations that do not suffer from schizophrenia. *Current Psychiatry Reports, 9*, 206-212.

Close, H., & Garety, P. (1998). Cognitive assessment of voices: Further developments in understanding the emotional impact of voices. *British Journal of Clinical Psychology, 37* 173-188.

Cornblatt, B., Lencz, T., & Obuchowski, M. (2002). The schizophrenia prodrome: Treatment and high-risk perspectives. *Schizophrenia Research, 54*, 177-186.

Cornblatt, B. A., Lencz, T., Smith, C. W., Olsen, R., Auther, A. M., Nakayama, E., et al. (2007). Can antidepressants be used to treat the schizophrenia prodrome? Results of a prospective, naturalistic treatment study of adolescents. *Journal of Clinical Psychiatry, 68*, 546-557.

Coryell, W., & Tsuang, M. T. (1985). Major depression with mood-congruent or mood-incongruent psychotic features: Outcome after 40 years. *American Journal of Psychiatry, 142*, 479-482.

Coryell, W., Tsuang, M. T., & McDaniel, J. (1982). Psychotic features in major depression. Is mood congruence important? *Journal of Affective Disorders, 4*, 227-236.

Cunningham, O. D., Miller, P., Lawrie, S., & Johnstone, E. (2005). Pathogenesis of schizophrenia: A psychopathological perspective. *British Journal of Psychiatry, 186*, 386-393.

Delespaul, P., deVries, M., & van Os, J. (2002). Determinants of occurrence and recovery from hallucinations in daily life. *Social Psychiatry and Psychiatric Epidemiology, 37*, 97-104.

Ensum, I., & Morrison, A. P. (2003). The effects of focus of attention on attributional bias in patients experiencing auditory hallucinations. *Behaviour Research and Therapy, 41*, 895-907.

Escher, S., Delespaul, P., Romme, M., Buiks, A., & Van Os, J. (2003). Coping defence and depression in adolescents hearing voices. *Journal of Mental Health (UK), 12*, 91-99.

Escher, S., Romme, M., Buiks, A., Delespaul, P., & van Os, J. (2002). Independent course of childhood auditory hallucinations: A sequential 3-year follow-up study. *British Journal of Psychiatry, 181*, 10-18.

Fennig, S., Bromet, E. J., Karant, M. T., Ram, R., & Jandorf, L. (1996). Mood-congruent versus mood-incongruent psychotic symptoms in first-admission patients with affective disorder. *Journal of Affective Disorders, 37*, 23-29.

Fialko, L., Freeman, D., Bebbington, P. E., Kuipers, E., Garety, P. A., Dunn, G., et al. (2006). Understanding suicidal ideation in psychosis: Findings from the Psychological Prevention of Relapse in Psychosis (PRP) trial. *Acta Psychiatrica Scandinavica, 114(3)*, 177-186.

Freeman, D., & Fowler, D. (2009). Routes to psychotic symptoms: Trauma, anxiety and psychosis-like experiences. *Psychiatry Research, 169*(2), 107-112.

Freeman, D., & Garety, P. A. (2003). Connecting neurosis and psychosis: The direct influence of emotion on delusions and hallucinations. *Behaviour Research and Therapy, 41*, 923-947.

Freeman, D., Garety, P. A., & Kuipers, E. (2001). Persecutory delusions: Developing the understanding of belief maintenance and emotional distress. *Psychological Medicine, 31*, 1293-1306.

Freud, S. (1924). The Loss of Reality in Neurosis and Psychosis. In J. Strachey (Ed.), *The standard edition of the complete psychological works of Sigmund Freud* (Vol. 19, pp. 181-188). London: Hogarth Press.

Frith, C. D. (1992). *The cognitive neuropsychology of schizophrenia*. Hove: LEA.

Gallagher, A. G., Dinan, T. G., Sheehy, N., & Baker, L. (1995). Chronic auditory hallucinations and suicide risk factors in schizophrenia. *Irish Journal of Psychology, 16*, 346-355.

Garca-Montes, J. M., Perez-Ãlvarez, M., & Fidalgo, Ã. M. (2003). Influence of the suppression of self-discrepant thoughts on the vividness of perception of auditory illusions. *Behavioural and Cognitive Psychotherapy, 31*, 33-44.

Garety, P. A., Kuipers, E., Fowler, D., Freeman, D., & Bebbington, P. E. (2001). A cognitive model of the positive symptoms of psychosis. *Psychological Medicine, 31*, 189-195.

Gelder, M., Gath, D., & Mayou, R. (1993). *Oxford textbook of psychiatry* (2nd ed.). Oxford: Oxford University Press.

Gillibert, J. (1968). Thoughts on hallucination. *Interpretation, 2*, 65-79.

Goodwin, R. D., Fergusson, D. M., & Horwood, L. J. (2004). Panic attacks and psychoticism. *American Journal of Psychiatry, 161*, 88-92.

Gross, J. J. (1998). The emerging field of emotion regulation: An integrative review. *Review of General Psychology, 2*(3), 271-299.

Guillem, F., Pampoulova, T., Stip, E., Lalonde, P., & Todorov, C. (2005). The relationships between symptom dimensions and dysphoria in schizophrenia. *Schizophrenia Research, 75*, 83-96.

Haddock, G., McCarron, J., Tarrier, N., & Faragher, E. B. (1999). Scales to measure dimensions of hallucinations and delusions: The psychotic symptom rating scales (PSYRATS). *Psychological Medicine, 29*, 879-889.

Hafner, H., Maurer, K., Trendler, G., an der Heiden, W., Schmidt, M., & Konnecke, R. (2005). Schizophrenia and depression: Challenging the paradigm of two separate diseases--A controlled study of schizophrenia, depression and healthy controls. *Schizophrenia Research, 77*, 11-24.

Hardy, A., Fowler, D., Freeman, D., Smith, B., Steel, C., Evans, J., et al. (2005). Trauma and hallucinatory experience in psychosis. *Journal of Nervous and Mental Disease, 193*, 501-507.

Hamner, M. B. (1997). Psychotic features and combat-associated PTSD. *Depression and Anxiety, 5*, 34-38.

Hamner, M. B., Frueh, B., Ulmer, H. G., Huber, M. G., Twomey, T. J., Tyson, C., et al. (2000). Psychotic features in chronic posttraumatic stress disorder and schizophrenia: Comparative severity. *Journal of Nervous and Mental Disease, 188*, 217-221.

Hayward, M. (2003). Interpersonal relating and voice hearing: To what extent does relating to the voice reflect social relating? *Psychology and Psychotherapy, 76*, 369-383.

Hayward, M., Overton, J., Dorey, T., & Denney, J. (2009). Relating therapy for people who hear voices: A case series. *Clinical Psychology and Psychotherapy, 16(3),* 216-227.

Herz, M. I., & Melville, C. (1980). Relapse in schizophrenia. *American Journal of Psychiatry, 137*, 801-805.

Honig, A., Romme, M. A., Ensink, B. J., Escher, S. D., Pennings, M. H., & deVries, M. W. (1998). Auditory hallucinations: A comparison between patients and nonpatients. *Journal of Nervous and Mental Disease, 186*, 646-651.

Huppert, J. D., & Smith, T. E. (2001). Longitudinal analysis of subjective quality of life in schizophrenia: Anxiety as the best symptom predictor. *Journal of Nervous and Mental Disease, 189*, 669-675.

Hustig, H. H., & Hafner, R. J. (1990). Persistent auditory hallucinations and their relationship to delusions and mood. *Journal of Nervous and Mental Disease, 178*, 264-267.

Johns, L. C., Hemsley, D., & Kuipers, E. (2002). A comparison of auditory hallucinations in a psychiatric and non-psychiatric group. *British Journal of Clinical Psychology, 41*, 81-86.

Johns, L. C., Nazroo, J. Y., Bebbington, P., & Kuipers, E. (1998). Occurrence of hallucinations in a community sample. *Schizophrenia Research, 29*, 23-23.

Johns, L. C., Rossell, S., Frith, C., Ahmad, F., Hemsley, D., Kuipers, E., et al. (2001). Verbal self-monitoring and auditory verbal hallucinations in patients with schizophrenia. *Psychological Medicine, 31*(4), 705-715.

Johnson, J., Horwath, E., & Weissman, M. M. (1991). The validity of major depression with psychotic features based on a community study. *Archives of General Psychiatry, 48*, 1075-1081.

Jones, P., Rodgers, B., Murray, R., & Marmot, M. (1994). Child development risk factors for adult schizophrenia in the British 1946 birth cohort. *Lancet, 344*, 1398-1402.

Kapsambelis, V. (2005). Is hallucination an external excitation? *Revue Francaise de Psychanalyse, 69*, 137-157.

Kastelan, A., Franciskovic, T., Moro, L., Roncevic-Grzeta, I., Grkovic, J., Jurcan, V., et al. (2007). Psychotic symptoms in combat-related post-traumatic stress disorder. *Military Medicine, 172*, 273-277.

Kendler, K. S., Gallagher, T. J., Abelson, J. M., & Kessler, R. C. (1996). Lifetime prevalence, demographic risk factors, and diagnostic validity of nonaffective psychosis as assessed in a US community sample. The National Comorbidity Survey. *Archives of General Psychiatry, 53*, 1022-1031.

Krabbendam, L., Janssen, I., Bak, M., Bijl, R. V., de Graaf, R., & van Os, J. (2002). Neuroticism and low self-esteem as risk factors for psychosis. *Society of Psychiatry and Psychiatric Epidemiology, 37*, 1-6.

Krabbendam, L., Myin-Germeys, I., Hanssen, M., de Graaf, R., Vollebergh, W., Bak, M., et al. (2005). Development of depressed mood predicts onset of psychotic disorder in individuals who report hallucinatory experiences. *British Journal of Clinical Psychology, 44*, 113-125.

Krabbendam, L., & van Os, J. (2005). Affective processes in the onset and persistence of psychosis. *European Archives of Psychiatry and Clinical Neuroscience, 255*, 185-189.

Kuipers, E., Fowler, D., Garety, P., Chisholm, D., Freeman, D., Dunn, G., et al. (1998). London-east Anglia randomised controlled trial of cognitive-behavioural therapy for psychosis. III: Follow-up and economic evaluation at 18 months. *British Journal of Psychiatry, 173*, 61-68.

Kuipers, E., Garety, P., Fowler, D., Freeman, D., Dunn, G., & Bebbington, P. (2006). Cognitive, emotional, and social processes in psychosis: Refining cognitive behavioral therapy for persistent positive symptoms. *Schizophrenia Bulletin, 32*, S24-31.

Leudar, I., Thomas, P., McNally, D., & Glinski, A. (1997). What voices can do with words: Pragmatics of verbal hallucinations. *Psychological Medicine, 27*, 885-898.

Limosin, F., Loze, J.-Y., Philippe, A., Casadebaig, F., & Rouillon, F. (2007). Ten-year prospective follow-up study of the mortality by suicide in schizophrenic patients. *Schizophrenia Research, 94*, 23-28.

Ohayon, M. M. (2000). Prevalence of hallucinations and their pathological associations in the general population. *Psychiatry Research, 97*, 153-164.

Ohayon, M. M., & Schatzberg, A. F. (2002). Prevalence of depressive episodes with psychotic features in the general population. *American Journal of Psychiatry, 159*, 1855-1861.

McCarley, R. W., Wible, C. G., Frumin, M., Hirayasu, Y., Levitt, J. J., Fischer, I. A., et al. (1999). MRI anatomy of schizophrenia. *Biological Psychiatry, 45*, 1099-1119.

McGee, R., Williams, S., & Poulton, R. (2000). Hallucinations in nonpsychotic children. *Journal of the American Academy of Child and Adolescent Psychiatry, 39*, 12-13.

Morrison, A. P. (1998). A cognitive analysis of the maintenance of auditory hallucinations: Are voices to schizophrenia what bodily sensations are to panic? *Behavioural and Cognitive Psychotherapy, 26*, 289-302.

Morrison, A. P. (2001). The interpretation of intrusions in psychosis: An integrative cognitive approach to hallucinations and delusions. *Behavioural and Cognitive Psychotherapy, 29*, 257-276.

Morrison, A. P., & Haddock, G. (1997). Cognitive factors in source monitoring and auditory hallucinations. *Psychological Medicine, 27*, 669-679.

Morrison, A. P., Nothard, S., Bowe, S. E., & Wells, A. (2004). Interpretations of voices in patients with hallucinations and non-patient controls: A comparison and predictors of distress in patients. *Behaviour Research and Therapy, 42*, 1315-1323.

Morrison, A., & Petersen, T. (2003). Trauma, metacognition and predisposition to hallucinations in non-patients. *Behavioural & Cognitive Psychotherapy, 31*, 235-246.

Morrison, A. P., & Wells, A. (2003). A comparison of metacognitions in patients with hallucinations, delusions, panic disorder, and non-patient controls. *Behaviour Research and Therapy, 41*, 251-256.

Myin-Germeys, I., Delespaul, P., & deVries, M. W. (2000). Schizophrenia patients are more emotionally active than is assumed based on their behavior. *Schizophrenia Bulletin, 26*

Myin-Germeys, I., Delespaul, P., & van Os, J. (2005). Behavioural sensitization to daily life stress in psychosis. *Psychological Medicine, 35*, 733-741.

Myin-Germeys, I., Marcelis, M., Krabbendam, L., Delespaul, P., & van Os, J. (2005). Subtle fluctuations in psychotic phenomena as functional states of abnormal dopamine reactivity in individuals at risk. *Biological Psychiatry, 58*, 105-110.

Nayani, T. H., & David, A. S. (1996a). The auditory hallucination: A phenomenological survey. *Psychological Medicine, 26*, 177-189.

Nayani, T. H., & David, A. S. (1996b). The neuropsychology and neurophenomenology of auditory hallucinations. In C. Peantelis, H. E. Nelson & T. R. E. Barnes (Eds.), *Schizophrenia: A neuropsychological perspective* (pp. 345-369). New York: John Wiley & Sons Ltd.

Norman, R. M., & Malla, A. K. (1991). Dysphoric mood and symptomotology in schizophrenia. *Psychological Medicine, 21*, 897-903.

Norman, R. M., Malla, A. K., Cortese, L., & Diaz, F. (1998). Aspects of dysphoria and symptoms of schizophrenia. *Psychological Medicine, 28*, 1433-1441.

Norman, R. M. G., & Malla, A. K. (1994). Correlations over time between dysphoric mood and symptomatology in schizophrenia. *Comprehensive Psychiatry, 35*, 34-38.

Nothard, S., Morrison, A. P., & Wells, A. (2008). Identifying specific interpretations and exploring the nature of safety behaviours for people who hear voices: An exploratory study. *Behavioural and Cognitive Psychotherapy, 36*, 353-357.

Paulik, G., Badcock, J. C., & Maybery, M. T. (2006). The multifactorial structure of the predisposition to hallucinate and associations with anxiety, depression and stress. Personality and Individual Differences, 41(6), 1067-1076.

Paulik, G., Badcock, J. C., & Maybery, M. T. (2007). Poor intentional inhibition in individuals predisposed to hallucinations. Cognitive Neuropsychiatry, 12(5), 457-470.

Perona-Garcelan, S., Cuevas-Yust, C., Garca-Montes, J., Perez-Ãlvarez, M., Ductor-Recuerda, M. J. s., Salas-Azcona, R., et al. (2008). Relationship between self-focused attention and dissociation in patients with an without auditory hallucinations. *Journal of Nervous and Mental Disease, 196*, 190-197.

Paulik, G., Badcock, J. C., & Maybery, M. T. (2009). Intentional cognitive control impairments in schizophrenia: Generalised or specific? *Journal of International Neuropsychological Society, 15*, 982-989.

Raij, T. T., Valkonen-Korhonen, M., Holi, M., Therman, S., Lehtonen, J., & Hari, R. (2009). Reality of auditory verbal hallucinations. *Brain: A Journal of Neurology, 132*, 2994-3001.

Read, J., van Os, J., Morrison, A. P., & Ross, C. A. (2005). Childhood trauma, psychosis and schizophrenia: A literature review with theoretical and clinical implications. *Acta Psychiatrica Scandinavica, 112*, 330-350.

Romme, M. A., Honig, A., Noorthoorn, E. O., & Escher, A. D. (1992). Coping with hearing voices: An emancipatory approach. *British Journal of Psychiatry, 161*, 99-103.

Ross, C. A. (2007). Dissociation and psychosis: Conceptual issues. *Journal of Psychological Trauma, 6*(2-3), 21-34.

Sanjuan, J., Gonzalez, J. C., Aguilar, E. J., Leal, C., & van Os, J. (2004). Pleasurable auditory hallucinations. *Acta Psychiatrica Scandinavica, 110*, 273-278.

Sartorius, N., Shapiro, R., & Jablensky, A. (1974). The international pilot study of schizophrenia. *Schizphrophrenia Bulletin, 8*, 21-34.

Seal, M. L., Aleman, A., McGuire, P. K., & Seal, M. L. (2004). Compelling imagery, unanticipated speech and deceptive memory: Neurocognitive models of auditory verbal hallucinations in schizophrenia. *Cognitive Neuropsychiatry, 9*(1-2), 43-72.

Shevlin, M., Murphy, J., Dorahy, M. J., & Adamson, G. (2007). The distribution of positive psychosis-like symptoms in the population: A latent class analysis of the National Comorbidity Survey. *Schizophrenia Research, 89*, 101-109.

Sidgewick, H., Johnson, A., Myers, F. W. H., et-al. (1894). Report on the census of hallucinations. *Proceedings of the Society for Psychiatric Research, 26*, 259-394.

Siris, G. G. (1995). Depression and schizophrenia. In S. R. Hirsch & D. R. Weinberger (Eds.), *Schizophrenia* (pp. 128–146). Oxford: Blackwell Science Ltd.

Slade, P. D. (1972). The effects of systematic desensitisation on auditory hallucinations. *Behaviour Research and Therapy, 10*, 85-91.

Slade, P. D. (1973). The psychological investigation and treatment of auditory hallucinations: A second case report. *British Journal of Medical Psychology, 46*, 293-296.

Slade, P. D. (1976b). An investigation of psychological factors involved in the predisposition to auditory hallucinations. *Psychological Medicine, 6*, 123-132.

Slade, P. D. (1976a). Towards a theory of auditory hallucinations: Outline of an hypothetical four-factor model. *British Journal of Social and Clinical Psychology 15*, 415-423.

Slade, P. D., & Bentall, R. P. (1988). *Sensory deception: A scientific analysis of hallucination*. London: Croom Helm.

Smith, B., Fowler, D. G., Freeman, D., Bebbington, P., Bashforth, H., Garety, P., et al. (2006). Emotion and psychosis: Links between depression, self-esteem, negative schematic beliefs and delusions and hallucinations. *Schizophrenia Research, 86*, 181-188.

Soppitt, R. W., & Birchwood, M. (1997). Depression, beliefs, voice content and topography: A cross-sectional study of schizophrenic patients with auditory verbal hallucinations. *Journal of Mental Health, 6*, 525-532.

Svirskis, T., Korkeila, J., Heinimaa, M., Huttunen, J., Ilonen, T., Ristkari, T., et al. (2005). Axis-I disorders and vulnerability to psychosis. *Schizophrenia Research, 75,* 439-446.

Taylor, K. N., Harper, S., & Chadwick, P. (2009). Impact of mindfulness on cognition and affect in voice hearing: Evidence from two case studies. *Behavioural and Cognitive Psychotherapy, 37*(4), 397-402.

Tibbo, P., Swainson, J., Chue, P., & LeMelledo, J. M. (2003). Prevalence and relationship to delusions and hallucinations of anxiety disorders in schizophrenia. *Depression and Anxiety, 17,* 65-72.

Tien, A. Y. (1991). Distribution of hallucinations in the population. *Psychiatric Epidemiology, 26,* 287-292.

Tien, A. Y., & Eaton, W. W. (1992). Psychopathologic precursors and sociodemographic risk factors for the schizophrenia syndrome. *Archives of General Psychiatry, 49,* 37-46.

Vaughan, S., & Fowler, D. (2004). The distress experienced by voice hearers is associated with the perceived relationship between the voice hearer and the voice. *British Journal of Clinical Psychology, 43,* 143-153.

Walsh, E., Harvey, K., White, I., Manley, C., Fraser, J., Stanbridge, S., et al. (1999). Prevalence and predictors of parasuicide in chronic psychosis. UK700 group. *Acta Psychiatrica Scandinavica, 100,* 375-382.

Waters, F. A. V., Badcock, J. C., & Maybery, M. T. (2006). The 'who' and 'when' of context memory: Different patterns of association with auditory hallucinations. *Schizophrenia Research, 82*(2-3), 271-273.

Waters, F. A. V., Badcock, J. C., Maybery, M. T., & Michie, P. T. (2003). Inhibition in schizophrenia: Association with auditory hallucinations. *Schizophrenia Research, 62*(3), 275-280.

Wiersma, D., Jenner, J. A., van de Willige, G., Spakman, M., & Nienhuis, F. J. (2001). Cognitive behaviour therapy with coping training for persistent auditory hallucinations in schizophrenia: A naturalistic follow-up study of the durability of effects. *Acta Psychiatrica Scandinavica, 103*(5), 393-399.

Winokur, G., Scharfetter, C., & Angst, J. (1985). The diagnostic value in assessing mood congruence in delusions and hallucinations and their relationship to the affective state. *European Archives of Psychiatry and Neurological Sciences, 234,* 299-302.

Wright, I. C., Rabe-Hesketh, S., Woodruff, P. W., David, A. S., Murray, R. M., & Bullmore, E. T. (2000). Meta-analysis of regional brain volumes in schizophrenia. *American Journal of Psychiatry, 157,* 16-25.

Yung, A. R., Buckby, J. A., Cosgrave, E. M., Killackey, E. J., Baker, K., Cotton, S. M., et al. (2007). Association between psychotic experiences and depression in a clinical sample over 6 months. Schizophrenia Research, 91(1-3), 246-253.

Yung, A. R., & McGorry, P. D. (1996). The prodromal phase of first-episode psychosis: Past and current conceptualizations. *Schizophrenia Bulletin, 22,* 353-370.

Yung, A. R., Phillips, L. J., Yuen, H. P., Francey, S. M., McFarlane, C. A., Hallgren, M., et al. (2003). Psychosis prediction: 12-month follow up of a high-risk ("prodromal") group. *Schizophrenia Research, 60,* 21-32.

In: Hallucinations: Types, Stages and Treatments
Editor: Meredith S. Payne, pp. 79-96
ISBN: 978-1-61728-275-1
© 2011 Nova Science Publishers, Inc.

Chapter 4

Hallucinations and Intrusive Thoughts

M. F. Soriano and Teresa Bajo
Hospital de Día de Salud Mental, Hospital San Agustín, Linares &
Departamento de Psicología Experimental, Universidad de Granada, Granada, Spain

Abstract

Hallucinations have traditionally been conceptualized as a perceptual disorder. However, several lines of research have recently highlighted the similarity between hallucinations and intrusive thoughts. For example, Morrison and Baker (2000) have shown that patients who experience hallucinations also have more intrusive thoughts than patients who do not hallucinate. Similarly, Moritz and Laroi (2008) examined the cognitive and sensory characteristics of thoughts, intrusions and hallucinations, and they did not find a specific profile for hallucinations, compared to intrusions and normal thoughts. From this view, perceptual abnormalities would not be central to the experience of hearing voices, but an interpretation of cognitive intrusions.

Recently, we have found (Soriano, Román, Jiménez & Bajo, 2009) that schizophrenic patients with hallucinations showed impairments in intentional inhibition in memory, compared to schizophrenics without hallucinations, and healthy controls. We have hypothesized that both hallucinations and intrusive thoughts could be partly due to difficulties to inhibit mental events, so that unwanted or repetitive thoughts or images intrude into consciousness. Consistent with this idea, Verwoerd, Wessel and de Jong (2009) have found a relationship between individual differences in inhibitory control and the frequency of experiencing intrusive memories. Interestingly, intrusive thoughts and images were only related to cognitive inhibition (measured as resistance to proactive interference), but not to response inhibition. Therefore, we suggest that inhibitory difficulties may underlie the frequency of intrusions, whereas the interpretation of these intrusions might lead to the experience of them as voices, intrusions-obsessions, or normal thoughts. As Morrison (2001) has proposed, in hallucinating patients, metacognitive beliefs would induce the erroneous attribution of intrusions to external sources, producing the hallucinatory experience.

This view has important consequences in the conceptualization of mental disorders. Hallucinations have been considered a cardinal symptom in schizophrenia, while intrusions are a common symptom of various mental disorders, such as obsessive-compulsive disorder, generalized anxiety, or post-traumatic stress disorder. The parallelism between hallucinations and intrusions may support the idea that differences between schizophrenia and other anxiety disorders are more quantitative than qualitative, and that certain common basic cognitive dysfunctions underlie mental disorders in general.

Hallucinations: Definition and Characteristics

Hallucinations are defined as false perceptions occurring in the absence of identifiable external stimulus. They are normally considered to have qualities of real perception, in that they must be vivid, substantial, and located in external objective space. In this sense, they have been considered to have four cardinal characteristics (the four As of hallucinations): they have to be Acoustic, Autonomous (beyond subjective control), Alien (strange to the self), and Authentic (similar to a real voice) external events (Moritz and Laroi, 2008). From this view, hallucinations are similar to real perceptions. However, this conceptualization has often been questioned, since there are demonstrations that these characteristics are neither necessary nor sufficient to account for the hallucinatory experience. That is, hallucinations may vary in their degree of resemblance to real voices: sometimes, voice hearers report they perceive their voices inside their own head, and they even can modulate their presence or frequency. On the other hand, other mental events, such as intrusive thoughts or images, can be experienced as autonomous and alien to the own self.

Hallucinations have been traditionally regarded as a central feature of schizophrenia. Schneider (1959) judged auditory hallucinations, together with delusions, as first-rank symptoms of schizophrenia. According to this author, first-rank symptoms are especially important for diagnostic distinctions between schizophrenic and other psychotic and affective disorders. This view has influenced more recent classifications, so that hallucinations are now considered one of the main diagnostic criteria for the illness both in the ICD-10 and the DSM-IV-R. Nevertheless, it has been shown that hallucinations and delusions may not have such a high diagnostic value as had been previously thought. Hallucinations have been observed in several mental disorders, especially in dissociative, affective and personality disorders; and they can also appear in organic diseases (Ohayon, 2000). And even a relatively high percentage of normal non-clinical population report hearing voices (Johns and van Os, 2001).

Hallucinations can be experienced in any sensory modality, but auditory hallucinations are the more commonly reported type in mental disorders. Olfactory hallucinations are also frequent and they are followed in frequency by the taste and tactile modalities. Visual hallucinations are more often observed in organic and drug-induced illnesses.

1. Models of the Hallucinatory Experience

1.1. The Perceptual Account

As we have seen, most definitions of the hallucinatory experience emphasize its perceptual characteristics. Schneider (1959) considered them abnormalities of perception that are *sensed*; he stressed the fact that they are the experience of sensing (and not only believing) something that is not really there. For Jaspers (1962) hallucinations are, in fact, false perceptions and not distortions of real perceptions. They appear on their own as something new, and they occur simultaneous to and alongside real perceptions. Jaspers accentuated the *reality* and *externality* of auditory hallucinations; that is, they arise with a quality of concrete reality, and they are located in the external objective space. These perceptual views have inspired the definition offered by the DSM-IV-R, which asserts that auditory hallucinations are experienced as voices that are perceived as different from the person's own thoughts.

Since hallucinations have been defined as perceptual experiences, with similar characteristics totrue perceptions, early explanations of the phenomena have stressed this perceptual dimension, and a number of sensory-perceptual models have been proposed. According to these models, dysfunctions of the sensory input would lead to perceptual entries that are erroneously (but reasonably) interpreted as externally generated. For example, it has been proposed that auditory hallucinations are derived from the subvocal speech of the individual. This inner speech would not be recognized as internal; instead, it would be perceived as coming from an external agent (Frith and Done, 1987). This misattribution would be caused by a failure in the perceptual feedback from self-generated actions. In normal conditions, a corollary discharge would act to disambiguate perceptions from self-generated and external signals. Executive mechanisms would activate cortical areas involved in perceptual processing, and an efference copy or corollary discharge of the motor command would be sent to the awareness area. For example, when an individual perceives his hand moving, this mechanism would be responsible for making him/her know whether he/she has moved it or it has been moved by someone else. From this view, hallucinations are due to abnormalities in the integration of the efference copy and the perceptual entries: in this case the perceptual activities registered by the corollary discharge would not match the self-generated signals (Li, Chen, Yang, Chen, and Tsay, 2002).

This view has received support mainly from neuroimaging studies. A number of studies (McGuire, Shah, and Murray, 1993; Suzuki, Yuasa, Minabe, Murata, and Kurachi, 1993) has reported activation in the primary and secondary auditory cortex, as well as language related areas, especially Broca's area (involved in speech production), in patients while they are experiencing hallucinations. These findings suggest that a dysfunctional activation in primary and secondary sensory areas may create the experience of vivid perceptions in the absence of real sensory stimuli.

However, other studies have shown that, in addition to sensory cortical areas, hallucinations are associated with reduced activation in the dorsolateral prefrontal cortex, the dorsal anterior cingulate, supplementary motor area and cerebellum (see Allen, Laroi, McGuire, & Aleman, 2008, for a revision). That is, brain networks involved in emotional, attentional and memory functions also seem to contribute to hallucinations. Based on these findings, Allen et al. (2008) have proposed a model in which bottom-up and top-down processes interact. The dysfunctional activation in sensory areas would act together with a weakening of top-down control from the cingulate, prefrontal, premotor and cerebellar areas, which are thought to be responsible for monitoring, volitional and emotional processes. Hence, perceptual characteristics of hallucinations would depend on alterations in brain sensory areas, whereas alterations in the top-down network would account for the emotional content, sense of externality and non-volition that also characterizes the hallucinatory experience.

1.2. The Interpretative Account

The interpretation-based explanation of the hallucinatory experience that has received more support has been provided by Morrison (2001). This author proposed that the underlying cause of hallucinations is related to the interpretation of intrusive thoughts. Hallucinations are considered as internal mental events (thoughts, images, impulses) that are misattributed to an external source. According to this author, this misattribution is the result of certain metacognitive beliefs about our own thoughts. For example, metacognitive beliefs about the controlability and acceptability of our own thoughts play a fundamental role in misattributing them to external sources. When a person has certain metacognitive beliefs, such as "I always must control my own thoughts", or "My thoughts can never be disagreeable", the experience of unwanted intrusive thoughts produces dissonance. This dissonance is a source of great distress, and the individual reduces this distress by attributing the intrusive thoughts to an external agent.

Several lines of research give support to this proposal. Morrison and Baker (2000) have shown that patients who experience hallucinations have also more intrusive thoughts than patients who do not hallucinate. More interestingly, hallucinating patients experience their intrusive thoughts as more distressing, uncontrollable and unacceptable than patients without hallucinations and healthy participants. In another study, Morrison and Wells (2003) also reported that psychotic patients with hallucinations have more dysfunctional metacognitive beliefs than patients with panic disorders and healthy controls. Specifically, the groups differed on beliefs about uncontrollability, danger, superstition, punishment and responsibility.

A recent study from Moritz and Laroi (2008) has also highlighted the similarities between hallucinations and intrusive thoughts. Moritz and Laroi (2008) examined the cognitive and sensory characteristics of thoughts, intrusions and hallucinations. Intrusions are cognitive events (thoughts, images or impulses) that are normally unwanted, and are experienced as non-volitional, egodystonic (inconsistent with the person beliefs), discomforting, and difficult to control. Intrusions are frequent in a wide range of disorders, especially obsessive-compulsive disorder (OCD), anxiety generalized disorder, and depression. Moritz and Laroi (2008) surveyed a sample of schizophrenic patients, OCD (obsessive-compulsive disorder) patients, and healthy controls. 82% of the schizophrenic patients reported hearing voices, but also a 15% of OCD patients and a similar rate of healthy controls acknowledged having hallucinatory experiences. Voice-hearers, irrespective of the diagnostic status, had thoughts and intrusions of greater acoustic qualities than participants who did not hear voices. In some respect this is congruent with Morrison and Baker's (2000) findings that hallucinating patients perceived their intrusions as more uncontrollable than healthy people. Only a minority of voice-hearers reported that their voices were as loud as external voices. Thus, only 12,5% of OCD patients and one third of schizophrenic patients and healthy participants who had hallucinations could not differentiate them from real voices. On the other hand, very few participants indicated that they could fully control their normal thoughts. Interestingly, the degree of subjective control was lower for patients reporting intrusions (particularly OCD patients) than for patients reporting auditory hallucinations.

It is interesting to note that even when a proportion of healthy participants reported that their voices were loud, they considered them more unreal and were less disturbed by them than schizophrenics. This supports the view that metacognitive beliefs, and not the perceptual qualities of the voices, were the responsible of the consideration of voices as external events. On the other hand, most OCD patients defined their intrusions as alien, autonomous and somewhat acoustic, but they did not tend to attribute them to external agents.

These results challenge the resemblance between hallucinations and real perceptions, showing that hallucinations are not always acoustic, autonomous, alien and authentic external events, while intrusions, and even normal thoughts, can be experienced as alien, autonomous, and acoustic. Therefore, Moritz and Laroi (2008) conclude that differences between hallucinations and thoughts seem to be more quantitative than qualitative.

In this line, Jones and Fernyhough (2009) have proposed that rumination would be related to hallucination-proneness, due to tendency for ruminations to cause cognitive intrusions. They defined rumination as an individual's tendency to focus on their own thoughts due to negative affect and anxiety. They tested this model by exploring self-reports from a normal population. Consistent with their hypothesis, they found that rumination was related to hallucination-proneness through the mediating variable of intrusive thoughts. In addition, they found that reflection, considered as self-consciousness of one's thought because of curiosity or epistemological reasons and not because of emotional reasons, was also related to hallucinations. These results suggest that any form of self-focus on the own thoughts increases the probability of hallucinatory experiences. They also are consistent with the proposal of some authors (Ensum and Morrison, 2003; Perona, 2004) that self-focused attention on private events contribute to the maintenance of hallucinations. When a person directs his attention towards self-generated information more than to external information coming from sensory organs, he/she becomes extremely aware of his own private events, such as intrusive thoughts, memories, images; and this awareness, together with the associated emotional distress, may trigger the hallucinatory experience.

The view that hallucinations result mainly from erroneous interpretations of intrusive thoughts receive additional support from studies that show a relationship between emotional factors and the experience of hearing voices. It has been shown that hallucinations have normally an emotional content: threat, abuse, criticism, or command. Distress caused by voices is usually related to the emotional content of them. Even more, it has been observed that emotional disturbances usually precede the occurrence of hallucinations, suggesting that emotions have an important role in triggering hallucinatory experiences (Freeman and Garety, 2003).

Thus, emotions might act as a mediating variable between traumatic experiences and the development of hallucinations. Traumatic experiences have long been associated to persistent and distressing intrusions; in fact, intrusions and flashbacks are among the diagnostic criteria for PTSD (post-traumatic stress disorder). Recently, some studies have explored how trauma also increases the likelihood of hallucinations. For example, Freeman and Fowler (2009) have explored the association between a history of trauma and both hallucinations and persecutory delusions. They found that a history of trauma was independently associated with the occurrence of auditory hallucinations. The occurrence of at least one lifetime traumatic event was associated with a 4.8 times greater risk of having experienced any form of verbal hallucination. Traumatic experiences also influenced persecutory ideas, but only indirectly, through the mediational variable of anxiety. Hence, having suffered traumatic events can result in the occurrence of both intrusions and hallucinations. Probably, trauma is related to repeated, intrusive and distressing recollections of stressing events, which may include images, thoughts and perceptions. The interpretation of these recollections, and the degree of associated distress, would lead to the experience of hallucinations in a minority of individuals.

In summary, hallucinations and intrusive thoughts are similarly perceived as alien, involuntary and uncontrollable by the individual experiencing them. They are also similarly influenced by self-focus attention, emotional factors, and traumatic events. Although most studies have focused on auditory hallucinations and intrusive thoughts, we think that the similarity may extend to visual hallucinations, and intrusive images. Rachman (2007) has described intrusive images, stating that they share some properties with intrusive thoughts and impulses: they interrupt the ongoing cognitive flow, are unexpected, unselected and normally unwelcome by the individual. But, unlike intrusive thoughts, intrusive images are usually vivid, and they tend to emerge fully formed, which makes them even more uncontrollable and inescapable than the formers, causing great distress and resistance. According to Rachman (2007), when an unwanted image is catastrophically misinterpreted as being of great and negative personal significance, it is likely that it turn into an obsessive image. We can further assume that, if the individual thinks that a "normal" person can never have dangerous or uncontrollable images, he/she could interpret that he/she is actually seeing things, and not only imagining them.

The great majority of research supporting interpretative accounts of hallucinatory experiences has employed self-report measures, and correlational analyses. Although this research has provided interesting findings about the qualities of individual internal experiences, experimental studies are needed to test specific hypotheses about the origin and nature of the hallucinatory phenomena. In the next section, we will focus on some of the results coming from experimental research.

2. Do Hallucinations Derive from Intrusive Thoughts? Insights from Experimental Psychology

From an experimental cognitive point of view, we think that the parallelism between intrusive thoughts and hallucinations can be understood by assuming that inhibitory dysfunctions are the underlying cause of both of them. Some authors have pointed out that deficits in inhibitory functioning, especially in the attentional domain, could be related to schizophrenia. Hemsley (2005) has proposed that hallucinations might be related to an inhibitory dysfunction that would result in the emergence of redundant or irrelevant material from long term memory into awareness. Several models of normal cognition suggest that awareness of redundant information is inhibited to reduce information processing demands on a limited capacity system. According to Hemsley, in schizophrenia there is a disruption of performance by the intrusion of redundant or non-significant aspects of the environment into awareness.

From our view, intrusive thoughts can be partly due to difficulties to inhibit mental events, so that unwanted or repetitive thoughts or images intrude frequently into consciousness. The individual tries to somewhat suppress these intrusions, but he/she is unable to do it.

Inhibitory problems have been extensively studied from experimental perspectives. Inhibitory control has been considered to be involved in numerous tasks and situations. Deficits in inhibitory control have been observed in children, in normal aging, and in a number of neuropsychological diseases, such as Alzheimer's disease (Collette, Schmidt, Scherrer, Adama, and Salmon, 2009; Lechuga, Moreno, Pelegrina, Gómez-Ariza and Bajo, 2006).

Inhibitory dysfunctions have also been detected in schizophrenia. Schizophrenic patients have been shown to exhibit difficulties to ignore irrelevant targets (Park, Püschel, Sauter, Rentsch and Hell, 2002) and to suppress dominant responses (Weisbrod, Kiefer, Marzinzik and Spitzer, 2000). But these deficits have rarely been linked to specific symptoms. Even more, few studies have examined the inhibitory processes that act specifically on memory representations in schizophrenia; that is, the inhibitory processes needed to suppress intrusive or unwanted thoughts, distractive memories or interfering mental images.

One of these few studies is the pioneering work from Waters, Badcock, Maybery and Michie (2003), who explored the relationship between inhibitory processes in memory and hallucinations. They employed two tasks that assessed the intentional suppression of conscious mental representations: the Hayling Sentence Completion Test (HSCT) and the Inhibition of Currently Irrelevant Memories task (ICIM). In the HSCT, participants have to complete sentences with single words that have to be unrelated to the meaning of the sentences. This task requires the ability to voluntarily suppress the related word that automatically would come to mind when the sentence is read. Thus, in order to perform the task correctly, it is necessary to inhibit the mental representations from semantic memory. In the ICIM, animal pictures are presented in four runs. Some pictures are repeated 8 times within each run. Participants are asked to identify which pictures are repeated, but only within each run, and they should forget the pictures that they have seen in previous runs. To do that, participants have to use active suppression of recently learned information that is no longer relevant for the current trial; that is, they have to suppress mental representations from episodic memory. Waters and colleagues found that schizophrenic patients performed significantly worse than control participants on these inhibitory tasks. More interestingly, there was a significant correlation between severity of hallucinations and inhibitory deficits. This relationship was specific, in the sense that impaired inhibition was not associated with general, positive, or negative symptoms. These results suggest that difficulties to intentionally inhibit mental representations in memory may underlie hallucinations.

We have further explored the relationship between inhibitory processes in memory and hallucinations (Soriano, Jiménez, Román and Bajo, 2009). In two studies, we have replicated and extended the findings from Waters et al. (2003) with different experimental tasks.

In our first experiment, we investigated inhibitory processes in episodic memory with a directed forgetting (DF) paradigm (Basden & Basden, 1998). Participants (schizophrenic patients with hallucinations, schizophrenic patients without hallucinations, and healthy controls) were presented with a set of items to be studied for later recall. After presentation of the first list, participants in the forget condition were instructed to forget the items they had just learned. Following these instructions, a second list was presented, and participants were required to learn these new items. At recall, they were asked to remember the items from both lists. As a control, in a remember condition, participants were presented the two lists and they were instructed to remember both. That is, participants in the remember condition also learned the two lists but they were not instructed to forget the first before presentation of the second list. Normally in a typical DF experiment, participants in the forget condition remember fewer items from List 1 than from List 2, and they remember fewer List 1 items in the forget condition than in the remember condition. These directed forgetting effects are considered to be the result of inhibitory processes (Basden & Basden, 1998; Bjork & Bjork, 1996). The instructions to forget, following the presentation of the first list of items, trigger inhibitory processes that decrease the accessibility of these items in episodic memory.

If hallucinations are associated with difficulties to suppress mental representations, we would expect to find smaller DF effects in schizophrenic patients with hallucinations. Moreover, we hypothesized to find an inverse relation between the magnitude of the DF effect and the severity of hallucinations.

Results were consistent with our predictions. Healthy controls and patients without hallucinations showed a reliable DF effect that was evident when we compared List 2 and List 1 recall in the forget condition, and List 1 recall in the remember and forget condition. In contrast, hallucinating patients did not show a DF effect: their recall was not affected by instructions to forget. Interestingly, patients with and without hallucinations did not differ in their general recall. This finding indicates that the difference between patients with and without hallucinations was specific to their ability to suppress irrelevant memory information, so that other memory processes involved in episodic recall were similar in both groups. Finally, we found a significant inverse correlation between the magnitude of the DF effect and the severity of hallucinations: the greater the intensity and frequency of hallucinations, the smaller the DF effect.

In our second experiment, we investigated inhibitory deficits in working memory (WM), with an updating task. WM is the memory system responsible for temporal maintenance and on-line manipulation of task-relevant information. Inhibitory processes are crucial to the correct functioning of WM (Baddeley, 1986). Inhibition is needed to control access to working memory by suppressing distracting and no-longer relevant information (Lustig, Hasher and Tonev, 2001). We employed the updating procedure by Palladino, Cornoldi, De Beni and Pazzaglia (2001). We asked participants to listen to a list of words, and then recall only the smaller objects or animals. Intrusions errors in this task (recall of large animals or objects) would signal difficulties in inhibiting irrelevant information. Items corresponding to larger objects have to be suppressed from WM as the items corresponding to smaller objects appear in the list; if they are not suppressed, they would be recalled, leading to intrusions errors. Hence, intrusions errors can be considered as indicators of inhibitory failures.

Results showed that patients with hallucinations committed more intrusions than patients without hallucinations and healthy controls, indicating that patients with hallucinations have difficulties to suppress irrelevant information from working memory. Again, there was no difference between patients with and without hallucinations in their percentage of recall. And we found a significant correlation between number of intrusions and severity of hallucinations.

Finally, we correlated our inhibitory indexes (magnitude of DF effect in our first experiment and the number of intrusions in our second experiment) with several demographic variables and cluster of symptoms. Results indicated that the relationship between inhibitory function on memory and hallucinations is highly specific, since we found no relationship between these inhibitory indexes and other symptoms, clusters of symptoms, or demographic variables.

This pattern of results reveals that hallucinating patients are particularly impaired in their ability to intentionally inhibit memory representations, and not in general memory processes. Hence, our results support Waters et al. claim that inhibitory deficits in suppressing irrelevant information is specifically linked to hallucinations, and they strengthen the parallelism between hallucinations and cognitive intrusions.

More recently, Verwoerd, Wessel, & de Jong (2009) explored whether poor inhibitory control acts as a vulnerability factor for the persistence of intrusive memories after traumatic events. They asked normal people to complete a self-report questionnaire on intrusive memories, and to perform three experimental tasks. The first task was designed to assess the participants' resistance to proactive interference in memory; that is, they try to evaluate the ability to inhibit previously learned but no longer relevant information. The other tasks involved response inhibition and assess the ability to suppress predominant responses. Results showed a significant relationship between inhibitory function in memory (measured by the resistance to proactive interference) and the frequency of intrusive memories. However, no relation was found between response inhibition performance and intrusive memories. Hence, it seems that the ability to inhibit interference from irrelevant information in memory is linked with the experience of undesirable intrusive memories after a traumatic event.

The findings from Verwoerd, Wessel & de Jong (2009) showing a relationship between inhibitory difficulties in memory and intrusive thoughts resemble our results concerning inhibitory difficulties and hallucinations, and they support again the parallelism between hallucinations and cognitive intrusions.

3. The Relationship between Inhibitory Dysfunctions, Intrusions and Hallucinations: A Cognitive Model

Before discussing a plausible model to account for the appearance and maintenance of hallucinations, we want to focus on the distinction between cognitive deficits and cognitive bias (Ensum and Morrison, 2003; Perona, 2004). Cognitive deficit refers to a basic cognitive dysfunction that can be evaluated with objective tasks and neutral material, whereas cognitive bias refers to the differential or preferential processing of certain material in relation to the specific cognitive schemas of the individual. For example, memory problems in Alzheimer disease can be considered stable cognitive deficits, independent on the context and testing material. In contrast, some attention-concentration difficulties in anxiety disorder are a result of certain biases, related to an excessive vigilance and erroneous appraisal of certain information; hence, these difficulties reflect cognitive biases because they can be influenced by a variety of contextual and emotional factors.

Interpretative models of hallucinations focus on cognitive biases as the main factor influencing hallucinatory experiences. Thus, this proposal successfully predicts the presence of incorrect attributions in hallucinatory experiences. Metacognitive beliefs, and the associated cognitive dissonance, are probably underlying the misattribution of private events to external agents. Emotional distress, and self-focused attention, would contribute to the maintenance and resistance to change of hallucinatory experiences.

Indeed, other processes that have also been associated to the hallucinatory phenomena can be also understood in terms of cognitive biases. For example, studies have consistently shown that hallucinating patients have poorer performance on source monitoring tasks than non-hallucinating patients and controls. Source monitoring tasks evaluate the ability to differentiate between the source of our memories: for example, a word we have listened to, as opposed to a word we have read (this would be the case of two external sources: acoustic versus visual); or a stimulus that we have seen, as opposed to one that we have imagined (this would be the case of an external source versus an internal one). Several studies have demonstrated that schizophrenic patients have difficulties to differentiate the source of their memories. More interestingly, only hallucinating patients show a deficit to distinguish between external and internal sources: they tend to attribute internally generated memories to external sources (Brunelin, Combris, Poulet, Kallel, D'Amato, Dalery, and Saoud, 2006; López-Frutos and Ruiz-Vargas, 1999)

These findings have lead to the proposal that source monitoring difficulties underlie hallucinations. However, poor performance in source monitoring tasks can be due to different factors. It can be caused by difficulties in managing contextual memory information, but source monitoring problems can also be the result of judgment biases.

From our point of view, data are more consistent with this second explanation. For example, Allen, Johns, Fu, Broome, Vythelingum, and McGuire (2004), asked participants to listen to recorded words emitted by themselves or by other person, and to judge the source of the recording. Schizophrenic patients with hallucinations tended to erroneously classify their own recorded words as produced by other person. As this task does not imply memory processes, findings suggest that hallucinating patients have a bias in their judgment processes. Similarly, these results indicate that hallucinations are not caused by a dysfunctional perception of the own inner speech, because in this task perceptual feedback of inner speech was not involved.

Consistent with this explanation, Ensum and Morrison (2003) have shown that the poor performance of hallucinating patients in source monitoring tasks depends on the emotional salience of the material, and on the attentional focus. When the material had an emotional content, and the participant's attention was self-focused, hallucinating patients produced more errors than when other type of material and attentional conditions were present. These results imply that difficulties in source monitoring in hallucinating patients reflect cognitive attributional bias that can fluctuate, and not a stable cognitive deficit.

However, we believe that attributional biases are not sufficient to explain the hallucinatory phenomena. Cognitive biases account for the erroneous interpretation and attribution of private events (thoughts, images, impulses...). But, for example, they cannot explain why hallucinating patients experience more intrusions than patients who do not hallucinate (Morrison & Baker, 2000). Taking into account the complete pattern of experimental data, we propose that the frequency of intrusions is caused by dysfunctions in inhibiting memory representations. Several findings have shown a relationship between difficulties to intentionally suppress memory representations and both hallucinations (Soriano et al., 2009; Waters et al., 2003), and intrusions (Verwoerd, Wessel and de Jong, 2009).

Thus, our proposal is that hallucinations result from the interaction of two main factors: a basic cognitive deficit in inhibitory control, and certain attributional biases. Patients with hallucinations have impairments in intentional inhibition in memory; consequently, irrelevant or unwanted images and thoughts would frequently intrude into their consciousness.

Metacognitive beliefs and processes would induce erroneous attributions of these unwanted and repetitive thoughts to external sources, producing hallucinatory experiences. That is, deficits in intentional inhibition in memory would underlie the greater occurrence of intrusive thoughts, whereas metacognitive beliefs would contribute to the incorrect attribution of these thoughts. As Morrison (2001) has proposed, the dissonance between the intrusions and certain metacognitive schemas (related mainly with the controllability and acceptability of the own thoughts) would finally make the internal thoughts being experienced as external voices. Thus, hallucinations would be the result of the mixed influence of inhibitory impairments and incorrect attributions. Emotional factors and self-focused attention would contribute to the pervasive maintenance of the phenomena.

Inhibitory dysfunctions can also underlie other psychotic symptoms. But the basic idea is that inhibitory difficulties would produce that irrelevant mental events emerge into awareness, producing the repeated and disturbing experience of cognitive intrusions. If the individual has certain metacognitive beliefs, such as "I must always control my own thought", or "I can never have disagreeable or dangerous thoughts", recurrent intrusions become unacceptable, and they would be source of great distress. These intrusions would be experienced as voices, reducing the dissonance associated to them. On the other hand, intruding mental representations that reach awareness (even previously neutral or irrelevant) may acquire a special meaning for the individual, if awareness of the intruding information is continuous. This special meaning could produce the development of delusional beliefs. For example, the repeated recollection of a message from a friend would lead to think that this message has significant and personal meanings, that it might be interpreted as a warning or a threat. These interpretations could easily lead to delusional beliefs. Finally, frequent intrusions can interfere with goal maintenance during thinking or during overt discourse, producing a disorganized and circumstantial speech.

4. Implications

4.1. Schizophrenia and Other Mental Disorders

The consideration of hallucinations as intrusive thoughts that are attributed to an external source has relevant consequences for our view of different mental disorders. As we mentioned previously, hallucinations are considered relevant diagnostic symptoms for schizophrenia and other psychotic illnesses. On the other hand, intrusions are frequently observed in several anxiety and affective disorders. They are even diagnostic criteria for some of them, such as OCD and PTSD. If hallucinations are only quantitatively different from cognitive intrusions, the distinction between psychotic and other mental disorders might be more subtle than previously thought.

The empirical evidence reviewed above suggests that hallucinations are not qualitatively different from normal experiences. If psychotic disorders are characterized by the presence of psychotic symptoms, specifically delusions and hallucinations, and such symptoms are associated to biases and dysfunctions in psychological processes that are similar to those involved in some neurotic disorders (i.e. OCD, PTSD), then, it is not clear that a sharp distinction between psychosis and neurosis should be drawn. This position has recently been defended by Freeman and Garety (2003). They argued that the frequent occurrence of emotional disorders prior to and accompanying psychosis indicates that neurosis contributes to the development of the positive symptoms present in psychotic patients. Similarly, they argued that processes traditionally associated to the maintenance of anxiety disorders, such as self-focus and safety behaviors, might also be maintaining positive symptoms in psychotic disorders. This suggests that there is not a clear distinction between neurotic and psychotic disorders, neither in terms of etiology, maintenance, symptoms, or psychological treatment. However, Freeman and Garety (2003) conclude that there might be some differences between psychotic and neurotic individuals in cognitive processing, in the sense that psychosis are associated to basic cognitive disturbances while neuroses are not. However, in view of the evidence discussed above, we think this is an erroneous conclusion because cognitive abnormalities seem to be linked to specific symptoms, more than to specific disorders.

We agree with the several authors (Bentall, 1990; Peters, Pickering, Kent, Glasper, Irani, David, Day, & Hemsley, 2000) who have emphasized the utility of a symptom-based approach in investigating cognitive deficits in schizophrenia. If we consider the symptomatic heterogeneity of some disorders, as schizophrenia, and the similarity between these heterogeneous symptoms and those in different mental disorders, as we have repeatedly shown in this chapter, it is difficult to defend that there are basic cognitive deficits that are common to all psychotic patients. In fact, the search of a basic cognitive dysfunction in schizophrenia has not proved fruitful so far.

The finding of inhibitory deficits underlying hallucinations and cognitive intrusions highlights the importance of this symptom–based approach. In agreement with this approach, we have previously found (Soriano, Jiménez, Román and Bajo, 2008) that inhibition in semantic memory was related to the presence of Formal-Thought Disorder (FTD) in schizophrenic patients, and not to the presence of hallucinations. In Experiment 2, participants were required to name pictures that were preceded by related or unrelated word primes. The interference effect that is typically observed when pictures are preceded by semantically related primes is explained as due to inhibitory processes from the word prime to the related picture target (Macizo & Bajo, 2004). The results indicated that non-FTD and control participants showed normal interference/inhibition effects from the related prime words, whereas patients with FTD showed similar performance for pictures preceded by related word than for pictures preceded by unrelated words. This last finding supports the hypothesis that abnormalities in inhibitory processes in semantic memory underlie FTD. Hence, if we take these findings together with evidence concerning hallucinations, it would be possible to conclude that specific symptoms can be related to specific inhibitory processes: patients with hallucinations show deficits in intentional episodic or working memory inhibition, whereas patients with FTD show the inhibitory deficit in task related to semantic memory.

Kerns and BerenBaum (2002; Berenbaum, Kerns, Vernon and Gomez, 2008) have also studied cognitive deficits in schizophrenia from a symptom-based perspective. They focus on how different symptoms of the disorder are associated to different cognitive deficits. These authors have defended the need to develop and test specific hypotheses about individual symptoms of schizophrenia, instead of focusing on cognitive deficits related to schizophrenia in general. Consistent with our results, they showed that hallucinations are specially related with difficulties in managing representations in episodic memory.

The advantages of a symptom-based approach versus a diagnostic approach also shows in the findings of inhibitory deficits in memory across different disorders where intrusions are frequently observed. For example, it has been shown that PTSD patients, when compared with healthy controls, have greater difficulties to inhibit previously learned information (Cottencin, Vaiva, Huron, Devos, Ducrocq, Jouvent, Goudemand, and Thomas, 2006). These difficulties could be a vulnerability factor, leading to a greater frequency and severity of intrusive memories in individuals exposed to traumatic events. In a similar vein, results from Verwoerd, Wessel and de Jong (2009) show the parallel between the experience of intrusive memories and inhibitory deficits in normal population.

Many studies have explored inhibitory function in OCD patients, both at a cognitive (Enright and Beech, 1993) and response level (Penadés, Catalán, Rubia, Andrés, Salamero, and Gastó, 2007), and in general, results indicate that OCD is characterized by impaired inhibition. It has been suggested that this inhibitory deficit may explain the difficulties that OCD patients have in suppressing intrusive thoughts, images or impulses. For example, Badcock, Waters and Maybery (2007) have reported difficulties to intentionally suppress memory information in OCD patients. Although many of these studies has not examined the relationship between inhibitory dysfunctions and the severity of intrusions.

Inhibitory dysfunctions have also been found in other disorders, but again they have not been related to specific symptoms. For example, Larson, Shear, Krikorian, Welge, and Strakowski (2005) have demonstrated that bipolar patients have poor performance in a response inhibition task. This deficit was observed in bipolar patients in maniac and euthymic phases, but the authors did not explore whether it was related to specific symptomatology. It makes sense that a dysfunctional inhibitory control in bipolar patients is related to the impulsive behavior usually observed in these patients, but results do not guaranty this conclusion. On the other hand, inhibitory processes in memory in bipolar disorder have been scarcely studied. Although a percentage of bipolar patients suffer from hallucinations, especially when they are in manic or depressive phases, the relationship between hallucinations in bipolar disorder and inhibition in memory has not been explored so far.

Finally, inhibitory deficits have also been reported in organic diseases such as Alzheimer's disease. Collette et al., (2009) have demonstrated that participants with Alzheimer's disease showed deficits in most tasks designed to measure inhibitory processes in memory. Normal elderly participants had difficulties only in tasks that required a more controlled and voluntary suppression of information. These inhibitory difficulties may explain why Alzheimer patients, and also some elderly individuals, suffer from a greater number of intrusions and perseverations in their memories, or in their normal speech. It would be interesting to investigate whether these inhibitory deficits are accentuated in more advanced stages of Alzheimer's disease, when hallucinations usually appear.

4.2. Implications for Treatment

The model that we have outlined regarding origin and maintenance of hallucinations has also relevant implications for intervention. If we consider hallucinations are the mixed result of inhibitory deficits and attributional biases, a successful treatment should address both factors.

In regard with the first of them, cognitive rehabilitation programs, specially focused on inhibitory functions in memory, should be developed. Nowadays, most rehabilitation programs used in mental patients have been designed for the treatment of brain damage, or for mental training in children and adolescents. The discovery of cognitive deficits linked to specific symptoms highlights the need to create rehabilitation programs, specifically designed to train memory dysfunctions. These programs should be based on theoretical models about normal cognitive functioning.

On the other hand, attributional biases should be addressed through therapy, but having in mind inhibitory deficits that are influencing symptoms. Cognitive-behavior therapy is already successfully used in the treatment of hallucinations and delusions. Emotional factors, and metacognitive beliefs, need to be specially taken into account in this type of therapy. But the consideration of hallucinations as cognitive intrusions can highlight other important aspects of any therapy designed to reduce the distress associated with hearing voices.

For example, it has been discovered that trying to suppress cognitive intrusions is a counterproductive technique in OCD (Najmi, Riemann, and Wegner, 2009). Attempts to suppress intrusions led to an increase in the associated distress. On the contrary, focused distraction (asking participants to focus on other specific thoughts; for example, a weekend they have recently enjoyed or they plan to enjoy in the near future), and acceptance (asking participants to passively observe their unwanted intrusions without trying to suppress or change them) significantly reduced the distress caused by intrusions. Acceptance techniques also reduced the frequency of intrusions in the short term.

Suppression efforts also have negative effects on intrusions in PTSD. Vázquez, Hervás and Pérez-Sales (2008) have shown that thought suppression is related to the severity of PTSD symptoms. In their study, they examined posttraumatic stress-related symptoms, coping strategies, and chronic attempts to avoid intrusive thoughts in a normal population after a traumatic event (terrorist attack in Madrid). They found that chronic thought suppression, and avoidance coping strategies, were related to greater severity of PTSD symptoms.

A possible explanation of the counterproductive effect of suppression for managing intrusions may lay in the inhibitory difficulties that underlie the symptom. Possibly, OCD patients are ineffective in suppressing their intrusions although they may try to actively suppress them. In the case of PTSD, inhibitory difficulties could be a vulnerability factor for the appearance of trauma-related symptoms in individuals exposed to a traumatic event. As Vázquez, Hervás and Pérez-Sales (2008) suggest, people with inhibitory deficits would experience more intrusive thoughts which might, in turn, lead to an intensified tendency to suppress such thoughts.

Acceptance techniques have recently been proposed for the treatment of hallucinations. For example, Perona (2004) has defended the idea that therapy should help subjects accept voices and avoid fighting and directly confronting them. Therapeutic techniques should help patients to adjust to their environment, independently of whether they continue hearing voices. Even more, techniques should encourage patients to accept and experience directly their private events.

Recent developments from a behavioral perspective are in this direction. It is suggested that individuals should stop efforts actively directed to suppress or change their symptoms. Instead, they are encouraged to observe and accept their symptoms, while trying to focus on their main values and goals in life. From this perspective, symptoms are important not because of the suffering they cause in the individual, but because they prevent individuals from achieving their life goals. Patients are encouraged to weigh the importance of their symptoms versus the importance of their values and goals, and to move towards their objectives despite their symptoms. To do this, they have to accept that a certain amount of suffering is going to be present in their daily lives. It is assumed that, when people accept their symptoms and stop fighting them, their frequency and severity would diminish. And that is so because the distress derived from metacognitive beliefs, self-focused attention and safety behaviors maintains and exacerbates symtomatology in any disorder. When the individual accepts their symptoms, these factors start to slowly reduce their influence. We strongly believe that this type of approach could be suitable for the treatment of hallucinations.

References

Allen, P. P., Johns, L. C., Fu, C. H. Y., Broome, M. R., Vythelingum, G. N. & McGuire, P. K. (2004). Misattribution of external speech in patients with hallucinations and delusions. *Schizophrenia Research, 69*, 277-287.

Allen, P., Laroi, F., McGuire, P. K. & Aleman, A. (2008). The hallucinating brain: A review of structural and functional neuroimaging studies of hallucinations. *Neuroscience and Biobehavioral Reviews, 32*, 175-191.

Badcock, J. C., Waters, F. A. V. & Maybery, M. (2007). On keeping (intrusive) thoughts to one's self: Testing a cognitive model of auditory hallucination. *Cognitive Neuropsychiatry, 12*, 78-89.

Baddeley, A. (1986). *Working memory*. Claredon Press. Oxford.

Basden, B. H. & Basden, D. R. (1998). Directed Forgetting: A Contrast of Methods and Interpretations. In: J. M. Golding, & C. M. MacLeod, (Eds.), *Intentional forgetting: Interdisciplinary Approaches* (139-173). *Lawrence Erlbaum Associates*. London.

Bentall, R. P. (1990). The illusion of reality: A review and integration of psychological research on hallucinations. *Psychological Bulletin, 107*, 82-95.

Berenbaum, H., Kerns, J., Vernon, L. & Gomez, J. (2008). Cognitive correlates of schizophrenia signs and symptoms: III. Hallucinations and delusions. *Psychiatry research, 159*, 163-166.

Bjork, E. L. & Bjork, R. A. (1996). Continuing influences of to-be-forgotten information. *Consciousness and Cognition, 5*, 176-196.

Brunelin, J., Combris, M., Poulet, E., Kallel, L., D'Amato, T., Dalery, J. & Saoud, M. (2006). Source monitoring deficits in hallucinating compared to non-hallucinating patients with schizophrenia. *European Psychiatry, 21*, 259-261.

Collette F., Schmidt, C., Scherrer, C., Adama, S. & Salmon, E. (2009). Specificity of inhibitory deficits in normal aging and Alzheimer's disease. *Neurobiology of Aging, 30*, 875-889.

Cottencin, O., Vaiva, G., Huron, C., Devos, P., Ducrocq, F., Jouvent, R., Goudemand, M. & Thomas, P. (2006). Directed forgetting in PTSD: a comparative study versus normal controls. *Journal of Psychiatric Research, 40*, 70-80.

Enright, S. J. & Beech, A. R. (1993). Reduced cognitive inhibition in obsessive-compulsive disorder. *British Journal of Clinical Psychology, 32*, 67-74.

Ensum, I. & Morrison, A. P. (2003). The effects of focus of attention on attributional bias in patients experiencing auditory hallucinations. *Behaviour Research and Therapy*, *41*, 895-907.

Freeman, D. & Garety, P. A. (2003). Connecting neurosis and psychosis: the direct influence of emotion on delusions and hallucinations. *Behaviour Research and Therapy*, *41*, 923-947.

Freeman, D. & Fowler (2009). Routes to psychotic symptoms: Trauma, anxiety and psychosis-like experiences. *Psychiatry Research*, *169*, 107-112.

Frith, C. D. & Done, D. J. (1987). Towards a cognitive neuropsychology of schizophrenia. *British Journal of Psychiatry*, *153*, 437-443.

Hemsley, D. R. (2005). The development of a cognitive model of schizophrenia: Placing it in context. *Neuroscience and Biobehavioral Reviews*, *29*, 977-988.

Jaspers, K. (1962). *General Psychopathology*. Manchester University Press, Manchester.

Johns, L. C. & van Os, J. (2001). The continuity of psychotic experiences in the general population. *Clinical Psychological Review*, *21*, 1125-1141.

Jones, S. R. & Fernyhough (2009). Rumination, reflection, intrusive thoughts, and hallucination-proneness: Towards a new model. *Behaviour Research and Therapy*, *47*, 54-59.

Kerns, J.G. & Berenbaum, H. (2002). Cognitive Impairments associated with formal thought disorder in people with schizophrenia. *Journal of Abnormal Psychology*, *111*, 211-224.

Larson, E. R., Shear, P. K., Krikorian, R., Welge, J. & Strakowski, S. M. (2005). Working memory and inhibitory control among manic and euthymic patients with bipolar disorder. *Journal of the International Neuropsychological Society*, *11*, 163-172.

Lechuga, M. T., Moreno, V., Pelegrina, S., Gómez-Ariza, C. J. & Bajo, M. T. (2006). Age differences in memory control: Evidence from updating and retrieval-practice tasks. *Acta Psychologica, 123*, 279-298.

Li, C. R., Chen, M-C., Yang, Y-Y., Chen, M-C. & Tsay, P-K. (2002). Altered performance of schizophrenia patients in an auditory detection and discrimination task: exploring the "self-monitoring" model of hallucination. *Schizophrenia Research*, *55*, 115-128.

López-Frutos, J. M. & Ruiz-Vargas, J. M. (1999). Presencia de alucinaciones y déficit en monitorización de las fuentes de los recuerdos en la esquizofrenia. *Archivos de Neurología*, *62*, 313-333.

Lustig, C., Hasher, L. & Tonev, S. T. (2001). Inhibitory control over the present and the past. *European Journal of Cognitive Psychology*, *13*, 107-122.

Macizo, P. & Bajo, M.T. (2004). Semantic facilitation and lexical competition in picture naming. *Psicológica*, *25*, 1-22.

McGuire, P.K., Shah, G.M. & Murray, R.M. (1993). Increased blood flow in Broca's area during auditory hallucinations in schizophrenia. *Lancet*, *342*, 703-706.

Moritz, S. & Laroi, F. (2008). Differences and similarities in the sensory and cognitive signatures of voice-hearing, intrusions and thoughts. *Schizophrenia Research 102*, 96-107.

Morrison, A. P. (2001). The interpretation of intrusions in psychosis: an integrative cognitive approach to psychotic symptoms. *Behavioural and Cognitive Psychotherapy, 29*, 257-276.

Morrison, A. P. & Baker, C. A. (2000). Intrusive thoughts and auditory hallucinations: a comparative study of intrusions in psychosis. *Behaviour Research and Therapy, 38*, 1097-1106.

Morrison, A. P. & Wells, A. (2003). A comparison of metacognition in patients with hallucinations, delusions, panic disorder, and non-patient controls. *Behaviour Research and Therapy, 41*, 251-256.

Najmi, S., Riemann, B. & Wegner, D. M. (2009). Managing unwanted intrusive thoughts in obsessive–compulsive disorder: Relative effectiveness of suppression, focused distraction, and acceptance. *Behaviour Research and Therapy, 47*, 494-503.

Ohayon, M. M. (2000). Prevalence of hallucinations and their pathological associations in the general population. *Psychiatry Research, 97*, 153-164.

Palladino, P., Cornoldi, c., De Beni, R. & Pazzaglia, F. (2001). Working memory and updating processes in reading comprehension. *Memory & Cognition, 29*, 344-354.

Park, S., Püschel, J., Sauter, B. H., Rentsch, M. & Hell, D. (2002). Spatial selective attention and inhibition in schizophrenia patients during acute psychosis and at 4-month follow-up. *Biological Psychiatry, 51*, 498-506.

Penadés, R., Catalán, R., Rubia, K., Andrés, S., Salamero, M. & Gastó, C. (2007). Impaired response inhibition in obsessive-compulsive disorder. *European Psychiatry*, 22, 404–410.

Perona, S. (2004). A psychological model for verbal auditory hallucinations. *International Journal of Psychology and Psychological Therapy, 4*, 1. 129-153.

Peters, E. R., Pickering, A. D., Kent, A., Glasper, A., Irani, M., David, A. S., Day, S. & Hemsley, D. R. (2000). The relationship between Cognitive Inhibition and psychotic symptoms. *Journal of Abnormal Psychology, 109*, 3, 386-395.

Rachman, S. (2007). Unwanted intrusive images in obsessive compulsive disorders. *Journal of Behavior Therapy and Experimental Psychiatry, 38*, 402-410.

Schneider, K. (1959). *Clinical psychopathology*. Grune and Stratton, Nueva Cork.

Soriano, M. F., Jiménez, J. F., Román, P. & Bajo, M. T. (2008). Cognitive Substrates in Semantic Memory of Formal Thought Disorder in Schizophrenia. *Journal of Clinical and Experimental Neuropsychology, 30*, 70-82.

Soriano, M. F., Jiménez, J. F., Román, P. & Bajo, M. T. (2009). Intentional inhibition in memory and hallucinations: Directed forgetting and updating. *Neuropsychology, 23(1)*, 61-70.

Suzuki, M., Yuasa, S., Minabe, Y., Murata, M. & Kurachi, M. (1993). Left superior temporal blood flow increases in schizophrenic and schizophreniform patients with auditory hallucination: a longitudinal case study using 123I-IMP SPECT. *European Archives of Psychiatry and Clinical Neuroscience, 242*, 257-261.

Vázquez, C., Hervás, G. & Pérez-Sales, P. (2008). Chronic thought suppression and posttraumatic symptoms: Data from the Madrid March 11, 2004 terrorist attack. *Journal of Anxiety Disorders, 22*, 1226-1236.

Verwoerd, J., Wessel, I. & de Jong, P. J. (2009). Individual differences in experiencing intrusive memories: The role of the ability to resist proactive interference. *Journal of Behavior Therapy and Experimental Psychiatry, 40*, 189-201.

Waters, F. A. V., Badcock, J. C., Maybery, M. T. & Michie, P. T. (2003). Inhibition in schizophrenia: association with auditory hallucinations. *Schizophrenia Research, 62*, 275-280.

Weisbrod, M., Kiefer, M., Marzinzik, F. & Spitzer, M. (2000). Executive control is disturbed in schizophrenia: evidence from event-related potentials in a Go-noGo task. *Biological Psychiatry, 47*, 51-60.

In: Hallucinations: Types, Stages and Treatments
Editor: Meredith S. Payne, pp. 97-112

ISBN: 978-1-61728-275-1
© 2011 Nova Science Publishers, Inc.

Chapter 5

Charles Bonnet Syndrome

*Chris Plummer**
[1]St Vincent's Hospital Centre for Neurosciences and Neurological Research, Melbourne, Australia
[2]Department of Medicine, University of Melbourne, Melbourne, Australia.

Abstract

Charles Bonnet Syndrome (CBS) is a fascinating disorder that is generally defined as the presence of visual hallucinations (simple or complex) in patients who meet two additional clinical criteria i) visual impairment is due to eye disease and ii) higher cognitive function is intact. The condition is most commonly encountered in elderly patients with advanced, age-related macular degeneration. The prevalence of the disorder is almost certainly under-estimated; this is because patients are typically reluctant to reveal their symptoms for fear of being labelled insane or demented. This underscores the importance of improved patient and physician awareness of CBS as its incidence is only likely to rise in an ever increasingly aged population. It is perhaps ironic that despite the major advances in neuroimaging technology over recent years, we have not moved so far from Bonnet's original insightful discourse on the possible pathogenesis of the disorder – the first recognized account of hallucinatory phenomena in the scientific literature. CBS still has much to teach us about the complexity of the visual association cortex in man.

A. Introduction

This chapter deals with the nature, epidemiology, pathophysiology, and treatment of Charles Bonnet Syndrome (CBS). It is important to appreciate that CBS is not actually a 'hallucinatory' disorder in the strictest sense, but rather a 'pseudo-hallucinatory' one based on the fact that the sufferer is mindful of the unreality of the visions so perceived. Moreover, the sufferer does not attach meaning to the visions, an important feature that sets CBS apart from the types of hallucinations that may be experienced by sufferers of psychiatric illness. The chapter begins with a working definition of CBS – 'working' because there is no universal agreement on this point – and goes on to document the historical aspects of the disorder. Particular attention is paid to the man after whom the disorder was named. The detailed clinical histories of two patients with CBS are then given followed by a review of the epidemiology and currently recognized risk factors. The as yet unresolved pathophysiology of CBS is discussed after outlining the neuro-anatomical pathways held to be central to the disorder's pathogenesis. Important differential diagnoses are described. The chapter concludes with a note on the disease course and management.

B. Definition and Syndrome Origins

Charles Bonnet Syndrome (CBS) is a widely under-recognized and under-diagnosed disorder that typically manifests as sudden onset, repetitive visual hallucinations (simple or complex) in the visually impaired. There are several characteristic features of the condition that support the diagnosis and help the physician distinguish it from other disorders that give rise to hallucinatory phenomena. The hallucinatory content in CBS is purely visual[1] (there are no olfactory, auditory, or other special sensory features); the sufferer's level of awareness is not impaired during the course of the hallucinatory episode; and, importantly, the sufferer realizes that the hallucinations are neither real or meaningful. By virtue of this latter point, CBS hallucinations are strictly pseudo-hallucinations because insight into their illusory nature is maintained. The lack of an attached meaning to the hallucinations serves to set them apart from the hallucinations associated with psychiatric illness (e.g., schizophrenia, major depression).

The syndrome of Charles Bonnet was eponymously coined by de Morsier[2] in 1936 in honour of the Swiss naturalist and philosopher who first documented the disorder in 1760. In what is widely held to be the first description in the scientific literature of hallucinatory phenomena in the psychologically normal[3], Bonnet's account relates a series of simple and complex images perceived by his then 89 year old grandfather, Charles Lullin, who had bilateral cataract disease[4]. While keenly aware that his hallucinations were not real, Lullin 'saw' people, carriages, birds, tapestries, and buildings. It was recently noted[5] that Bonnet somewhat underplayed the sophistication of his grandfather's visions in his original publication. We know this from Fluornoy's essay[6] published in 1902 (over a century after Bonnet's death) on the subject of Lullin's hallucinations. The essay relates, in exquisite detail, the personal account given by Lullin to his grandson[7]. Lullin's "women" were actually young dancing girls "dressed in yellow silks with rose coloured ribbons, pearl collars, golden buckles, and diamond pendants", and Lullin's "carriage" was "a coach complete with drivers and horses, expanded in correct proportion to the size of a house"[5]. To this day, CBS is known for this very flavour of imagery – extended landscapes, human and animal figures, and ornate structures. Colour, movement, and unusual detail appear to be common themes. Simpler images include lines, dots, and geometric patterns.

The intriguing story of Charles Bonnet – the man – was recently reviewed by Hedges[7]. Ironically, it seems that Bonnet himself experienced visual hallucinations as his vision dimmed with age[8]. In fact, his vision was first noted to be deteriorating when he was only 22 years-old for reasons that remain unclear. This must have been especially frustrating to

Bonnet because his first great passion was entomology, a discipline that demanded constant use of the microscope[7]. In spite of this disability, he went on to detail the respiratory apparatus of caterpillars and butterflies. This work, along with his ground-breaking discovery of parthenogenesis (embryogenesis from an unfertilized egg) in an aphid species, won him membership to the prestigious Royal Society of London in 1743[7]. Over the next ten years, while his vision continued to deteriorate to the point where it precluded his use of the microscope altogether, his intellectual curiosity never waned as evidenced by the lucid description and interpretation of his grandfather's peculiar symptoms.

"I should tell you about a strange case that would be considered fabulous if not supported by testimonies of the highest credibility. I will simply say that I know a respectable man full of health, of ingenuousness, judgement, and memory, who, completely alert and independently from all outside influences, sees from time to time, in front of him, figures...getting closer, going away, fleeing, diminishing or increasing in size, appearing or disappearing; he sees buildings rise in front of his eyes and a display of all the outside construction material. The tapestries in his apartment appear to change suddenly; these tapestries cover themselves with painting displaying different landscapes. Another day, instead of the tapestries and furniture it is only the naked walls with an assembly of raw materials. All these visions appear to him in perfect clarity and affect him as strongly as if the objects themselves were present. However, these are only paintings because the men and women do not talk and no noise comes to his ear"[4, 7]. And in an extraordinary display of scientific thought 200 years before the advent of neuroimaging of any kind, he goes on to say: "All of this appears to have a seat in the part of the brain that commands the sense of sight. It is not difficult to imagine physical causes, strong enough to shake sensitive bundles of fibres that will produce in the mind, the picture of various objects with as much veracity as if the objects themselves had stimulated the fibres. And if the fibres used for thought are not involved but remain in their natural state, the mind will not confuse vision with reality"[4, 7]. What makes this extraordinary is the fact that we haven't moved much closer to the pathogenesis of visual hallucinations in the sight impaired. Bonnet's 250 year old hypothesis remains on the table.

Since Bonnet's description, and with the development of computerized tomography and magnetic resonance imaging (MRI), CBS-like hallucinations have been associated with lesions seated anywhere along the central visual pathway – from the orbit to the calcarine fissure, which houses the primary visual cortex. This has contributed to a now 70 year-long[5] controversy surrounding the definition of CBS based on the localization of the inciting pathology. In deference to Bonnet's original case description and given that the key studies in CBS are based on patients with ocular disease, 'CBS' herein refers to patients with visual hallucinations (simple or complex) associated with pathology of the eye.

C. Hallucinatory Content

To illustrate the nature of the hallucinations experienced by CBS sufferers in greater detail, two particularly instructive examples of the syndrome now follow. Both patients had severe visual impairment from end-stage, age related macular degeneration (AMD). This is one of the more common ocular pathologies associated with CBS[9, 10].

Case 1: A 73 year-old woman who lived alone presented with anxiety provoking visual hallucinations. Hundreds of black ants, some up to an inch in length, scurried across her kitchen floor, walls, windows, and curtains. In desperation, she started spraying insecticide throughout the house. She ran next-door for help. Her neighbour, whose features were also seemingly masked by the insects, called an ambulance. Floating sea horses and featherless chickens joined the colonies of ants in the casualty ward of the local hospital. A Roman chariot, the rider dressed in gold, the horses dressed in silks, flashed across the curtain several times. On the ward, tropical vines grew from the foot of her bed and appeared to tower towards and then project through the ceiling. A man stood with thick brown tree trunks for legs and thick green branches for arms. Nurses' heads would slowly shrink and then expand before melting into the floor. Brightly coloured fairies carrying wands nodded and smiled, seemingly wanting to invite her for long walks around the hospital grounds. She once caught herself telling them to get off a road at which point they donned diamond coats, jumped into a wooden carriage, and rode up to her bedside. Ants in the mirror were at times replaced by an enormous elephant trunk blotting out half her face. Her hair in the reflection flowed with cobwebs and the basin was matted with hair and whiskers. Cobwebs spilled from her cereal bowl at breakfast. The bathroom floor was covered with water that vanished whenever she tried to mop it up. The carpet in the room would lift away from the floor, roll up in the form of a snake, and slither out the door. A little girl and boy with a black and white dog stood next to the bed, as did extraterrestrial-like beings with large domed shaped heads and slitted black eyes. Twisted heads with grotesque faces and bulbous eyes peered out from the wall, while little red carriages, trains and push bikes disappeared into it. Further history revealed an experience of similar black ant hallucinations four months previously but the images disappeared after two weeks. She did not seek medical advice at that time fearing that she might be considered "a bit odd". Throughout the hospital admission she was rarely hallucination-free and would repeatedly ask for reassurance from medical and nursing staff that she was not "going mad". Two months after discharge the hallucinations were still active. She owned a small black dog but would see several dogs resembling oversized greyhounds with unusually long snouts in her daughter's yard. A man and a large goat, both wearing grey hats and overcoats, often stood beside her before wandering off together down a crooked road. She grew accustomed to seeing a baby seated on the lounge chair wearing grey clothes. She did not recognize the child. It smiled but made no sounds. Rainbow-coloured caterpillars and green tree frogs began joining her for the evening bath. She began to notice that distractions, such as listening to the radio and attending to household chores, dampened the hallucinations while solitude and fatigue tended to heighten them. At follow up one year later, she was experiencing very much the same hallucinations but was more cognisant of their unreality and less anxious as a result. The only new hallucination that had since appeared was that of a bright kaleidoscopic array which would transiently emanate from her central field of vision. By this time she had tried various medications without effect. They included sodium valproate, carbamazepine, and diazepam.

Case 2: A 90 year-old man who lived with his wife woke to find a bright pink handkerchief on the floor of his bedroom. He tried to retrieve it but every time he leant over to pick it up it seemed to move beyond his reach. He followed it from room to room but was distracted by the appearance of rows of bearded human faces with bulging eyes jutting out from the lounge-room wall. Through the window he saw a large brown Ayrshire cow in the front yard and, beyond it, made out a red sports car racing up the street towards his house. He opened the front door only to be greeted by a trio of policeman dressed like American highway patrol officers toting large guns. Fearing at this point that he was losing his faculties he summoned his wife and an ambulance was called. In the casualty room of the local hospital he saw a draught horse pulling a cart loaded with wooden logs. The cart transformed into a Roman chariot and sped across the hospital curtain with a rider at the helm. Large tree trunks appeared at the foot of the bed and began cracking down the middle one by one. The cubicle curtain was replaced by rows of neatly arranged wooden palings. He was soon convinced that the visions were imagined and his anxiety was replaced by a sense of amusement. At follow up two years later the patient was still experiencing frequent visual hallucinations. Grazing Ayrshire cows continued to appear in the front yard. Little children in red outfits ran playfully around the house. Oddly shaped people of varying sizes wore raincoats and trudged through pools of water inside the house. Three years later he was virtually hallucination-free, reporting only very occasional episodes of visions of cows and children. Carbamazepine was initially trialled without benefit. He had concurrent cataract disease but surgery (12 months after presentation) made no definitive impact on the course of his symptoms.

D. Image Categorization

The case histories are characteristic of the vivid and often bizarre images that may be perceived by patients with CBS. The images of CBS range from simple (lines, dots, basic shapes) to complex (faces, people, vehicles). Simple forms are more commonly encountered in practice than the latter but both forms can co-exist. Images can also change from simple to complex (and vice-versa) over time. Despite the remarkable detail and variety of images reported by many patients, common themes and figures emerge. In the present examples we have Roman chariots, grotesque faces, tree trunks, and pools of water. Until recently, categorization of the hallucinatory phenomena encountered in CBS has been hampered by two factors – the limited number of published cases (as few as 46 cases were counted in the literature from the time of Bonnet's original description through to 1989)[11], and the limited detail given by many authors on the nature of the hallucinations experienced (not unlike Bonnet's landmark paper). Clearly the latter is made difficult by the surreal characteristics of the images, rendering description by the elderly patient challenging at best. And, while the proverbial picture may 'paint a thousand words', any attempt by the patient to sketch such images is often precluded by the very factor that triggers them – poor visual acuity. Both patients featured in the case descriptions above were unable to reproduce their hallucinations on paper with any measure of accuracy because visual acuity was limited to finger counting.

The 1996 case series by Teunisse and colleagues[9], still the largest to date, represents the first dedicated attempt to elucidate the clinical spectrum of CBS. Features of the images reported by the 60 patients (drawn from 505 individuals recruited for the study based on the presence of significant visual impairment secondary to eye disease) varied greatly in terms of colour, movement, clarity, and bizarreness. Examples cited included a dragon, a shining angel, and a humorous police arrest played out in miniature. Additional sensory phenomena such as auditory and olfactory hallucinations were invariably absent. Subsequently published case reports[12-16] re-iterated the range of hallucinations encountered in CBS. Ffytche and Howard[17], in a novel approach, separated their patients' hallucinations into eight categories based on the central distinguishing feature: tessellopsia (regular, overlapping patterns), hyperchromatopsia (vivid colours), prosopometamorphopsia (facial distortion), dendropsia (branching forms), perseveration (palinoptic forms that persist as the gaze moves), illusory visual spread (patterned forms that move or spread to cover neighbouring objects), polyopia (multiple identical forms, often in rows and columns), and micro/macropsia (very small/very large sized forms). The potential clinical utility of this schema rests with the notion that it captures not only the range of hallucinations experienced by the individual patient, but also the themes common to hallucinations across the disorder. To illustrate, the presently described patients' visual experiences match this system of classification well: tessellopsia (cobwebs, rows of trees), hyperchromatopsia (caterpillars, kaleidoscopes, bright red vehicles, gold chariots), prosopometamorphopsia (grotesque faces, extraterrestrial-like heads), dendropsia (vines, roads), polyopia (ant colonies, wooden palings), micropsia (trains, push-bikes, fairies) and macropsia (greyhounds, nurses' heads). Indeed, a similar case might be made for the categorization of Lullin's 'visions' as described by Bonnet. While the clinical validity of this classification system is yet to be established, it does go some way in respecting the known specialization of the visual association cortex as discussed later.

E. Clinical factors

The images of CBS have been described as tending to appear within the boundaries of the negative scotoma in the partially sighted[18]. The predominantly central projection of imagery in patients with AMD is in keeping with the central field loss typical of macular disease. However, it should be appreciated that in clinical practice patients are seldom able to accurately delineate scotoma margins (if indeed they appreciate a scotoma exists at all); further, macula vision so dominates the binocular field that the patient's impression of a centrally projected hallucination need not imply a topographical link between the two (personal communication J. O'Day, 2009). A recent review has also highlighted the lack of association between scotoma size and risk of developing CBS[19]. Dimly lit conditions, states of drowsiness and physical isolation, and circumstances of relative social isolation have been noted as factors favouring the recurrence of hallucinations[9]. Whereas rapid blinking, sustained eye closure, diversionary activities, or simply walking away may relieve them[9]. Faces are genuinely foreign[19]; it is rare for family members or friends to feature in hallucinatory episodes. Sufferers typically regard themselves as the onlooker and it is unusual for them to feel as though they are part of the panorama. The first patient's impression of being invited to tour the hospital grounds by fairies might therefore be considered atypical. However, it is clear that she was initially drawn in by the life-like nature of the images. This initial deception is not uncommon[3] and patients do ultimately appreciate that the visions are not real such that, with time, the emotional response elicited by these images tends to be neutral. In these circumstances it is not uncommon for CBS patients to turn out phrases like: "Yes, my little friends are still there, popping in and out whenever it pleases them" (personal observation). Understandably, at least 30% of sufferers experience significant distress with the initial hallucinatory experience[20], particularly if the images are complex, highly intrusive and frequent. The situation is made more problematic because sufferers generally remain quite reluctant to report their symptoms for fear of being labelled mad or demented[3, 9]. Indeed, patients with CBS have been erroneously admitted to psychiatric institutions on one level[21], while on another, have had their experiences dismissed as 'silly' by medical practitioners[9]. This is a cause for concern because it is widely anticipated that the incidence and the prevalence of CBS will increase in an ever-increasingly aged population.

F. Epidemiology

Suspicion that CBS prevalence estimates are spuriously low has as much to do with the sufferer's fear of being labelled insane upon symptom disclosure, as with a lack of awareness of the disorder in the broader medical community[3, 9]. Estimates have ranged widely from 0.4% to 63% in the visually impaired[3, 9, 18, 22]. A clearer view of the epidemiology is also hamstrung by sub-specialty recruitment bias, prevalence findings varying across the disciplines of geriatric medicine, neurology, ophthalmology, and psychiatry[18, 23-25]. Elements of this bias might relate to potentially different pathogenetic contributions made by acuity loss, field loss, or even contrast sensitivity loss to the definition of any individual's summated CBS risk. Another confounding factor in regard to the prevalence data is the manner in which sight impaired patients are questioned about hallucinatory episodes. Unless specifically reassured that hallucinations can occur in acquired visual loss, and that such hallucinations are not a harbinger of psychiatric or neurodegenerative illness, many sufferers tend not to disclose such experiences[3]. The relative import of the ageing brain on the genesis of hallucinations is also unclear. Mean age-of-onset data from larger series demonstrate clustering across the eighth and ninth decades[3, 9, 22, 24, 25], by which time age-related cerebral atrophy and small vessel cerebrovascular ischaemic disease have also usually developed. The mini-mental state exam score[26], used as evidence against dementia in many CBS studies, may not detect subtler higher order cognitive deficits. De Morsier himself stressed the potential contribution of age to syndrome onset and actually de-emphasised visual loss as a diagnostic pre-requisite[8]. Indeed, the man who coined the syndrome later confessed that it was never his intention to link the symptoms to eye disease. De Morsier strenuously argued until his death that his later reference to CBS as a "senile syndrome with lesions of the eyes" was misconstrued but the connection had already stuck[5]. It seems then that the eponym was fraught with confusion from the outset. Nonetheless, the general consensus currently held in the literature is that CBS is the triad of visual (pseudo)-hallucinations (simple or complex), visual impairment due to ocular disease (irrespective of the specific aetiology), and intact cognition. Based on this definition, the two largest epidemiological studies carried out to date on visually impaired subjects determined that the prevalence of CBS was 12% from a cohort of 505 patients[9], and 27% from a cohort of 360 patients[27]. The higher prevalence rate found in the latter study must partly relate to the fact that the cohort was restricted to patients with end-stage AMD; in the former study, only half the patients experiencing hallucinations had AMD, and even then recruitment was not limited to advanced macular pathology.

G. Anatomical Considerations

Before embarking on a discussion of the theorized pathophysiology of CBS, it is prudent to give a brief overview of the normal visual cortical pathways in man[28]. The visual cortex is anatomically and functionally divided into primary visual cortex (V_1) and visual association cortex (V_{2-5}). V_1 is seated at the medial surface of the occipital lobe over the calcarine gyrus, Brodmann area (BA) 17, and receives input from the lateral geniculate nucleus (LGN) whose fibres originate in the retina. Cortical representation is retinotopic such that fibres that subserve macula (central) vision project to the posterior part of V_1, while peripheral retinal fibres project to the anterior part of V_1. There are two output pathways (or streams) from V_1 – the dorsal stream that projects to occipito-parietal cortex (the 'where' pathway) and the ventral stream that projects to occipito-temporal cortex (the 'what' pathway)[28].

Abutting the primary visual cortex is the visual association cortical region comprising multiple, functionally discrete anatomical subunits. While the primary visual cortex is dedicated to the processing of simpler visual stimuli, such as straight lines, the visual association cortex is responsible for the processing of higher order visual stimuli, such as colour and movement. V_2 (BA 18) is also retinotopic and, together with V_3 (BA 19), projects to parietal and inferotemporal cortex to subserve the appreciation of spatial form and depth. V_2 and V_3 receive the majority the output from V_1 and are therefore also referred to as secondary visual cortex. V_4 is the main functional subunit dealing with colour recognition; it is seated at the inferior occipito-temporal cortex adjacent to BA 37 (occipito-temporal junction). BA 37 is important for facial recognition. V_5 is reserved for the appreciation of movement[28].

The primary visual cortex is also referred to as striate cortex (of Genari). This stems from its appearance as a thick white band in freshly sectioned cortex. Genari was the young medical student who first described the pattern in 1782[28]. Visual association cortex is therefore synonymous with extrastriate cortex. It is important to appreciate that much of our current knowledge of the various functions of the visual association cortex stem from electrophysiological studies in animals, more particularly primates. The second major source of our current understanding of these higher order visual subunits is from lesional case studies. For instance, lesions of the inferior occipito-temporal cortex will typically lead to an inability to perceive colour (achromatopsia) and familiar faces (prosopagnosia). This is because V_4 and BA37 are very closely positioned anatomically. Lesions of V_5 will result in an inability to appreciate movement (akinetopsia)[28]. While current-day non-invasive neuroimaging methods show great promise in helping to elucidate the pathophysiology of CBS, and while it is nice to speculate on the underlying mechanisms driving the disorder, it must be acknowledged that a significant stumbling block for current-day researchers is the fact that our knowledge of the structure and function of higher-order visual pathways *in health* is not yet complete.

H. Pathophysiology

While preserved insight into the illusory nature of the hallucinations is a consistently acknowledged feature of CBS, less agreed upon is the specification that the primary pathology be restricted to the eye as previously noted. While AMD is the most commonly cited ocular pathology in CBS[9, 10], in terms of the pathogenesis of visual hallucinations in general, it may not be the nature of the visual pathology, the lesion site, or even the severity of visual acuity impairment[29] that confers the major risk, but rather the rate of development of that visual impairment[15, 30]. In this context, accelerated acuity loss in the setting of retinal epithelial detachment in neovascular ('wet') AMD has been documented as a forerunner to CBS [18, 31]. Laser photocoagulation, a recognized treatment for AMD, has also been cited as a potential precipitant[32]. Sudden severe anaemia in three patients with pre-existing eye disease has also been described as a trigger[33]. Haemoglobin levels ranged from 78 to 86 g/L. With correction of the anaemia following blood transfusion and with the subsequent restoration of pre-morbid visual acuity, CBS symptoms were rapidly abolished in each case. A more recent proposition by Jackson and colleagues is that contrast sensitivity is a more reliable marker of CBS risk than acuity per se[34]. They examined a cohort of 225 patients with low visual acuity, most of whom had AMD (63%). A total of 78 patients (35%) from the group described visual hallucinations. Based on multiple logistic regression analysis, they found that contrast sensitivity (ability to distinguish between shades of grey) was strongly related to the presence of CBS. The lower the contrast sensitivity score, the higher the likelihood that CBS symptoms were present. Visual acuity, by comparison, was actually less predictive of CBS symptoms. As Ffytche points out[19], this finding should be taken into account in the design of future studies that look to address the pathophysiology of CBS.

Less frequently reported ocular pathologies associated with CBS have included glaucoma[9], central retinal artery occlusion[13], temporal arteritis[35] and optic neuritis[36]. Extra-ocular central visual axis pathologies associated with CBS-like hallucinations have included chiasmal and pituitary lesions[37] and occipital stroke[38, 39]. As Manford and Andermann indicate[40], John Hughlings Jackson's original concept of the 'dissolution of the central nervous system'[41] might well reconcile the often remarkable similarity of certain hallucinatory percepts (as complex as they may be) with the multiplicity of pathologies (for aetiology and location) giving rise to such experiences.

There is little doubt though that central to the genesis of complex visual forms in man is the visual association (extrastriate) cortex[10, 40]. In a prospective study of 32 patients with ischaemic stroke of the retrochiasmal visual pathways, Valphiades and colleagues[1] noted that patients with large territory ischaemic lesions involving anterior visual association cortex never experienced visual hallucinations. Perhaps more convincing though was the landmark functional magnetic resonance imaging (fMRI) study by Ffytch and colleagues published two years later[17]. This group was the first to investigate a potential correlation between specific hallucinatory episodes and specific functional and anatomical subunits within the visual association cortex in patients with CBS. From a group of eight visually impaired patients with eye disease, they were able to link certain regions of fMRI signal activation to specific hallucinatory experiences: the inferior occipito-temporal region to hallucinations featuring scenic landscapes and small costumed figures; the fusiform face area to hallucinations featuring cartoon-like facial images; and the posterior fusiform gyrus (V_4, colour) to hyperchromatic hallucinations. Between hallucinatory episodes, there appeared to be a tonic increase in signal activity in the region of the ventral extrastriate cortex. In the three patients with AMD, this tonic activity corresponded to area V_4. A more recent neuroimaging study by Kazui and colleagues[42] used single photon emission tomography (SPECT) to map the regional cortical activation in two CBS patients. Marked reductions in regionalized cerebral blood flow were noted in both patients corresponding to the ventral regions of BA 17 and BA 18. While there was an absence of hypoperfusion in the visual association cortical regions (BA 19, BA 37) for both patients, it is unclear whether the patients were actively hallucinating during the SPECT recording (if they were, one might have anticipated a relative increase in perfusion to these areas). A follow-on study using magnetoencephalography (MEG) was carried out on the same two patients, only one of whom returned a sufficiently artefact-free recording. The patient was indicated to have hallucinated during only part of the recording. Hallucinatory content included white clouds, black smoke, and sea bream all moving in a left to right direction. A commonly applied source localization technique known as synthetic aperture magnetometry (SAM) was used to analyse and compare the MEG recordings taken with and without active hallucination. During hallucinatory events, the recordings pointed to a strong suppression of 4-8 Hz band background activity at BA 37 unilaterally with a weak concurrent suppression at BA 19 bilaterally. The authors posited that this reflected cortical activation of those areas during hallucinatory episodes[42].

While the demonstration of increased extrastriate cortical activity in CBS is satisfying, there is no clear explanation for it. As previously alluded to, we are only beginning to understand the intricacies of the sub-specialised regions of the extrastriate cortex (V_2-V_5) along with their respective anatomical and functional connections to the primary visual or striate cortex (V_1)[43], thalamus, and brainstem as regards normal visual perception – let alone the abnormal.

One of the earliest hypotheses raised to explain the phenomenon of complex visual hallucinations is Cogan's 1973 analogy to West's perceptual release theory – that a loss of visual input decreases cortical inhibition and 'releases' visual hallucinations[44]. This idea has largely been superseded by the more neurophysiologically robust principle of 'de-afferentation' – that the denervation or de-afferentation of a neuron leads to an increase in its degree of hyper-excitability. Much has been written about this concept and, outside the visual system, the effects of de-afferentation have been demonstrated in the auditory, vestibular, somatosensory, and motor systems[10]. As reviewed by Burke[10], neuronal de-afferentation leads to two important sets of changes at the synaptic level. First, several molecular changes occur at the presynapse. These include increases in bouton size, vesicle number, and probability of neurotransmitter release. Post-synaptically, there is an increase in receptor number and a step up in the membrane response to an applied current. Second, biochemical changes occur at the synapse. These include an increase in the glutaminergic n-methyl-d-aspartate (NMDA) response and a decrease in $GABA_A$ (gamma-aminobutyric acid) and $GABA_B$ responses. Hence, loss of the normal inhibitory tone on extrastriate cortex might understandably result from direct interruption of cortico-cortical fibres from striate cortex, such as in occipital stroke with sparing of visual association cortex[29, 40].

How then might ocular disease lead to CBS given that the retino-thalamic pathway is essentially excitatory? Interruption of thalamic afferents to the lateral geniculate nucleus (LGN) has been shown to result in membrane hyperpolarisation and to the subsequent generation of low-threshold calcium spike bursts[10, 45, 46]. 'Positive' visual symptoms might thereby arise from propagation of this burst activity to the visual cortex via thalamo-cortical pathways[47]. Hyperperfusion of the thalamus, inferior lateral temporal cortex, and striatum has been captured by SPECT in a group of five CBS patients who were experiencing visual hallucinations during the scanning procedure[48]. Intimate connections between the thalamus and the reticular formation may underpin the observation that visual hallucinations tend to flourish during states of drowsiness, particularly during evening hours[10, 40].

Although less well understood, the lateral pulvinar nucleus of the thalamus may serve a more direct role than the LGN in the elaboration of visual hallucinations as it more specifically innervates extra-striate cortex[40]. Along these lines, the cone photoreceptor loss (retino-thalamic de-afferentation) that occurs in AMD might well lead to a functional de-afferentation of V_4 cortex[49] with the subsequent manifestation of 'positive' hyperchromatic hallucinations. In a group of 97 patients with CBS secondary to end-stage AMD[27], close to three-quarters of the images were coloured, around 85% of the images were 'seen' centrally, and the most common images involved people (20%). It has been noted that patients tend to hallucinate in a dominant colour or in a limited colour spectrum. In an interesting study of ten CBS patients who were experiencing hyperchromatic hallucinations[50], it was shown that the dominant colour featured in the hallucination was the within the spectrum associated with a lower colour-contrast threshold. Hence, dominant red-green hallucinators returned red-green/blue-yellow colour-contrast threshold ratios less than 1.0, while dominant blue-yellow hallucinators returned threshold ratios greater than 1.0. Intermediate ranges were given by CBS patients who hallucinated in purple. The authors proposed that their study was the first to evidence cerebral hyper-excitability in AMD manifesting as a reduction in colour contrast thresholds[50].

Despite the intuitiveness of de-afferentation as a unifying explanation for the genesis of visual hallucinations in eye disease, (and notwithstanding methodological issues related to estimates of CBS prevalence in epidemiological studies), the hypothesis falls short in accounting for the sizeable number of patients who have major visual impairment without CBS[19]. Further neuroimaging studies on larger cohorts of visually impaired patients (with and without visual hallucinations) might be sufficiently geared to address this problem. Such studies might incorporate newer non-invasive imaging modalities such as diffusion tensor imaging and magnetic resonance spectroscopy in a way that helps delineate de-afferented occipital cortical and subcortical pathways in CBS.

I. Disease Course and Management

The management of CBS centres on patient reassurance that the condition is not rare and that it is not a marker of psychiatric or neurodegenerative illness. The unpredictable course of the disorder can frustrate patients and physicians alike. Just as hallucinatory episodes can last from seconds to hours and even days, the duration of CBS may extend from days to years[9]. Indeed, two CBS cohort studies, one longitudinal[51] and one cross-sectional[27] arrived at the conclusion that around 40% of CBS patients are still experiencing hallucinations two to three years after onset. Clustering of episodes across days or weeks is not uncommon and recurrence after a prolonged symptom free interval can occur. Patients have also reported permanent remissions occurring in tandem with ongoing visual decline[15, 23, 52]. The reason why this might occur is still not clear. The combined effect of these factors has rendered it especially difficult to judge the efficacy of any given treatment strategy, medical or surgical. In fact, to date, no randomised therapeutic trial for CBS has been done. Based on the few case reports that examine the effects of drug initiation, cessation, and re-challenge on hallucination frequency, sodium valproate[53], gabapentin[54], olanzapine[55, 56] and carbamazepine[57] have demonstrated some efficacy. Aggravation with the drug levetiracetam has also been reported[58]. The minimization or avoidance of medications that are known to be potentially hallucinogenic (sedatives, dopamine agonists) is also prudent. Amelioration of the patient's visual deficit where possible, as with cataract and laser surgery, has benefited anecdotally[59]. Other non-pharmacological interventions worth pursuing are the minimization of any potential aggravating factors. Limiting exposure to dim lighting, strengthening social networks, and engaging in distracting activities may therefore help[9]. Treatment of a complicating mood disturbance, such as depression or anxiety, is clearly important.

J. Differential Diagnosis

Migraine, occipital seizures, hypnagogic hallucinations, peduncular hallucinosis, drug induced states, and psychiatric disease form part of the differential diagnosis in patients presenting with visual hallucinations. Migraine as a cause of complex hallucinations is quite uncommon unless the history suggests familial hemiplegic migraine or migraine coma[40]. The seizures of temporal lobe epilepsy and occipital lobe epilepsy can feature simple or complex visual auras but there is usually greater stereotypy and fragmentation of the imagery than that encountered in CBS[40]. Additional post-ictal features may also be present such as drowsiness and disorientation. Peduncular hallucinosis, typically from rostral brainstem ischaemic infarction, tends to be associated with impaired consciousness and usually displays a diurnal pattern, hallucinations being entirely limited to the evening hours. In contradistinction to CBS, tactile and auditory hallucinations also occur in this condition[40] [60]. Hypnagogic hallucinations occur with sleep onset, have a consistently brief duration (seconds to minutes), and may co-exist with an underlying sleep disorder such as narcolepsy or cataplexy[40, 60].

Conclusion

Charles Bonnet Syndrome (CBS) is an under-diagnosed, yet not uncommon, disorder typically characterised by visual hallucinations (simple or complex) in the visually impaired. Prevalence is highest in the elderly, cognitively intact population. There are several important distinguishing features of the condition – the hallucinatory content is purely visual (there are no olfactory, auditory, or other special sensory features), the sufferer's level of awareness is unaffected during the course of the episode, and the sufferer realizes that the hallucinations are not real (they are therefore pseudo-hallucinations in the strictest sense). More recent neuroimaging studies, particularly those that have applied fMRI techniques, have lent support to the hypothesis that CBS hallucinations arise from particular regions of the visual association cortex as a consequence of 'de-afferentation' from primary visual cortical pathways. Treatment, if required, is largely symptomatic. Interventions aimed at improving the visual deficit have had mixed success, as have variously tried anti-epileptic and antipsychotic medications. Treatment validation studies have been hampered by evidence that

CBS can remit spontaneously, often – and perhaps ironically – in concert with any further deterioration of the patient's vision. Indeed, a cornerstone in the management of patients with CBS is reassurance that the condition is not a marker of psychiatric or neurodegenerative disease. In an ever-expanding aged population, it goes without saying that both public and physician awareness of the condition must increase. For its part, CBS promises to teach us much about the pathophysiology of visual hallucinations and, more specifically, about the extraordinary complexity of the human visual cortex.

References

[1] Vaphiades, MS; Celesia, GG; Brigell, MG. Positive spontaneous visual phenomena limited to the hemianopic field in lesions of central visual pathways. *Neurology*, 1996, 47(2), 408-17.

[2] de Morsier, G. Les automatismes visuals. (Hallucinations visuelles retrochiasmatiques). *Schweiz Med Wschr*, 1936, 66, 700-703.

[3] Menon, GJ. Complex visual hallucinations in the visually impaired: a structured history-taking approach. *Arch Ophthalmol*, 2005, 123(3), 349-55.

[4] Bonnet, C. Essai analytique sur les facultes d l'ame. Copenhagen: *Philibert*, 1760.

[5] Ffytche, DH. Visual hallucinations and the charles bonnet syndrome. *Curr Psychiatry Rep*, 2005, 7(3), 168-79.

[6] Flournoy, T. Le cas de Charles Bonnet. Hallucinations visuelles chez un vieillerd opera de la cataracte. *Arch de Psychologie (Geneve)*, 1902, 1, 1-23.

[7] Hedges, TR. Charles Bonnet, his life, and his syndrome. *Survey of Ophthalmology*, 2007, 52(1), 111-114.

[8] de Morsier, G. Le syndrome de Charles Bonnet: hallucinations visuelles des vieillards sans deficience mentale. *Ann Med Psychol (Paris)*, 1967, 2(5), 678-702.

[9] Teunisse, RJ; Cruysberg, JR; Hoefnagels, WH; Verbeek, AL; Zitman, FG. Visual hallucinations in psychologically normal people: Charles Bonnet's syndrome. *Lancet*, 1996, 347(9004), 794-7.

[10] Burke, W. The neural basis of Charles Bonnet hallucinations: a hypothesis. *J Neurol Neurosurg Psychiatry*, 2002, 73(5), 535-41.

[11] Podoll, K; Osterheider, M; Noth, J. Das Charles Bonnet Syndrom. *Fortschr Neurol Psychiatr*, 1989, 57(2), 43-60.

[12] Jacob, A; Prasad, S; Boggild, M; Chandratre, S. Charles Bonnet Syndrome--elderly people and visual hallucinations. *Bmj*, 2004, 328(7455), 1552-4.

[13] Tan, CS; Sabel, BA; Goh, KY. Visual hallucinations during visual recovery after central retinal artery occlusion. *Arch Neurol*, 2006, 63(4), 598-600.

[14] Needham, WE; Taylor, RE. Atypical Charles Bonnet hallucinations: an elf in the woodshed, a spirit of evil, and the cowboy malefactors. *J Nerv Ment Dis*, 2000, 188(2), 108-15.

[15] Shiraishi, Y; Terao, T; Ibi, K; Nakamura, J; Tawara, A. Charles Bonnet Syndrome and visual acuity--the involvement of dynamic or acute sensory deprivation. *Eur Arch Psychiatry Clin Neurosci*, 2004, 254(6), 362-4.

[16] Nixon, PA; Mason, JO. 3rd. Visual hallucinations from age-related macular degeneration. *Am J Med*, 2006, 119(3), e1-2.

[17] Ffytche, DH; Howard, RJ; Brammer, MJ; David, A; Woodruff, P; Williams, S. The anatomy of conscious vision: an fMRI study of visual hallucinations. *Nat Neurosci*, 1998, 1(8), 738-42.

[18] Holroyd, S; Rabins, PV; Finkelstein, D; Nicholson, MC; Chase, GA; Wisniewski, SC. Visual hallucinations in patients with macular degeneration. *Am J Psychiatry*, 1992, 149(12), 1701-6.

[19] Ffytche, DH. Visual hallucinations in eye disease. *Current Opinion in Neurology*, 2009, 22(1), 28-35.

[20] Gilmour, G; Schreiber, C; Ewing, C. An examination of the relationship between low vision and Charles Bonnet Syndrome. Canadian *Journal of Ophthalmology-Journal Canadien D Ophtalmologie*, 2009, 44(1), 49-52.

[21] Hart, J. Phantom visions: real enough to touch. *Elder Care*, 1997, 9(1), 30-2.

[22] Tan, CS; Lim, VS; Ho, DY; Yeo, E; Ng, BY; Au Eong, KG. Charles Bonnet Syndrome in Asian patients in a tertiary ophthalmic centre. *Br J Ophthalmol*, 2004, 88(10), 1325-9.

[23] Fernandez, A; Lichtshein, G; Vieweg, WV. The Charles Bonnet Syndrome: a review. *J Nerv Ment Dis*, 1997, 185(3), 195-200.

[24] Norton-Willson, L; Munir, M. Visual perceptual disorders resembling the Charles Bonnet Syndrome. A study of 434 consecutive patients referred to a psychogeriatric unit. *Fam Pract*, 1987, 4(1), 27-35.

[25] Teunisse, RJ; Cruysberg, JR; Verbeek, A; Zitman, FG. The Charles Bonnet Syndrome: a large prospective study in The Netherlands. A study of the prevalence of the Charles Bonnet Syndrome and associated factors in 500 patients attending the University Department of Ophthalmology at Nijmegen. *Br J Psychiatry*, 1995, 166(2), 254-7.

[26] Folstein, MF; Folstein, SE; McHugh, PR. "Mini-mental state". A practical method for grading the cognitive state of patients for the clinician. *Journal of Psychiatric Research*, 1975, 12(3), 189-198.

[27] Khan, JC; Shahid, H; Thurlby, DA; Yates, JRW; Moore, AT. Charles Bonnet Syndrome in age-related macular degeneration: The nature and frequency of images in subjects with end-stage disease. *Ophthalmic Epidemiology*, 2008, 15(3), 202-208.

[28] Afifi, AKBR. Functional Neuroanatomy: Text and Atlas. 2 ed. New York: McGraw-Hill, 2005.

[29] Holroyd, S; Rabins, PV; Finkelstein, D; Lavrisha, M. Visual hallucinations in patients from an ophthalmology clinic and medical clinic population. *J Nerv Ment Dis*, 1994, 182(5), 273-6.

[30] Tan, CS; Sabel, BA. Dynamic changes in visual acuity as the pathophysiologic mechanism in Charles Bonnet Syndrome (visual hallucinations). *Eur Arch Psychiatry Clin Neurosci*, 2006, 256(1), 62-3, author reply 64.

[31] Nadarajah, J. Visual hallucinations and macular degeneration: an example of the Charles Bonnet Syndrome. *Aust N Z J Ophthalmol*, 1998, 26(1), 63-5.

[32] Cohen, SY; Safran, AB; Tadayoni, R; Quentel, G; Guiberteau, B; Delahaye-Mazza, C. Visual hallucinations immediately after macular photocoagulation. *Am J Ophthalmol*, 2000, 129(6), 815-6.

[33] Kaeser, PF; Borruat, FX. Acute reversible Charles Bonnet Syndrome precipitated by sudden severe anemia. *European Journal of Ophthalmology*, 2009, 19(3), 494-495.
[34] Jackson, ML; Ferencz, J. Charles Bonnet Syndrome: visual loss and hallucinations. *Canadian Medical Association Journal*, 2009, 181(3-4), 175-176.
[35] Sonnenblick, M; Nesher, R; Rozenman, Y; Nesher, G. Charles Bonnet Syndrome in temporal arteritis. *Journal of Rheumatology*, 1995, 22(8), 1596-1597.
[36] Komeima, K; Kameyama, T; Miyake, Y. Charles Bonnet Syndrome associated with a first attack of multiple sclerosis. *Jpn J Ophthalmol*, 2005, 49(6), 533-4.
[37] Lepore, FE. Spontaneous visual phenomena with visual loss: 104 patients with lesions of retinal and neural afferent pathways. *Neurology*, 1990, 40(3 Pt 1), 444-7.
[38] Flint, AC; Loh, JP; Brust, JC. Vivid visual hallucinations from occipital lobe infarction. *Neurology*, 2005, 65(5), 756.
[39] Ashwin, PT; Tsaloumas, MD. Complex visual hallucinations (Charles Bonnet Syndrome) in the hemianopic visual field following occipital infarction. *J Neurol Sci*, 2007, 263(1-2), 184-6.
[40] Manford, M; Andermann, F. Complex visual hallucinations. Clinical and neurobiological insights. *Brain*, 1998, 121 (Pt 10), 1819-40.
[41] Taylor, JHG; Walshe, FMR. Evolution and dissolution of the nervous system. In: Taylor J HG, Walshe FMR, editor. Selected writings of John Hughlings Jackson. London: *Hodder and Stoughton*, 1932, 3-120.
[42] Kazui, H; Ishii, R; Yoshida, T; Ikezawa, K; Takaya, M; Tokunaga, H; et al. Neuroimaging studies in patients with Charles Bonnet Syndrome. *Psychogeriatrics*, 2009, 9(2), 77-84.
[43] Goebel, R; Muckli, L; Kim, DS. Visual System. In: G; Paxinos, J; Mai, editors. The Human Nervous System. second ed. San Diego: *Elsevier Academic Press*, 2004.
[44] Cogan, DG. Visual hallucinations as release phenomena. *Albrecht Von Graefes Arch Klin Exp Ophthalmol*, 1973, 188(2), 139-50.
[45] Malcolm, LJ; Bruce, IS; Burke, W. Excitability of the lateral geniculate nucleus in the alert, non-alert and sleeping cat. *Exp Brain Res*, 1970, 10(3), 283-97.
[46] Jeanmonod, D; Magnin, M; Morel, A. Low-threshold calcium spike bursts in the human thalamus. Common physiopathology for sensory, motor and limbic positive symptoms. *Brain*, 1996, 119 (Pt 2), 363-75.
[47] Ffytche, DH; Howard, RJ. The perceptual consequences of visual loss: 'positive' pathologies of vision. *Brain*, 1999, 122 (Pt 7), 1247-60.
[48] Adachi, N; Watanabe, T; Matsuda, H; Onuma, T. Hyperperfusion in the lateral temporal cortex, the striatum and the thalamus during complex visual hallucinations: Single photon emission computed tomography findings in patients with Charles Bonnet Syndrome. *Psychiatry and Clinical Neurosciences*, 2000, 54(2), 157-162.
[49] Santhouse, AM; Howard, RJ; ffytche, DH. Visual hallucinatory syndromes and the anatomy of the visual brain. *Brain*, 2000, 123, (Pt 10), 2055-64.
[50] Madill, SA; Lascaratos, G; Arden, GB; Ffytche, DH. Perceived color of hallucinations in the Charles Bonnet Syndrome is related to residual color contrast sensitivity. *Journal of Neuro-Ophthalmology,* 2009, 29(3), 192-196.
[51] Holroyd, S; Rabins, PV. A three-year follow-up study of visual hallucinations in patients with macular degeneration. *J Nerv Ment Dis*, 1996, 184(3), 188-9.

[52] White, NJ. Complex visual hallucinations in partial blindness due to eye disease. *Br J Psychiatry*, 1980, 136, 284-6.
[53] Hori, H; Terao, T; Shiraishi, Y; Nakamura, J. Treatment of Charles Bonnet Syndrome with valproate. *Int Clin Psychopharmacol*, 2000, 15(2), 117-9.
[54] Paulig, M; Mentrup, H. Charles Bonnet's syndrome: complete remission of complex visual hallucinations treated by gabapentin. *Journal of Neurology Neurosurgery and Psychiatry*, 2001, 70(6), 813-814.
[55] Coletti Moja, M; Milano, E; Gasverde, S; Gianelli, M; Giordana, MT. Olanzapine therapy in hallucinatory visions related to Bonnet syndrome. *Neurol Sci*, 2005, 26(3), 168-70.
[56] Alao, AO; Hanrahan, B. Charles Bonnet Syndrome: Visual hallucination and multiple sclerosis. *International Journal of Psychiatry in Medicine*, 2003, 33(2), 195-199.
[57] Chaudhuri, A. Charles Bonnet Syndrome: an example of cortical dissociation syndrome affecting vision. *J Neurol Neurosurg Psychiatry*, 2000, 69(5), 704-5.
[58] Segers, K. Charles Bonnet Syndrome disappearing with carbamazepine and valproic acid but not with levetiracetam. *Acta Neurologica Belgica*, 2009, 109(1), 42-43.
[59] Rovner, BW. The Charles Bonnet Syndrome: a review of recent research. *Curr Opin Ophthalmol*, 2006, 17(3), 275-7.
[60] Cascino, GD; Adams, RD. Brainstem auditory hallucinosis. *Neurology*, 1986, 36(8), 1042-7.

Chapter 6

Assessing Anomalous Perceptions in Youths: A Preliminary Validation Study of the Cardiff Anomalous Perceptions Scale (CAPS)

Martin Debbané[1,2*]*, Maude Schneider*[2]*, Stephan Eliez*[2,4]*, and Martial Van der Linden*[3]

[1]Adolescent Clinical Psychology Unit, Faculty of Psychology and Educational Sciences, University of Geneva, Switzerland
[2]Office Médico-Pédagogique, Department of Psychiatry, Faculty of Medicine, University of Geneva, Switzerland
[3]Cognitive Psychopathology and Neuropsychology Unit, Faculty of Psychology and Educational Sciences, University of Geneva, Switzerland
[4]Department of Genetic Medicine and Development, Faculty of Medicine, University of Geneva, Switzerland

Abstract

Survey studies indicate that hallucinations and other anomalous perceptions constitute relatively common mental events in adults, yet they remain poorly characterized in younger individuals. Information about the factor structure of anomalous perceptions or information on their frequency in the general and clinical youth populations are still incomplete. Recent epidemiological studies have provided the most consistent data, suggesting that some early anomalous perceptions such as auditory hallucinations can be predictive of later psychiatric illness during adulthood. Would this be true of other anomalous perceptions? Longitudinal studies also observe that the intrusive quality of early hallucinations combined to emotional distress in young voice-

---

[*] Corresponding author: Faculty of Psychology and Educational Sciences, University of Geneva, 40 Boulevard du Pont d'Arve, Switzerland, Tel : 0041 22 379 94 18, E-mail : martin.debbane@unige.ch

hearers sustain the expression and development of auditory hallucinations. If perceived distress and intrusiveness contribute to the potential unfolding of hallucinations, how do they relate to other anomalous perceptions? The first step to answer these questions is to provide a psychometric instrument that could assess the variety of anomalous perceptions in youths, combined with subjective ratings of frequency, distress and intrusiveness. This chapter presents preliminary data on the validation of a self-report instrument shown to reliably measure anomalous perceptions and their experiential dimensions in adults. The current study introduces a validation of the Cardiff Anomalous Perception Scale adapted for francophone youths. The results demonstrate its usefulness in characterizing the multifactorial nature of anomalous perceptions in youths. Further, the analyses support the pertinence of this instrument as an assessment tool for psychosis-proneness in young samples. Finally, the study highlights significant associations between specific anomalous perceptions and self-reported anxiety and depression ratings. The CAPS adaptation for youths thus contains the features required for the advancement of research on anomalous perceptions in young individuals.

1. Introduction

Anomalous perceptions can trigger a host of different subjective experiences, ranging from pleasant bewilderment to terrifying horror. The terrifying anomalous perceptions are less likely to be shared openly, and can represent very disturbing experiences that induce a sense of vulnerability in a child or adolescent prone to such unusual perceptions. Beyond the emotional implications anomalous perceptions may bear on youths, epidemiological surveys suggest that certain types of anomalous perceptions, such as auditory hallucinations, can predict later unfolding of psychosis (Chapman et al. 1994; Miller et al. 2002). Furthermore, cognitive psychopathology studies find that emotional and appraisal factors promote the maintenance and potential exacerbation of anomalous perceptions (Freeman et al. 2002; Morrison et al. 2007). Therefore, studies on anomalous perceptions in youths suggest that hallucinations hold predictive value for later psychotic psychopathology, and that emotional distress and appraisal mechanisms sustain their maintenance and potential exacerbation (Debbané et al. 2009). There remains a number of limitations to the available data on anomalous perceptions in youths. First, it is unclear whether anomalous perceptions regroup into a single factor, or whether a multifactorial structure would better account for such manifestations in youths. Second, most assessment tools examine the frequency of anomalous perceptions, without probing more experiential dimensions such as distress and intrusiveness. Finally, the available empirical data on anomalous perceptions in youths fail to characterize the clinically relevant associations between discrete manifestations of anomalous perceptions and the need for psychological assistance. The current chapter presents a study that aims to provide preliminary data on these three points through a validation study of the Cardiff Anomalous Perceptions Scale (CAPS) (Bell et al. 2006) with francophone youths.

Prediction and Persistence of Anomalous Perceptions in Youths

Not until recently, hallucinations and other anomalous perceptions were not considered to be common experiences in children and adolescents (Altman et al. 1997). These experiences, when considered, were not taken seriously until Poulton and collaborators' seminal study demonstrated the predictive power of psychotic-like symptoms during childhood (Poulton *et al.* 2000). This longitudinal prospective study followed a birth cohort of 761 participants who, at age 11 years, filled a self-report questionnaire including four questions on positive schizotypy (hallucinations and delusional beliefs). Participants underwent psychiatric follow-up evaluations at age 26. Results showed that endorsing at least 2 positive schizotypy items at age 11 increased by 16.4 times the odds of developing a schizophreniform disorder at follow-up. Additionally, 90% of members endorsing two or more items experienced occupational or social dysfunction at follow-up. Furthermore, participants endorsing only one item were also more likely to develop schizophreniform disorders compared to the no-symptom group. Finally, participants endorsing at least 1 item showed increased risk to develop anxiety disorders. These results not only suggest that anomalous perceptions hold predictive power of future psychotic disorders, but they also put forward a significant association between early anomalous perceptions and unfolding of emotional disorders during adulthood.

Interestingly, another group of epidemiologists that prospectively followed young voice-hearers evidenced the crucial link between emotional distress and hallucinations. In their series of studies, Escher and colleagues recruited 80 adolescents, ages 8-19 years, all of which were hearing voices (Escher 2004; Escher *et al.* 2002). The study proposed an examination of the factors associated with the persistence of verbal auditory hallucinations over a 3-year period. The cumulative incidence of discontinuation of hallucinations was 60%. For those still experiencing hallucinations, several factors were identified as predicting the persistence of voices during the 3-year period. First, the authors found that hallucinations judged as intrusive or "omnipotent" were more likely to persist. Also, the hallucinations' lack of an environmental trigger was associated with the persistence of the hallucinatory phenomena. Finally, participant ratings of psychological distress dimensions of anxiety and depression were associated with the perseverance of auditory hallucinations. These observations helped illustrate that some anomalous perceptions, namely auditory hallucinations, are more likely to persist in the presence of emotional distress (Dhossche *et al.* 2002).

Appraisal Contributes to the Maintenance of Anomalous Perceptions through the Promotion of Emotional Distress

Interestingly, Escher et al.'s longitudinal examinations also suggest that the appraisal of the hallucinations' intrusive character represents an additional maintenance factor in hallucination-prone adolescents. Concurrently to these epidemiological findings, contemporary cognitive models of auditory hallucinations put a major emphasis on one's appraisal when experiencing such anomalous perceptions. Morrison and collaborators argue that auditory hallucinations, much like intrusive thoughts in obsessive compulsive disorders, are common mental events that occur in a significant proportion of the general population (Morrison 2001). This account argues that neither auditory hallucinations nor intrusive thoughts *in themselves* create the distress associated with their expression in clinical populations. Rather, it is argued that faulty appraisal (interpretations) of these mental contents bread emotional distress that impede the individual's psychological functioning (Chadwick & Birchwood 1994; Morrison *et al.* 1995). Supporting evidence for this account can be found in recent literature on the maintenance of auditory hallucinations. The first point concerns the frequency of auditory hallucinations in the general population. Several survey studies demonstrate that in approximately 10 to 30% of general population samples report auditory hallucinations at least once in their lifetime (Larøi & Van der Linden 2005). Another study reports that more than a third of a sample of 173 voice-hearers do not require psychiatric care (Romme et al. 1992). These observations support the notion that auditory hallucinations constitute common experiences that do not necessarily imply clinically relevant emotional distress. Secondly, cognitive psychopathology studies have identified several factors that contribute to faulty appraisal of auditory hallucinations through their promotion of anxious psychological states. These factors include self knowledge and metacognitive beliefs (Lyon et al. 1994; Morrison 2001), beliefs about voices (Morrison et al. 2000), early trauma (Shevlin et al. 2007) and information processing biases (Garety et al. 2001). These factors promote faulty appraisal mechanisms that contribute to the emotional distress associated to hallucinations (Freeman & Garety 2003). In sum, the contemporary cognitive models of auditory hallucinations skilfully demonstrate the role of appraisal in triggering emotional distress during episodes of hallucinations, and such a conceptualization may serve as guide to understand the *anomalous* or *psychotic* quality of unusual perceptions in general.

Attention and the Intrusiveness of Some Anomalous Perceptions

Building on Escher et al.'s reports on young voice-hearers, we note that the intrusive quality of auditory hallucinations constitute a predictor of their maintenance during adolescent development. Intrusiveness may be conceptualized in psychological terms as a hostile takeover of attentional resources by irrelevant and somewhat uncontrollable mental content. The experience of an auditory hallucination may serve as an illustration, as it implies increased focused attention on the internal voice that may be reported as an anomalous verbal content that does not originate from oneself (Frith 1992). Several contemporary theories on positive symptoms of psychosis try to capture the specific contribution of attention in the experience of hallucinations and other anomalous perceptions. For example, some argue that personality traits such as self-absorption can directly predispose an individual to experience hallucinations (Glicksohn et al. 1999). Other theories concentrate on neurophysiological mechanisms (Behrendt & Young 2004) or on the neurobiological effects of dopamine (Kapur et al. 2005) underpinning the potential action of attentional processes in the expression of hallucinations. The common base of these theories is to argue for a top-down influence that disrupts the balanced distribution of attentional resources to external and internal stimuli in favour of an exaggerated and somewhat forced focus on internal perceptions. Through this process the internal stimuli acquire aberrant salience thought to underlie the sense of realness in anomalous perceptions such as hallucinations (see Aleman & Larøi 2008 for a full discussion of this issue). The data available on hallucinations in youths strongly argue in favour of including the voice hearer's intrusiveness rating when assessing auditory hallucinations. Whether this is also true for other anomalous perceptions will be tested in the present study.

To recapitulate the literature surveyed above, we first reviewed studies reporting the types and frequencies of anomalous perceptions in youth and adult samples. These data suggest that anomalous perceptions such as hallucinations during childhood and adolescence are predictive psychiatric disorder development during adulthood, and most importantly associated with the unfolding of psychotic disorders. Prospective longitudinal studies illustrate the necessity to provide more information on experiential dimensions, and more specifically on the relationship between emotional distress and appraisal of anomalous perceptions. Indeed, these epidemiological reports suggest that hallucinations during adolescence are more likely to persist when experienced as intrusive, and within a context of emotional distress. Emotional distress can be further exacerbated by faulty appraisal of anomalous perceptions that elicit increased affective turmoil which feeds into the vicious circle of emotionally unsettling anomalous perceptions. Finally, anomalous perceptions are also associated with a disturbance of attentional processes thought to convey the sense of "realness" of these internal mental events.

With this in mind, we sought to identify an instrument that could measure the frequency, emotional distress, and intrusiveness associated with anomalous perceptions during adolescence and into early adulthood, known as the high-risk period of psychosis unfolding. While there exists no validated self-report measure designed to capture the three critical dimensions of anomalous perceptions in youths, the recently validated Cardiff Anomalous Perception Scale (CAPS) (Bell *et al.* 2006) offers a promising psychometric instrument that may be adapted to younger age groups. The CAPS is a 32-item self-report questionnaire that seeks to account for the multiple-factor structure of anomalous perceptions. Each question is accompanied by a 5-point (1-5) Likert scale subjective evaluation of distress, intrusiveness and frequency dimensions. In their validation study on an adult sample of 336 participants and 20 psychotic inpatients, the authors report a factorial structure comprised of 3 components: clinical psychosis, temporal lobe disturbance, and chemosensation. The items loading on the clinical psychosis component evaluated Schneiderian first-rank symptoms such as auditory hallucinations or thought broadcasting. Temporal lobe disturbance items contained questions pertaining to seizure-like disturbances such as altered temporal perception. The third component regrouped chemosensation items assessing different sensory alterations in touch, taste or smell. Findings on the total score for the general population group revealed that 11% of the sample scored above the schizophrenia group mean. This result is in line with the argument put forth by Morrison and others, suggesting that anomalous experiences need not be pathological. Group comparisons between controls and schizophrenic patients showed that the latter clinical group obtained higher mean scores for total items, distress, intrusiveness and frequency. This finding sustains the significant implications of these three dimensions together with a greater variety of anomalous perceptions in clinical expressions of psychosis.

The current chapter introduces a preliminary validation study of a CAPS version adapted for francophone youths. The objectives of this study comprise three principal aims. Our first aim is to analyze the factorial structure of anomalous perceptions in youths. Second, we wish to provide preliminary data on the experiential dimensions of anomalous perceptions during adolescence and early adulthood, covering emotional distress, attentional disturbance (intrusiveness) and frequency. Finally, we wish to examine whether distress and intrusiveness linked to experiencing anomalous perceptions in youths correlate with anxiety and depression ratings.

Method

Participants

A total of 72 adolescents and young adults aged between 12 and 24 years old (m = 16.72, sd = 2.69, 39 females and 33 males) were included in the study. Typically developing adolescents (m = 17.06, sd = 3.52, 14 females and 14 males) screened for lifetime presence of neurological, psychiatric or learning issues (n = 28) participated to this study. Youths were also recruited through the child and adolescent community outpatient psychiatric service (m = 15.51, sd = 2.01, 25 females and 19 males) affiliated to the University of Geneva's Psychiatry Department and to the Canton of Geneva Education Department (n=44). The motive for recruiting adolescents from the community in combination with those seeking psychological help was to obtain a distribution representing the wide range of anomalous perception expression in our final youth sample.

Written informed consent was obtained from participants under protocols approved by the Institutional Review Board of the Department of Psychiatry of the University of Geneva Medical School.

Materials

Anomalous perceptions were investigated through the French translation of the Cardiff Anomalous Perception Scale (CAPS; (Bell *et al.* 2006).

The CAPS original version was first adapted for use with adolescents (M.D. and M. VDL). It was then translated from English into French using a forward (M.D, B.A, M.S, M.VDL) and a backward (P.D.) translation.

As in the original version, the 32 items yield a yes/no answer. Then, for all endorsed items, the participant is asked to rate the level of distress and intrusiveness associated with the manifestation, as well as its frequency on a 5-point Likert scale. In the original study of Bell and collaborators, three items were not included in the analysis due to an endorsement rate of less than 10% and 10 items didn't load on any factor.

Anomalous perceptions were also investigated through the French validated translation (Dumas *et al.* 2000) of the Schizotypal Personality Questionnaire (SPQ ; Raine 1991). The SPQ is a 74 dichotomous (yes/no) item questionnaire assessing three dimensions of schizotypy: positive (cognitive-perceptual), negative (interpersonal), and disorganization. In particular, the positive dimension evaluates ideas of reference, odd beliefs/magical thinking, unusual perceptual experiences, suspiciousness/paranoid ideation. The SPQ is appropriate for use with adolescents (Axelrod *et al.* 2001).

We also examined additional clinical characteristics in a subsample of participants. We used the French validated translation of the Child Depression Inventory (CDI; Saint-Laurent 1990)) to obtain an evaluation of self-reported depression. The 27 items of the CDI are composed of 3 sentences varying in severity (symptom absent, mildly severe, very severe) and the participant has to choose which sentence best describes his feelings within the last two weeks. This yields a global t-score of depression. We also examined self-reported anxiety using the Revised Children's Manifest Anxiety Scale (R-CMAS; Turgeon & Chartrand 2003). We used the French Canadian norms to obtain a total percentile score of anxiety.

To ensure that all participants understood the items, a trained psychologist supervised the questionnaire process.

Statistical Analyses

The use of classical exploratory factor analysis has been shown to be not suited for dichotomous items (Muthèn 1983). We thus transformed the CAPS yes/no response choice to include a frequency component by introducing a 6-point Likert scale, ranging from 0 (not present) to 5 (constantly present). This new variable can be considered continuous and suitable for an exploratory factor analysis. Based on the assumption that the extracted factors were not independent, we performed a promax rotation before analyzing the factor loadings. Because of the small sample size, we used a conservative factor loading threshold of .50.

We then performed Wilcoxon tests in the total sample to compare the mean distress, intrusiveness, and frequency of the extracted factors. We also performed group comparisons (clinical vs control) for the three dimensions of distress, intrusiveness and frequency using Mann-Whitney tests.

Finally, we examined the associations between the CAPS and other clinical characteristics using Spearman correlations. In particular we performed correlations with self-reported schizotypy (SPQ), anxiety (R-CMAS) and depression (CDI).

Results

Descriptive Statistics

On average, each participant endorsed 5.4 items (sd = 5.38, range: 0-25) (see Figure 1). Item 15 was the most endorsed (33.3%, "Do you ever find that sensations happen all at once and flood you with information") (see Table 1). As it was the case in the study of Bell *et al.* (2006), some items were endorsed by less than 10% of the sample and therefore removed from the factorial analysis. The removed items were the following: 10 ("Do you ever have the sensation that your limbs might not be your own or might not be properly connected to your body?"), 16 ("Do you ever find that sounds are distorted in strange or unusual ways?"), 19 ("Do you ever find the appearance of things or people seems to change in a puzzling way, e.g. distorted shapes or sizes or colour?"), 21 ("Do you ever think that food or drink tastes much stronger than it normally would?"), 25 ("Do you ever find that common smells sometimes seem unusually different?"), 28 ("Have you ever heard two or more unexplained voices talking with each other?"), and 31 ("Do you ever see things that other people cannot?").

Table 1. descriptive statistics for each item

	% endorsement	Mean distress (s.d.)	Mean intrusiveness (s.d.)	Mean frequency (s.d.)
Item 1	27.8	1.6 (0.88)	2.15 (1.09)	1.9 (0.72)
Item 2	22.2	2.31 (1.25)	2.87 (1.09)	1.75 (0.93)
Item 3	16.7	2.25 (1.06)	2.75 (0.97)	2.33 (1.16)
Item 4	13.9	1.4 (0.7)	1.9 (0.99)	1.8 (0.92)
Item 5	29.2	2.1 (1)	2.43 (1.08)	2.14 (0.73)
Item 6	16.7	1.75 (0.62)	2.17 (0.94)	2.08 (1.08)
Item 7	18.1	2.77 (1.17)	2.54 (1.33)	2.62 (1.12)
Item 8	18.1	1.69 (0.75)	2.15 (0.90)	1.69 (0.95)
Item 9	16.7	1.58 (1.17)	1.92 (1.17)	2.25 (0.75)
Item 10	5.6	2.75 (1.71)	2.25 (1.26)	2.75 (1.71)
Item 11	11.1	3.12 (1.55)	3 (1.31)	2.75 (1.39)
Item 12	16.7	1.92 (1)	2.17 (1.12)	1.67 (1.16)
Item 13	13.9	2.73 (1.42)	3 (1.34)	2.27 (0.79)
Item 14	20.8	1.43 (0.65)	2 (0.68)	1.5 (0.65)
Item 15	33.3	2.61 (0.99)	2.57 (1.16)	2.13 (0.97)
Item 16	9.7	1.29 (0.49)	1.86 (0.9)	1.86 (0.69)
Item 17	22.2	2.5 (1.21)	2.31 (0.79)	2.25 (1.18)
Item 18	15.3	1.5 (0.67)	1.58 (0.67)	1.75 (1.14)
Item 19	2.8	1.5 (0.71)	2 (0)	3 (1.41)
Item 20	25	1.44 (0.71)	1.89 (1.02)	1.94 (0.54)
Item 21	9.7	1.25 (0.46)	1.38 (0.52)	2.38 (1.41)
Item 22	19.4	2.21 (1.42)	2.29 (1.33)	2.29 (0.91)
Item 23	18.1	1.23 (0.44)	2.46 (0.97)	1.69 (0.86)
Item 24	16.7	1.58 (0.67)	1.83 (0.72)	1.75 (0.97)
Item 25	6.9	1.2 (0.45)	1.4 (0.55)	1.8 (0.84)
Item 26	13.9	2.3 (1.06)	2.7 (0.95)	2.5 (1.51)
Item 27	26.4	2.16 (1.21)	1.84 (0.77)	2.95 (1.03)
Item 28	5.6	3.25 (1.5)	3.25 (1.71)	2 (0.82)
Item 29	29.2	1.38 (0.81)	1.52 (0.81)	1.81 (0.98)
Item 30	13.9	1.90 (0.99)	1.9 (0.99)	2.2 (0.92)
Item 31	9.7	2.29 (1.38)	2.43 (0.98)	2.71 (1.38)
Item 32	15.3	1.45 (0.52)	2.09 (0.83)	2.18 (1.08)

Most items have a mean distress and intrusiveness score around 1 or 2, indicating relatively low severity (see Table 1). However, few items have a distress and/or intrusiveness score greater than or equal to 3, indicating symptoms of moderate intensity (items 11 "Do you ever hear voices commenting on what you are thinking or doing?", 13 "Do you ever hear voices saying words or sentences when there is no one around that might account for it?", and 28 "Have you ever heard two or more unexplained voices talking with each other?").

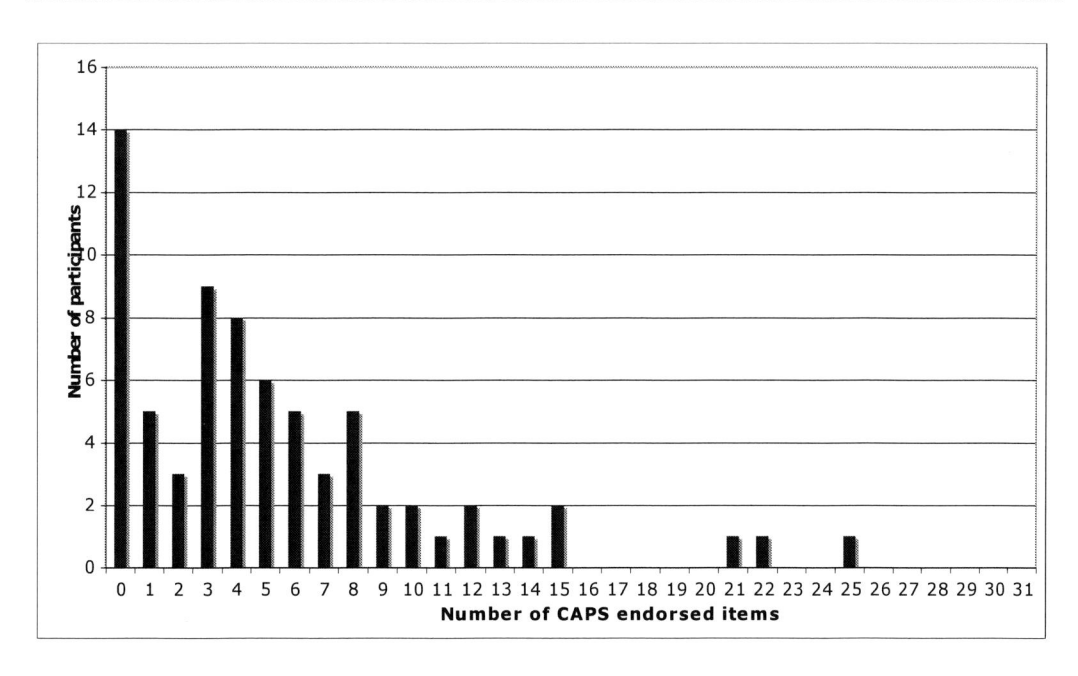

Figure 1. Total number of CAPS items endorsed by each participant

Exploratory Factor Analysis

An exploratory factor analysis was conducted on the total sample. It revealed the presence of 8 factors with eigenvalues above 1 (Kaiser-Guttman criterion). However, graphical analysis using the screeplot clearly indicated a 3 factor structure explaining 42.94% of the variance. A further factorial analysis with promax rotation was run with 3 factors. Using a conservative threshold of .50 for factor loadings, we were able to identify the following groupings (see Table 2): items 1, 14, 20, 27, and 30 loaded on the first factor labeled "perceptual distortions"; items 2, 3, 11, and 13 loaded on the second factor labeled "clinical psychosis"; and the last factor labeled "anomalous olfactory experience" consisted of items 12, 18, and 29. Thirteen items didn't load on any factor.

The three factors were moderately correlated with each other (correlations ranging from .300 to .444).

Intra-Group Comparisons

Based on the results from the factorial analysis, we computed a mean distress, intrusiveness and frequency score for each factor (perceptual distortions, clinical psychosis, and anomalous olfactory experience) (see Table 3). This enabled to examine if one factor was associated with higher symptom frequency or greater severity. The "clinical psychosis" factor was found to include manifestations of greater distress and intrusiveness than the "perceptual distortions" factor ($z = -2.028$, $p = .043$ and $z = -2.562$, $p = .010$, respectively) and the "anomalous olfactory experience" factor ($z = -2.233$, $p = .026$ and $z = -2.432$, $p = .015$, respectively). In addition, we observed that symptoms contained in the "perceptual distortions" factor were more frequent than those included in the "anomalous olfactory experience" factor ($z = -2.564, p = .010$).

Table 2. Factor loadings extracted from exploratory factor analysis with promax rotation. Loadings below .33 are not shown

	Factor 1	Factor 2	Factor 3
Item 14	.714		
Item 27	.615		
Item 1	.592		
Item 30	.592		
Item 20	.545		
Item 32	.452		
Item 6	.435		
Item 5	.416		
Item 22	.392	.370	
Item 4	.358	.350	
Item 7			
Item 15			
Item 9			
Item 11		.926	
Item 13		.763	
Item 2		.615	
Item 3		.516	
Item 8		.467	
Item 24		.463	
Item 23			
Item 17			
Item 29		-.340	.810
Item 18			.674
Item 12		.485	.642
Item 26			.466

Table 3. Mean (s.d.) distress, intrusiveness and frequency score by factor

	Distress	Intrusiveness	Frequency
Perceptual distortions	1.66 (0.75)	1.84 (0.82)	2.05 (0.75)
Clinical psychosis	2.40 (1.18)	2.83 (0.95)	1.96 (0.94)
Anomalous olfactory experience	1.53 (0.84)	1.72 (0.77)	1.67 (0.89)

Inter-Group Comparisons

Mann-Whitney tests revealed that clinical participants did not report a significantly higher number of symptoms ($p = .136$). However, the endorsed manifestations were experienced significantly more often by the group of help-seeking adolescents ($z = -2.549$, $p = .011$). More precisely, this difference of frequency was only observable for the items included in the « clinical psychosis » factor ($z = -2.601$, $p = .009$) but not in the two other factors ($z = -0.166$, $p = .868$ for perceptual distortions; $z = -0.361$, $p = .718$ for anomalous olfactory experience). Items contained in the "clinical psychosis" factor were also rated as more intrusive by clinical participants ($z = -2.071$, $p = .038$), which was not the case for the items included in the "perceptual distortion" ($z = -0.560$, $p = .576$) or "anomalous olfactory experience" ($z = -0.536$, $p = .592$) factors.

Association with Clinical Characteristics

The CAPS total score showed significant positive correlations with the SPQ total score ($r_s = .500$, $p < .001$), SPQ positive dimension ($r_s = .544$, $p < .001$), and SPQ unusual perceptual experiences ($r_s = .451$, $p < .001$). This suggests acceptable convergent validity between the CAPS and the SPQ.

SPQ total score was also positively and significantly associated with the mean distress ($r_s = .554$, $p = .003$), intrusiveness ($r_s = .538$, $p = .004$), and frequency ($r_s = .598$, $p = .001$) score of the "clinical psychosis" factor. It was not the case for the two other factors (all $p > .05$).

Furthermore, we examined associations between the CAPS extracted factors and self-reported anxiety and depression in a subsample of 51 participants (29 females and 22 males; 33 clinical and 18 control participants) aged between 12 and 18 years old (m = 15.52, sd = 1.68). We observed that the items loading on the clinical psychosis factor had a mean distress and intrusiveness score positively associated with depression ($r_s = .418$, $p = .053$, $r_s = .569$, $p = .006$, respectively) and anxiety ($r_s = .459$, $p = .031$, $r_s = .473$, $p = .026$, respectively). However, mean distress and/or intrusiveness scores of the items loading on the two other factors were not significantly associated with anxiety or depression (all $p > .05$). In addition, the number of CAPS endorsed items was positively associated with self-reported depression ($r_s = .429$, $p = .002$) and anxiety ($r_s = .458$, $p = .001$).

Conclusion

The objectives of this study were threefold. First, we wished to examine the factor structure of anomalous perceptions in a sample of youths. In doing so, we obtained a 3-factor structure comprising a *clinical psychosis* factor, a *perceptual distortion* factor, and a third factor called *olfactory distortions*. These findings will be discussed in comparison to the original Cardiff Anomalous Perception Scale (CAPS) validation study in adults (Bell et al. 2006). Our second objective was to provide preliminary data on the experiential dimensions of anomalous perceptions in youths, in terms of frequency, emotional distress and attentional intrusiveness. Approximately 80% of our sample endorsed at least one item on anomalous perceptions, with an average endorsement ratio of 5.4 out of 32 total items. These results combined to the other experiential dimensions of emotional distress and attentional intrusiveness will be further discussed in relationship to their distribution across the three different factors of the CAPS. More specifically, we will discuss the specificity of the experiential dimensions that characterize the clinical psychosis factor in our sample. Our third objective was to examine anxiety and depression self-ratings relate to the dimensions of emotional distress and attentional intrusiveness in youths' experience of anomalous perceptions. We find that emotional distress and attentional intrusiveness dimensions from the clinical psychosis factor correlate with self-ratings of anxiety and depression. These results will be discussed in terms of clinical relevance of anomalous perceptions and integrated into contemporary cognitive formulation of anomalous perceptions in youths.

The Multifactorial Structure of Anomalous Perceptions

The results presented in this study support the argument put forth by Bell and colleagues that anomalous perceptions cannot be apprehended as a single entity, rather they involve distinct subtypes. Our results further extend this proposition to adolescents. The present analyses also yield a 3-factor composition of anomalous perceptions that involve a *clinical psychosis* factor, yet in comparison to adults, we observe differences in the 2 remaining factors. Our youth sample presents a second factor that we termed *perceptual distortions*, which includes items that belong to both *chemosensation* and *temporal lobe* factors reported in the Bell et al. (2006) study. The underlying causes for this disparity may involve methodological differences of group composition, sample size, but may also result from developmental issues such as cerebral and cognitive maturation (Shaw *et al.* 2008). One could formulate the hypothesis that because of massive neuronal pruning and white matter maturation shaping cerebral connectivity during adolescence, the expression of perceptual distortions during this developmental stage differ from those emanating from adult brains, which appear to more clearly polarize into distinct clusters of chemosensations and seizure-like manifestations. The current validation of an instrument that can be employed in both adolescents and adults will benefit future longitudinal studies that will be better equipped to clarify the issue anomalous perception expression in relation to the developing brain.

Another important characteristic in our youth sample is the clustering on the third factor of items that target olfactory distortions. Although this result diverges from the original CAPS validation study in adults, it carries important implications for psychosis-proneness evaluation in youths. Indeed, there exists an extensive line of research on the olfactory function in schizophrenia (for a review, see Rupp, 2010). Most studies focus on the olfactory identification ability in individuals with schizophrenia, which appears to be impaired in both fist-episode and chronic patients (Brewer *et al.* 2001). Associations linking cognitive deficits in executive function, verbal ability, and memory functions to olfactory deficits in schizophrenia strengthen the case for involvement of faulty temporolimbic - prefrontal connectivity sustaining these impairments. The nature of these olfactory deficits may vary, however. Some findings report olfactory hypersensitivity (Sirota *et al.* 1999), while others observe normal (Striebel *et al.* 1999) or impaired olfactory identification ability (Turetsky *et al.* 2003). The discrepancy between results may be explained by impairments in olfactory discrimination (Rupp *et al.* 2005), and lead to inconsistencies in the experience of olfaction in individuals with psychosis. We note that impairments in olfactory discrimination do not correspond to olfactory distortions per se, as described in our youth sample. However, much like olfactory discrimination impairments (Brewer *et al.* 2003), deviant olfactory experiences in psychosis-prone individuals carry predictive value for the unfolding of psychosis (Mohr *et al.* 2002). A 10-year longitudinal study found that compared to students without deviant olfactory experiences, those participants reporting olfactory hallucinations obtained higher scores on psychosis measures upon follow-up evaluation (Kwapil *et al.* 1996). Thus, there is reason to believe that anomalous olfactory experiences constitute a trait-marker for psychosis in youths. As suggested by family and high-risk studies, future research will need to examine whether anomalous perceptions of olfaction represent genetically heritable impairments that can contribute to the early identification of psychosis-proneness in youths.

The Experiential Dimensions of Anomalous Perceptions in Youths

Previously published investigations on anomalous perceptions in youths mainly focused on hallucination and delusion-like phenomena (Sosland & Edelsohn 2005). Their main focus of interest was to assess the frequency of these phenomena in clinical and non-clinical populations (Larøi *et al.* 2006). The endorsement rate of self-report items on hallucinations and delusions in youth vary between 6 and 33% of the studied samples (Larøi *et al.* 2006). Our study included items on hallucinations and delusions, and extended to anomalous perceptions that targeted perceptual and olfactory distortions. This difference may explain why we find that almost 80% of our sample endorsed at least one anomalous perception item. The average participant in our sample reports almost 6 different anomalous perceptual experiences, supporting the claim of Morrisson and other authors that these phenomena common experiences in adults (Morrison 2001), to which we would now include youth populations. The current results bring further supporting evidence to the continuum hypothesis of anomalous perceptions expression in the general population. We show that anomalous perceptions in youths yield a continuous half-normal distribution comparable to that reported in adult samples (Johns & van Os 2001). The prevalence of anomalous perceptions in youths further suggest that the continuum of expression takes its roots during adolescence and perhaps in earlier developmental stages.

The examination of frequency, emotional distress and intrusiveness of anomalous perceptions in youths reveals very important distinctions between the three factors emerging from the CAPS self-report as perceptual distortions, olfactory distortions and clinical psychosis. Youths rate perceptual distortions as more frequent than olfactory distortions, and while they are on average more frequent than clinical psychosis perceptions, this difference is non-significant. Comparing CAPS factors on their experiential dimensions reveals that youths clearly identify anomalous perceptions of clinical psychosis as significantly more intrusive and emotionally distressing. This results contrasts with Bell et al. (2006) who fail to find significant differences between the experiential dimensions of anomalous perceptions in adults. The divergence of these results may be explained by several differences between studies. Firstly, aside from the clinical psychosis factor, the factorial solution differ between studies. Furthermore, our youth sample include help-seeking adolescents, who appear to experience anomalous perception as more intrusive. Finally, youths may be experiencing their "first" anomalous perceptions of clinical psychosis nature in their lifetime, which may leave a strong and sometimes overwhelming first subjective impression that somewhat fades over time and into adulthood. Nevertheless, with the available epidemiological data suggesting that maintenance of auditory hallucinations during adolescence is associated with their intrusive and distressing quality, the current findings should inform early psychosis-proneness assessment strategies. Indeed, when assessing anomalous perceptions related to clinical psychosis, it appears crucial to not only assess their frequency but also the intrusive and distressing quality with which they may be experienced. Also, early interventions on voices should aim to reduce the frequency of such anomalous perceptions by working on the mental representations and appraisal mechanisms that sustain their intrusive and emotionally disturbing quality. Already, cognitive therapy for young individuals at high-risk for developing psychosis integrate these principles with some success (Morrison et al. 2004). The use of mental imagery (Morrison et al. 2002) or mentalization-based treatment techniques (Brent 2009) represent contemporary psychotherapeutic innovations that may by successful in diminishing the intrusive and emotionally disturbing dimensions in patients experiencing anomalous perceptions by fostering alternative mental representations and adaptative appraisal mechanisms.

Anomalous Perceptions and Adolescents Seeking Psychological Help

Our final analyses were performed on a subgroup of our subjects ages 12 to 18 years for which self-report on anxiety and depression were available. We found that the total number of endorsed items on the CAPS, and more specifically, the experiential dimensions of clinical psychosis items to be significantly associated with self-reports of anxiety and depression. Indeed, those adolescents who reported clinical psychosis factors as more distressing and intrusive were also found to score higher on depression and anxiety measures. These results confirm that anomalous perception appraisal (distress and intrusiveness) are associated with greater psychological distress in everyday life. A longitudinal follow-up would be necessary to examine whether these adolescents' anomalous perceptions are more likely to persist during development. The association between psychological distress and distressing anomalous perceptions further support the usefulness of the clinical psychosis factor of the CAPS in the evaluation of psychosis-proneness in youths. Additionally, when comparing help-seeking adolescents to control adolescents, we note that the major difference can be found on the clinical psychosis factor. Adolescents seeking psychological help rated these items as more frequent and more intrusive. It is difficult to say whether baseline psychological distress augmented the frequency and intrusiveness of these anomalous perceptions in help-seeking adolescents, or if on the contrary these anomalous perceptions triggered further psychological distress. As reported elsewhere, we observe that anxiety and anomalous perceptions during adolescence entertain a reciprocal relationship (Debbané 2008). As concerns depression, different accounts conceptualize its association as either preceding (Krabbendam et al. 2005) anomalous perceptions, or rather as a consequence of perceptual aberrations (Birchwood et al. 2000). Our own data on adolescents seeking psychological help supports the latter view of depression resulting from the unfolding of anomalous perceptions such as hallucinations and also delusional thinking (Debbané 2008). The preliminary results from the current validation study, together with previously published research on the subject, favor the inclusion of an instrument such as the CAPS to assess the crucial experiential dimensions of anomalous perceptions when considering psychosis-proneness in the clinical domain.

Acknowledgments

The authors would like to thank the volunteer participants. Special thanks go to Philippe De Clercq for back translation of the scale. Additional thanks go to the Adolescent Outpatient Psychiatry Services, Drs Dario Balanzin and Serges Djapo-Yogwa, and Bertrand Auckenthaler. This work has been supported in part by he Gertrude Von Meissner Foundation (ME 7871) grant to S. Eliez and M. Debbané, and by the Swiss National Science Foundation (PP00B-102864) grants to S. Eliez.

References

Aleman, A. & Larøi, F. (2008). *Hallucinations: The science of idiosyncratic perception.* Washington: *American Psychological Association.*

Altman, H., Collins, M. & Mundy, P. (1997). Subclinical hallucinations and delusions in nonpsychotic adolescents. *Journal of Child Psychology and Psychiatry, 38(4)*, 413-420.

Axelrod, S. R., Grilo, C. M., Sanislow, C. & McGlashan, T. H. (2001). Schizotypal personality questionnaire-brief: Factor structure and convergent validity in inpatient adolescents. *J Personal Disord, 15(2)*, 168-179.

Behrendt, R. P. & Young, C. (2004). Hallucinations in schizophrenia, sensory impairment, and brain disease: A unifying model. *Behavioral and Brain Sciences, 27(6)*, 771-787; discussion 787-830.

Bell, V., Halligan, P. W. & Ellis, H. D. (2006). The Cardiff anomalous perceptions scale (Caps): A new validated measure of anomalous perceptual experience. *Schizophr Bull, 32(2)*, 366-377.

Birchwood, M., Meaden, A., Trower, P., Gilbert, P. & Plaistow, J. (2000). The power and omnipotence of voices: Subordination and entrapment by voices and significant others. *Psychol Med, 30(2)*, 337-344.

Brent, B. (2009). Mentalization-based psychodynamic psychotherapy for psychosis. *J Clin Psychol, 65(8)*, 803-814.

Brewer, W. J., Pantelis, C., Anderson, V., Velakoulis, D., Singh, B., Copolov, D. L., *et al.* (2001). Stability of olfactory identification deficits in neuroleptic-naive patients with first-episode psychosis. *Am J Psychiatry, 158(1)*, 107-115.

Brewer, W. J., Wood, S. J., McGorry, P. D., Francey, S. M., Phillips, L. J., Yung, A. R., *et al.* (2003). Impairment of olfactory identification ability in individuals at ultra-high risk for psychosis who later develop schizophrenia. *Am J Psychiatry, 160(10)*, 1790-1794.

Chadwick, P. & Birchwood, M. (1994). The omnipotence of voices. A cognitive approach to auditory hallucinations. *British Journal of Psychiatry, 164(2)*, 190-201.

Chapman, L. J., Chapman, J. P., Kwapil, T. R., Eckblad, M. & Zinser, M. C. (1994). Putatively psychosis-prone subjects 10 years later. *Journal of Abnormal Psychology, 103(2)*, 171-183.

Debbané, M. (2008). *Metacognitive processes and vulnerability to psychosis in adolescents.* Unpublished thesis. University of Geneva, Geneva.

Debbané, M., Van der Linden, M., Gex-Fabry, M. & Eliez, S. (2009). Cognitive and emotional associations to positive schizotypy during adolescence. *J Child Psychol Psychiatry, 50(3)*, 326-334.

Dhossche, D., Ferdinand, R., Van der Ende, J., Hofstra, M. B. & Verhulst, F. (2002). Diagnostic outcome of self-reported hallucinations in a community sample of adolescents. *Psychological Medicine, 32(4)*, 619-627.

Dumas, P., Bouafia, S., Gutknecht, C., Saoud, M., Dalery, J. & d'Amato, T. (2000). [validation of the french version of the raine schizotypal personality disorder questionnaire--categorial and dimensional approach to schizotypal personality traits in a normal student population]. *Encephale, 26(5)*, 23-29.

Escher, S. (2004). Determinants of outcome in the pathways through care for children hearing voices. *International Journal of Social Welfare, 13*(208-222).

Escher, S., Romme, M., Buiks, A., Delespaul, P. & Van Os, J. (2002). Independent course of childhood auditory hallucinations: A sequential 3-year follow-up study. *British Journal of Psychiatry - Supplements, 43*, s10-18.

Freeman, D. & Garety, P. A. (2003). Connecting neurosis and psychosis: The direct influence of emotion on delusions and hallucinations. *Behaviour Research and Therapy, 41(8)*, 923-947.

Freeman, D., Garety, P. A., Kuipers, E., Fowler, D. & Bebbington, P. E. (2002). A cognitive model of persecutory delusions. *British Journal of Clinical Psychology, 41*(Pt 4), 331-347.

Frith, C. D. (1992). *The cognitive neuropsychology of schizophrenia.* Hove: Psychology Press Ltd.

Garety, P. A., Kuipers, E., Fowler, D., Freeman, D. & Bebbington, P. E. (2001). A cognitive model of the positive symptoms of psychosis. *Psychological Medicine, 31(2)*, 189-195.

Glicksohn, J., Steinbach, I. & Elimalach-Malmilyan, S. (1999). Cognitive dedifferentiation in eidetics and synaesthesia: Hunting for the ghost once more. *Perception, 28(1)*, 109-120.

Johns, L. C. & van Os, J. (2001). The continuity of psychotic experiences in the general population. *Clinical Psychology Review, 21(8)*, 1125-1141.

Kapur, S., Mizrahi, R. & Li, M. (2005). From dopamine to salience to psychosis--linking biology, pharmacology and phenomenology of psychosis. *Schizophrenia Research, 79(1)*, 59-68.

Krabbendam, L., Myin-Germeys, I., Hanssen, M., de Graaf, R., Vollebergh, W., Bak, M.*, et al.* (2005). Development of depressed mood predicts onset of psychotic disorder in individuals who report hallucinatory experiences. *Br J Clin Psychol, 44*(Pt 1), 113-125.

Kwapil, T. R., Chapman, J. P., Chapman, L. J. & Miller, M. B. (1996). Deviant olfactory experiences as indicators of risk for psychosis. *Schizophr Bull, 22(2)*, 371-382.

Larøi, F. & Van der Linden, M. (2005). Nonclinical participants' reports of hallucinatory experiences. *Canadian Journal of Behavioural Science, 37(1)*, 33-43.

Larøi, F., Van der Linden, M. & Goëb, J.-L. (2006). Hallucinations and delusions in children and adolescents. *Current Psychiatry Reviews, 2(4),* 473-485.

Lyon, H. M., Kaney, S. & Bentall, R. P. (1994). The defensive function of persecutory delusions. Evidence from attribution tasks. *Br J Psychiatry, 164(5),* 637-646.

Miller, P., Byrne, M., Hodges, A., Lawrie, S. M., Owens, D. G. & Johnstone, E. C. (2002). Schizotypal components in people at high risk of developing schizophrenia: Early findings from the edinburgh high-risk study. *British Journal of Psychiatry, 180,* 179-184.

Mohr, C., Hubener, F. & Laska, M. (2002). Deviant olfactory experiences, magical ideation, and olfactory sensitivity: A study with healthy german and japanese subjects. *Psychiatry Res, 111(1),* 21-33.

Morrison, A. P. (2001). The interpretation of intrusions in psychosis: An integrative cognitive approach to hallucinations and delusions. *Behavioural and Cognitive Psychotherapy, 29,* 257-276.

Morrison, A. P., Beck, A. T., Glentworth, D., Dunn, H., Reid, G. S., Larkin, W., et al. (2002). Imagery and psychotic symptoms: A preliminary investigation. *Behaviour Research and Therapy, 40(9),* 1053-1062.

Morrison, A. P., French, P., Walford, L., Lewis, S. W., Kilcommons, A., Green, J., et al. (2004). Cognitive therapy for the prevention of psychosis in people at ultra-high risk: Randomised controlled trial. *British Journal of Psychiatry, 185,* 291-297.

Morrison, A. P., French, P. & Wells, A. (2007). Metacognitive beliefs across the continuum of psychosis: Comparisons between patients with psychotic disorders, patients at ultra-high risk and non-patients. *Behaviour Research and Therapy, 45(9),* 2241-2246.

Morrison, A. P., Haddock, G. & Tarrier, N. (1995). Intrusive thoughts and auditory hallucinations: A cognitive approach. *Behavioral and Cognitive Psychotherapy, 23,* 265-280.

Morrison, A. P., Wells, A. & Nothard, S. (2000). Cognitive factors in predisposition to auditory and visual hallucinations. *British Journal of Clinical Psychology, 39 (Pt 1),* 67-78.

Muthèn, B. O. (1983). Latent variable structural equation modeling with categorical data. *Journal of Econometrics, 22,* 43-65.

Poulton, R., Caspi, A., Moffitt, T. E., Cannon, M., Murray, R. & Harrington, H. (2000). Children's self-reported psychotic symptoms and adult schizophreniform disorder: A 15-year longitudinal study. *Archives of General Psychiatry, 57(11),* 1053-1058.

Raine, A. (1991). The spq: A scale for the assessment of schizotypal personality based on dsm-iii-r criteria. *Schizophrenia Bulletin, 17(4),* 555-564.

Romme, M. A., Honig, A., Noorthoorn, E. O. & Escher, A. D. (1992). Coping with hearing voices: An emancipatory approach. *British Journal of Psychiatry, 161,* 99-103.

Rupp, C. I. Olfactory function and schizophrenia: An update (2010). *Curr Opin Psychiatry, 23(2),* 97-102.

Rupp, C. I., Fleischhacker, W. W., Kemmler, G., Oberbauer, H., Scholtz, A. W., Wanko, C., et al. (2005). Various bilateral olfactory deficits in male patients with schizophrenia. *Schizophr Bull, 31(1),* 155-165.

Saint-Laurent, L. (1990). Etude psychometrique de l'inventaire de depression pour enfants de kovacs aupres d'un echantillon francophone [psychometric study of kovacs' children's depression inventory with a french-speaking sample]. *Canadian Journal of Behavioural Science, 22,* 377–384.

Shaw, P., Kabani, N. J., Lerch, J. P., Eckstrand, K., Lenroot, R., Gogtay, N., *et al.* (2008). Neurodevelopmental trajectories of the human cerebral cortex. *J Neurosci, 28(14)*, 3586-3594.

Shevlin, M., Dorahy, M. & Adamson, G. (2007). Childhood traumas and hallucinations: An analysis of the national comorbidity survey. *J Psychiatr Res, 41*(3-4), 222-228.

Sirota, P., Davidson, B., Mosheva, T., Benhatov, R., Zohar, J. & Gross-Isseroff, R. (1999). Increased olfactory sensitivity in first episode psychosis and the effect of neuroleptic treatment on olfactory sensitivity in schizophrenia. *Psychiatry Res, 86(2)*, 143-153.

Sosland, M. D. & Edelsohn, G. A. (2005). Hallucinations in children and adolescents. *Current Psychiatry Reports, 7(3)*, 180-188.

Striebel, K. M., Beyerstein, B., Remick, R. A., Kopala, L. & Honer, W. G. (1999). Olfactory identification and psychosis. *Biol Psychiatry, 45(11)*, 1419-1425.

Turetsky, B. I., Moberg, P. J., Arnold, S. E., Doty, R. L. & Gur, R. E. (2003). Low olfactory bulb volume in first-degree relatives of patients with schizophrenia. *Am J Psychiatry, 160(4)*, 703-708.

Turgeon, L. & Chartrand, E. (2003). Reliability and validity of the revised children's manifest anxiety scale in a french-canadian sample. *Psychol Assess, 15(3)*, 378-383.

In: Hallucinations: Types, Stages and Treatments
Editor: Meredith S. Payne, pp. 131-146

ISBN: 978-1-61728-275-1
© 2011 Nova Science Publishers, Inc.

Chapter 7

Psychotic-like Experiences in Nonclinical Adolescents

Eduardo Fonseca-Pedrero, Serafín Lemos-Giráldez[*],
Mercedes Paino and Susana Sierra-Baigrie
Department of Psychology. University of Oviedo, Spain, and Carlos III
Health Institute, Research Centre in the Mental Health Network (CIBERSAM), Spain

Interest in psychotic-like experiences (PLEs), such as magical thinking, delusional ideation or hallucinatory experiences, in general and clinical populations has recently increased in the scientific community. Psychotic symptoms, particularly in the context of schizophrenia-spectrum disorders, have traditionally been viewed as categorical phenomena (i.e., either present or absent in an individual). However, the literature shows that PLEs can be found in the general population, even during adolescence, becoming in this way even more prevalent than the clinical phenotype itself. Thus, PLEs are understood as alterations in how one perceives and thinks about reality, in such a way that the individuals who experience these would present a certain bizarreness of thought, characterized by non-conventional logic. This group of experiences, also known as positive schizotypy, can be found, therefore, below the clinical threshold without necessarily being associated to a psychological, medical or any other type of alteration (Nelson & Yung, 2009; Scott, Chant, Andrews, & McGrath, 2006; Verdoux & van Os, 2002). From a dimensional point of view, it is assumed that the psychotic phenotype is distributed in the general population along a *continuum* of severity, with the psychotic disorder at its extreme end (van Os, Hanssen, Bijl, & Ravelli, 2000; van Os, Linscott, Myin-Germeys, Delespaul, & Krabbendam, 2009). In this regard, the expression of the psychotic phenotype would fluctuate from a normal state of functioning, going from the apparition of intermediate transitory states that precede the development of subsyndromal psychotic symptoms, toward its clinical manifestation in the form of psychosis. PLEs would be, therefore, located on a point of the continuum next to the transitory intermediate states,

---

[*] Corresponding author: Department of Psychology, University of Oviedo, Plaza Feijoo, s/n, 33003 Oviedo, Spain, E-mail address: slemos@uniovi.es

being understood as subclinical processes. In this manner, PLEs could be seen as an "intermediate" phenotype qualitatively similar to the symptomatology found in patients with psychosis, but quantitatively less severe, showing lower intensity, persistence, frequency of symptoms and associated impairment (Dominguez, Wichers, Lieb, Wittchen, & van Os, in press; Scott, Martin, Welham, Bor, Najman, O'Callaghan et al., 2009; Yung, Nelson, Baker, Buckby, Baksheev, & Cosgrave, 2009).

From an epidemiological perspective, the presence of psychotic experiences in nonclinical populations may represent the phenotypic expression of the increased proneness or risk for the development of psychotic disorders. Follow up studies conducted in nonclinical adolescents and adults selected from the general population have shown that the presence of PLEs increases the future risk of transiting toward a schizophrenia-spectrum disorder (Chapman, Chapman, Raulin, & Eckblad, 1994; Gooding, Tallent, & Matts, 2005; Poulton, Caspi, Moffitt, Cannon, Murray, & Harrington, 2000; Welham et al., 2009) or predicts delusional-like experiences in adulthood (Scott, Martin, Welham, Bor, Najman, O'Callaghan et al., 2009). A continuous dose-response risk function exists between subclinical psychotic experiences and later clinical disorder (van Os et al., 2009). However, it is equally true that most of the participants who report PLEs may be experiencing a transitory state or may never progress to clinical psychotic disorder, or may develop other types of disorders (e.g., depression or substance abuse) (Dhossche, Ferdinand, van der Ende, Hofstra, & Verhulst, 2002; Hanssen, Bak, Bijl, Vollebergh, & Van Os, 2005; Verdoux, van Os, & Maurice-Tison, 1999). Specifically, between 10 and 25% of these subclinical psychotic experiences can interact synergetically or additively with other environmental factors (i.e., genetic, trauma, cannabis, urbanicity, victimization, etc.) increasing the persistence of psychotic experiences and consequently becoming abnormally persistent, clinically relevant and in need of care (Bendall, Jackson, Hulbert, & McGorry 2008; Cougnard et al., 2007; Freeman & Fowler, 2009; Kelleher, Harley, Lynch, Arseneault, Fitzpatrick, & Cannon, 2008; Kelly, O'Callaghan, Waddington, Feeney, Browne, Scully, et al., 2010; Larkin & Morrison, 2006; Morgan & Fisher 2007; Spauwen, Krabbendam, Lieb, Wittchen, & van Os, 2006; van Os, Hanssen, Bak, Bijl, & Vollebergh, 2003; van Os & Poulton, 2009). In this regard, the prompt detection of these individuals with PLEs, and subsequent implementation of prophylactic treatments in early prevention programs is of particular interest. Likewise, their study allows us to explore and improve the comprehension of the risk or vulnerability markers toward psychosis and its related disorders and offer more evidence in support of the dimensional models of psychosis.

The Explanation of Hallucinatory and Delusional Phenomena

The continuum model of PLEs is consistent with the symptom-based approach advocated by some researchers (Bentall, 2005), who argue that rather than approaching psychotic symptoms as expressions of a more general pathological process, they are best understood as discrete entities. The symptom-oriented approach implies that each symptom should be understood as an isolated complaint, with a focus on the pathogenesis of each individual complaint, possibly reflecting a core disturbance or a basic alteration of experience, or a basic disruption of the relationship with the self and the world (Nelson, Yung, Bechdolf, & McGorry, 2008; Nelson & Yung, 2009; Sass & Parnas, 2003).

Hallucinatory experiences and delusional thoughts are derived from the distortion in the processes of perception (hallucinations) and analysis of reality (delusion). If, as is known, perception is an active process which requires the focalization of attention, the automatic discrimination or deliberate selection of environmental stimuli, and the recognition or attribution of meaning to these, it is reasonable to think that any alteration that affects both the capacity of sensory processing (i.e., bottom-up mechanisms), and the recognition or inference of meaning to the stimuli (top-down inferences) may produce as a result, a perceptual distortion of reality. Likewise, it is assumed that both components of sensory processing and of attribution of meaning are also implicated in the origin of delusional beliefs. Human beings are characterized by the natural necessity of searching for explanation and meaning (search for meaning), and of interpreting or attributing meaning to the signals received from the external and internal environment itself. Nonetheless, the thought processes implicated in delusional beliefs are considered to be similar to those implicated in normal thought, differing from non-delusional beliefs only quantitatively in a spectrum of degree of resistance to the modification due to evidences and disconfirming events, which endorses the idea of a continuous distribution of these experiences.

It has also been verified that hallucinatory experiences (a) are usually more likely to be present during periods of anxiety and psychological stress, that is, after threatening experiences or intense emotional states; suggesting that they are related to fluctuations in psychophysiological activation; (b) can be influenced by environmental circumstances such as sensory deprivation or social isolation, the exposure to "white noise" or other forms of ambiguous or unstructured stimulation; (c) can be induced through suggestion, lack of sleep, reinforcement or motivational factors; (d) are occasionally present during stressful states, in the transition from vigilance to sleep or sleep to vigilance, as well as in diverse disorders of the central nervous system and organic diseases such as toxic states, cortical injuries, epilepsy, tumors, dementias, etc. ; and (e) are usually related to the concealed activity of the speech muscles or sub-vocalization, and can be blocked or inhibited by other concurrent tasks, such as reading, talking, singing, etc. (Morrison, Wells, & Nothard, 2000).

With regard to the mechanisms implicated, it is agreed that hallucinations take place when the experiences or private or mental events are not recognized as one's owns and originating from the inner domain, but rather, on the contrary, are attributed to an external source (mistakes in external attribution). This explains why the content of hallucinations holds such as strong relationship with the interests, concerns or conflicts of the person who is experiencing them. The explanation of the origin of hallucinations has led, however, to several probably complementary and not mutually exclusive theories that refer to the presence of *deficit* in the perceptual processes referred to (the abovementioned bottom-up influences) (Frith, 1992; Goldman-Rakic, 1991; Hemsley, 1994; Nuechterlein & Dawson, 1984; Posner, 1982), or the existence of cognitive *biases* which affect the interpretation of the phenomena of internal origin (or top-down influences) (Bentall, 2003; Bentall, Haddock, & Slade, 1994; Morrison, Haddock, & Tarrier, 1995).

Table 1. Prevalence of PLEs in adolescent populations according to studies

Study	Type	Sample N; M (SD)	Measurement instrument	Prevalence/results
(Wigman et al., in press)	T	1 = 5422; 14 years (1.3) 2 = 2230; 11.1 years (.6) Dutch	CAPE	1) 95% endorsed at least one psychotic experience at least "sometimes," 43% endorsed at least one experience "often" or "almost always." 2) 94% endorsed at least one CAPE experience at least "sometimes," 39% endorsed at least one experience "often" or "nearly always."
(Yung et al., 2009)	T	875; 15.6 years (.5) Australian	CAPE	Between 10.9%–91.5% reported some psychotic symptoms at least "sometimes" Between 0.9%–9.1% reported some psychotic symptoms "always/nearly always"
(Scott, Martin, Bor et al., 2009)	T	1261; 14.8 years (1.2) Australian	CBCL; YSR; DISC-IV	8.4 % of the adolescents experienced visual and/or auditory hallucinations
(Kelleher et al., 2008)	T	211; 12-15 years Irish	K-SADS	6.6% reported experiencing psychotic symptoms
(De Loore et al., 2008)	L	1903; 13-14 years Dutch	SDQ	5.3% reported baseline hallucinatory experiences, and 28.7% persisted after 2 years
(Horwood et al., 2008)	T	6455; 12.9 years English	12 items Halluc. Exp. DISC-IV	38.9% reported one or more psychotic symptoms in previous 6 months 18.2% reported more than two symptoms in previous 6 months 13.7% reported one or more symptoms observer-rated assessment
(Spauwen et al., 2006)	L	918; 15.1 years (1.1) German	M-CIDI; SCL-90-R	16% respond affirmatively to at least one item on the M-CIDI
(Yoshizumi et al., 2004)	T	791; 11-12 years Japanese	Ad hoc questionnaire of Halluc. Exp.	21.3% reported some hallucinatory experience 9.2% reported auditory hallucinations and 5.5% visual hallucinations 6.6% reported both hallucinatory experiences

T: Transversal; L: Longitudinal; CAPE: *Community Assessment* of Psychotic Experiences; CBCL: Child Behavior Checklist; YSR: Youth Self Report; DISC-IV: Diagnostic Interview Schedule for Children; K-SADS: Schedule for Affective Disorders and Schizophrenia for school-Age Children; M-CIDI: Munich-Composite International Diagnostic Interview; SDQ: Strengths Difficulties Questionnaire; SCL-90-R: Symptom Checklist-90-Revised. Halluc. Exp.: Hallucinatory experiences

In regard to delusional beliefs, the nature and content of these show great diversity in aspects such as the degree of conviction with which these are held, the cultural congruence, their systematization and structure, the concern they generate or the relevance they may have in an individual's life. For this reason, it is improbable that such phenomenological diversity can be explained by one single casual factor; consequently, it is necessary once again to consider several determinants which can be potentially present in their apparition. In addition to the explanations that presume the existence of possible cognitive deficits or neuropsychological anomalies implicated in the mere perception and interpretation of reality (Cummings, 1985; Gazzaniga, Ivry, & Mangun, 1998), the etiology of delusions has generally been attributed to "motivational" and "defectual" factors, without both points of view being mutually exclusive. The motivational explanations presuppose that delusions fulfill a function of compensating or balancing the emotional life of the person who holds them, as they arise due to a necessity of explaining bizarre experiences (e.g., hallucinations themselves), threatening events for the person's self-esteem, unpredictable or simply incomprehensible phenomena (Maher, 1992; Maher & Spitzer, 1993). The defectual explanations regarding the origin of delusions presume the existence of latent anomalies or cognitive-attentional deficits in reasoning or in the formation of beliefs and opinions, which would lead to a distorted interpretation of reality (Freeman & Fowler, 2009; Freeman, Garety, & Fowler, 2008; Garety, Kuipers, Fowler, Freeman, & Bebbington, 2001).

Prevalence of Psychotic-like Experiences in Nonclinical Adolescents

The expression of psychosis is more common in young people and declines with age, whether it be full-blown psychosis (prevalence 1%), isolated psychotic symptoms (prevalence around 5%) or broadly defined psychotic experiences (mean prevalence around 15%) (Cougnard et al., 2007; van Os et al., 2009). Therefore, this group of experiences constitutes a fairly common psychological phenomenon in the general population with prevalences ranging from 10% to 25% according to different studies (Aleman, Nieuwenstein, Boker, & De Haan, 2001; Scott et al., 2008; Tien, 1991; Verdoux & van Os, 2002; Young, Bentall, Slade, & Dewey, 1986).

In particular, the percentage of self-reported PLEs in adolescents is more prevalent than that found in studies with adults in both clinical and general population samples (Fonseca-Pedrero, Lemos-Giráldez, Paino, Sierra-Baigrie, Villazón-García, & Muñiz, 2009). As can be observed in Table 1, the prevalence of PLEs varies considerably across epidemiological studies. It must be mentioned that strict comparison among studies is limited by the type of instrument and the characteristics of the sample used as well as by the statistical criteria employed to determine the prevalence of these experiences. This consideration must be kept in mind when interpreting and comparing the results obtained in different investigations.

In this regard, Yung et al. (2009), using a sample of 875 Australian adolescents, found that around 28% of the assessed participants reported hearing voices sometimes, and 1.9% reported always or nearly always experiencing this. In another study, Scott et al. (2009), analyzing a sample of 1,261 Australian adolescents, found that 8.4% of these reported having experienced some visual or auditory hallucinatory experience on some occasion. On their part, Kelleher et al. (2008), using the *Schedule for Affective Disorders and Schizophrenia for school-Age Children* (K-SADS), in a sample of 211 Irish participants, found that 6.6% reported some psychotic symptom. In another investigation by De Loore and cols. (2008) conducted in a sample of 1,903 Dutch adolescents, the results showed that 5.3% of the participants reported some hallucinatory experience. Higher percentages were found in the study by Horwood and cols. (2008), who, using a sample of 6,455 English adolescents, found that 38.9% scored positively on more than one item regarding psychotic experiences, although when these experiences were assessed through an observer-rated method, the percentage decreased to 13.7%. Similarly, Spauwen et al. (2006), analyzing a sample of 918 German adolescents, found that 16% scored positively on at least one item regarding hallucinatory or delusional experiences. In another study conducted in a sample of 761 Japanese children (non-western society), Yoszhumi and cols. (2004) found that 21% of these reported some hallucinatory experience. Finally, Wigman et al. (in press) in two representative samples of Dutch adolescents ($n = 5422$; $n = 2230$), using the *Community Assessment of Psychotic Experiences* (CAPE), found that approximately 95% of both samples endorsed at least one positive psychotic experience at least "sometimes" and between 39-43% endorsed at least one experience at level "often" or "nearly always".

Recently, our research team has conducted an empirical study with the aim of examining the distribution of PLEs in a representative sample of the adolescent general population. In this investigation, a total of 1,438 students participated, 691 males (48.1%), belonging to 28 different high schools and 91 classrooms in the Principality of Asturias, a region in northern Spain, and selected using a stratified random sampling at classroom level. The mean age was 15.92 years ($SD = 1.17$), ranging from 14 to 18 years. Ten items included in the *Oviedo Questionnaire for Schizotypy Assessment* (ESQUIZO-Q) that assess aspects related to magical thinking, unusual perceptual experiences and paranoid ideation were used (Fonseca-Pedrero, Muñiz, Lemos-Giráldez, Paino, & Villazón-García, 2010). The ESQUIZO-Q is a questionnaire of recent construction for the assessment of schizotypal personality traits in adolescents. The number and percentage of participants who gave an "*I agree quite a bit*" (4) or "*Completely agree*" (5) answer to the 10 selected items in the ESQUIZO-Q are presented in Table 2. As can be seen, between 3.2 and 7.2% of the adolescents reported symptoms related to magical thinking (items 1 to 3); between 1.2 and 8.8% reported having experienced some Unusual perceptual experience (items 4 to 7); finally, between 1.3 and 13.2% of the studied adolescents were found to report paranoid ideation symptoms (items 8 to 10).

Influence of Gender and Age in the Expression of Psychotic-like Experiences

The phenotypic expression of PLEs in adolescents seems to vary as a function of gender or age. Regarding gender, and similarly to what happens in adults, adolescent females usually report a higher number of positive psychotic symptoms (e. g., ideas of reference or paranoid ideation) than males (Fonseca-Pedrero, Lemos-Giráldez, Paino, Villazón-García, Sierra-Baigrie, & Muñiz, 2009; Wigman et al., in press; Yung et al., 2009); however, other studies have found contradictory results, failing to find such association (Fonseca-Pedrero, Paino-Piñeiro, Lemos-Giráldez, Villazón-García, & Muñiz, 2009; Scott, Martin, Welham, Bor, Najman, & O'Callaghan, 2009), or even other studies have found that there is a greater percentage of males that report such experiences than females (Kelleher et al., 2008). In relation to age, younger participants usually obtain higher scores in measures of PLEs compared to older participants (van Os et al., 2009) although, when only groups of adolescents were compared, some studies did not confirm this finding (Scott, Martin, Welham, Bor, Najman, & O'Callaghan, 2009) or even obtained findings in the opposite direction (Fonseca-Pedrero, Lemos-Giráldez, Muñiz, García-Cueto, & Campillo-Álvarez, 2008). A global analysis of the different studies regarding the variability in PLEs as a function of gender and age, therefore, indicates that there are certain inconsistencies and incongruencies in the results. Thus, it would be interesting to continue examining the role played by these two sociodemographic variables in the expression of PLEs in the general adolescent population where developmental processes may be playing an interesting role.

Prediction and Temporal Persistence of PLEs in Adolescents across Longitudinal Studies

PLEs are risk or vulnerability markers for psychosis and its related disorders. Longitudinal studies using nonclinical adolescents have shown that the presence of these experiences at these ages increases the future risk of transiting toward a schizophrenia-spectrum disorder (Dominguez et al., in press; Poulton et al., 2000; Welham et al., 2009) or predicts delusional-like experiences in adulthood (Scott, Martin, Welham, Bor, Najman, O'Callaghan et al., 2009). Poulton et al. (2000), in a follow-up study conducted in New Zealand in a sample of children from the general population, found that more than 25% of the participants who had reported such experiences at the age of 11, developed a schizophreniform-type disorder at the age of 26. Similarly, Welham et al. (2009) also conducted a longitudinal study where information was obtained from both parents and adolescents at different moments, and found that the presence of auditory hallucinatory experiences was associated, after 14 years, to a greater risk for the later development of non-affective psychosis. More recently, Dominguez and cols. (in press), in an 8-year-longitudinal study conducted in a sample of 845 German adolescents, found that of the participants who had been considered as clinical cases of psychosis at the end of the assessment period, 38.3% had previously presented at least one psychotic experience, and 19.6% of these cases had been preceded by at least two subclinical-psychotic experiences.

In addition to the predictive validity of subclinical-psychotic experiences, another extremely interesting issue is to determine its degree of continuity and temporal persistence as well as delimit the factors that make these experiences transitory or, on the contrary, persistent over time evolving into a state of impairment and need for care. In general terms, the temporal persistence of these experiences during adolescence and adulthood is around 10-40% (De Loore et al., 2008; Dominguez et al., in press; van Os et al., 2009). For example, Loore and cols. (2008) examined a sample of 1,903 adolescents, and found that after 2 years, psychotic experiences persisted in 28.7% of the cases that had reported such experiences in the basal period (5.3% of the adolescents). However, Dominguez et al. (in press) found that in 30-40% of the cases, the attenuated-psychotic symptoms persisted and re-occurred over time; moreover, the greater the temporal persistence of the subclinical-psychotic symptoms was, the greater the risk of transiting toward a psychotic disorder after 8 years in a dose-response fashion.

Table 2. Number (and percentage) of participants who obtained high scores (values of 4 or 5 on the *Likert* scale) on ten items of the *Oviedo Questionnaire for Schizotypy Assessment* (ESQUIZO-Q) assessing PLEs

Items	Total (*n* = 1438)	Men (*n* = 691)	Women (*n* = 747)
1."I believe that the things that are on the radio or television have a special meaning to me, that my friends don't understand"	54 (3,8)	30 (4,3)	24 (3,2)
2."I think that there are some people who can read other people's minds"	96 (6,7)	50 (7,2)	46 (6,2)
3."I believe there are people who can control the thoughts of others"	94 (6,5)	40 (5,8)	54 (7,2)
4."Being alone at home, I have had the feeling that someone was talking to me"	86 (6,0)	40 (5,8)	46 (6,2)
5."I hear voices that others can't hear"	26 (1,8)	17 (2,5)	9 (1,2)
6."When I am alone, I have the feeling that someone is whispering my name"	38 (2,6)	16 (2,3)	22 (2,9)
7."I have thoughts which are so real that it seems as if someone was talking to me"	126 (8,8)	60 (8,7)	66 (8,8)
8."I think that someone is planning something against me"	83 (5,8)	50 (7,2)	33 (4,4)
9."Somebody has it in for me"	165 (11,5)	91 (13,2)	74 (9,9)
10."My classmates are against me"	21 (1,5)	11 (1,6)	10 (1,3)

As can be observed, the great majority of adolescents experience PLEs of a transitory nature and do not necessarily evolve toward a psychotic disorder; for only a small percentage of adolescents, these experiences evolve unfavorably and reach its clinical expression causing clinically significant impact and the need for care (Dominguez et al., in press; van Os et al., 2009; Welham et al., 2009). Specifically, these experiences have to interact in a synergic or additive manner with other early environmental (e.g., cannabis, urbanicity, traumatic events etc.), genetic (e.g., presence of first degree relatives with a psychotic disorder) and/or psychological factors (e.g., depression, coping strategies) to surpass the subclinical threshold and evolve into a psychotic disorder. In this regard, the possible evolutionary trajectories toward psychotic disorders may be heterogeneous and diverse, and therefore, the mere presence of PLEs at early stages does not necessarily implicate the apparition of a severe psychopathological alteration in the future.

Relationship between Psychotic-like Experiences and Other Clinical Symptoms in Adolescents

PLEs in adolescents have been linked to the presence of diverse psychological problems such as anxiety, dissociation, distress, depression, impaired social functioning (Scott, Martin, Bor et al., 2009; Wigman et al., in press; Yoshizumi et al., 2004; Yung et al., 2009), childhood trauma, and increased likelihood of receiving an Axis I psychiatric diagnosis (Kelleher et al., 2008). For example, Yoshizumi and cols. (2004) found that those participants with auditory and visual hallucinations scored significantly higher on measures of anxiety and dissociation compared to those who did not report said symptoms. On their part, Scott et al. (2009) found that those adolescents with auditory and/or visual hallucinations presented higher levels of depressive symptoms in comparison to the control group. Yung et al. (2009) found that a high presence of PLEs was associated to self-reported depressive symptomatology, as well as worse social functioning. On the other hand, in a study by Kelleher et al. (2008), a greater prevalence of physical and sexual abuse as well as a greater number of Axis psychiatric diagnoses, particularly depressive disorders, were found in adolescents with PLEs. These data suggest that nonclinical adolescents with PLEs frequently present, although to a lesser degree, affective and behavioral alterations similar to those found in patients with schizophrenia.

Gaps in Knowledge

The study of psychotic experiences is a field that is in clear expansion where several extremely interesting questions still remain unsolved. On the one hand, the role of PLEs at an early age in the prediction of psychotic disorders should continue to be explored in greater depth through independent longitudinal studies in both nonclinical adolescent populations and in adolescents at risk (e.g., offspring of one or two parents with schizophrenia). On the other hand, the exploration of the type of relationship that these psychotic experiences have with biochemical, physiological, environmental and psychosocial variables is also very interesting, as well as their interaction with several psychological variables such as depressive symptomatology or coping strategies, with a view to understanding which factors determine the transition or not toward a psychotic state.

Recent research from Nelson and Yung (2009) indicates that PLEs do not constitute a unitary phenomenon; in fact, it seems that there are different types of PLEs with different likely trajectories and underlying causes. Data from nonclinical samples and nonpsychotic clinical samples indicates that Bizarre Experiences, Perceptual Abnormalities and Persecutory Ideas may be more malignant forms of PLEs and confer a greater risk of developing psychotic disorder than Magical Thinking (Yung et al., 2009). Likewise, this research indicates that PLEs might either be: (a) an expression of meta-cognitive deficits in discriminating between self-generated and external sources of information, in combination with cognitive faults in self-monitoring, such as an underlying basic self-disturbance resulting in a person experiencing their body as an external object (Sass, 2003); (b) clinical "noise" around a non-psychotic syndrome and not necessarily associated with distress or disability (e.g., a patient with depression, who on questioning admits to hearing voices occasionally which do not bother him), and (c) present in nonclinical "normal" individuals, not associated with distress or disability or increased vulnerability to psychotic disorder.

A theoretical model of psychotic vulnerability was also proposed by Yung et al. (2007), indicating that, in terms of clinical care, PLEs belonging to a first category would be of greatest concern, probably belonging to a categorically separated class of psychopathology known as schizotaxia (Lenzenweger, 2006; Meehl, 1990), followed by PLEs in the second category; however, PLEs in the third category may reflect a form of "happy" or "benign" schizotypy (McCreery & Claridge, 2002), particularly prone to mystical experiences, lucid dreams and creativity, and probably do not warrant clinical attention. These authors consider that clinical attention for these forms of PLEs may have a counter-productive effect by raising anxiety about essentially benign experiences.

At present, the identification of which of the three subtypes of PLEs is manifested in different clinical presentations remains poor; this is reflected in our limited capacity to predict which at-risk individuals with attenuated psychotic symptoms will go on to develop full-blown psychotic disorders (Lemos-Giráldez et al., 2009). Central to the psychological approach is the notion that the response to PLEs is cognitively mediated by beliefs or appraisals. Thus, the mere experience of voices itself does not lead to full-blown psychotic symptoms, but attributing the voice to an external source and giving it personal significance does (Freeman, 2007).

Additionally, as previously mentioned, it may be that the presence of PLEs in combination with other factors, such as traumatic experiences (Larkin & Morrison, 2006), cannabis use (Henquet, Di Forte, Murray, & Van Os, 2008; Schiffman, Nakamura, Earleywine, & LaBrie, 2005; Weiser & Noy, 2005; Barkus & Murray, 2010), marked functional decline (Yung et al., 2006), high levels of distress (Hanssen, Krabbendam, de Graaf, Vollebergh, & van Os, 2005), maladaptive coping style (Krabbendam, Myin-Germeys, Bak, & van Os, 2005), self-disturbance (Nelson et al., 2008), depressed mood (Birchwood, Mason, MacMillan, & Healy, 1993; Smith et al., 2006), or low IQ (Horwood et al., 2008) may enhance an individual's risk of full-blown psychotic disorder. This may in turn shed light on the conceptual and construct validity of schizophrenia and other psychotic disorders, their essential psychopathological features, and phenotypic boundaries. However, a continuum-threshold approach to psychosis-proneness was proposed by Hafner (1992), assuming that PLEs exist along a continuum, but that at a certain level of intensity/severity beyond a critical threshold they are associated with clinical symptoms and functional decline, likely resulting in a psychotic disorder. In this regard, explanatory models in psychosis are still a topic for discussion (Linscott & van Os, 2010).

To Sum up

The study of PLEs in adolescence and their relationship to the subsequent risk for schizophrenia-spectrum disorders has become an area of interest within the current research. The study of PLEs opens the possibility of examining and understanding the possible risk or vulnerability markers prior to the clinical expression of the disorder with a view to improving early detection strategies and aiding in the possible implementation of prevention programs. In the present chapter we have had the opportunity to verify that: a) PLEs in adolescents are relatively common psychological phenomena and characteristic of the maturational processes of development; b) are not necessarily related to a psychopathological alteration or to subsequent greater risk for the development of psychotic disorders; c) most of these experiences are transitory and discontinuous although it is true that, in a small percentage of individuals, these experiences may persist or evolve unfavorably over time and that in their interaction with genetic, psychological and/or psychosocial variables may lead to a psychotic disorder; finally, d) the evidences indicate that the psychotic phenotype appears to be distributed along a severity continuum, at which extreme end we would find psychosis; this dimensional point of view seems to go beyond the frontiers proposed by the international classification systems given that only a part of this continuum is represented by the "clinical" case.

This continuum-threshold approach has not yet been contemplated in the international classification systems, however, the adequacy of including a *"Risk syndrome for psychosis"* category in future editions is currently a subject of debate (Carpenter, 2009; Woods et al., 2009), particularly when PLEs are a cause of distress, dysfunction and/or disability; said syndrome would therefore be characterized by symptoms such as bizarre perceptual experiences or delusional ideation (e.g., distrust/suspiciousness) in the absence of functional deterioration or dysphoria, and without meeting the criteria for a clinical disorder. Little is known, however, about the mechanisms that mediate the relationship between nonclinical psychotic experience and subsequent clinical disorder; but the interpretation, not the experience of voices themselves, probably causes the associated distress and disability, thereby increasing the risk of developing need for treatment.

References

Aleman, A., Nieuwenstein, M. R., Boker, K. B. E. & De Haan, E. H. F. (2001). Multidimensionality of hallucinatory predisposition: Factor structure of the Launay-Slade Hallucination Scale in a normal sample. *Personality and Individual Differences, 30,* 287-292.

Barkus, E. & Murray, R. M. (2010). Substance use in adolescence and psychosis: clarifying the relationship. *Annual Review of Clinical Psychology, 6,* 365-389.

Bendall, S., Jackson, H. J., Hulbert, C. A. & McGorry, P. D. (2008). Childhood trauma and psychotic disorders: A systematic, critical review of the evidence. *Schizophrenia Bulletin, 34,* 568-579.

Bentall, R. (2003). The paranoid self. In T. Kircher & A. David (Eds.), *The self in neuroscience and psychiatry* (293-318). Cambridge, UK: Cambridge University Press.

Bentall, R. P. (2005). *Madness explained.* London: Penguin.

Bentall, R. P., Haddock, G. & Slade, P. D. (1994). Cognitive behavior therapy for persistent auditory hallucinations: From theory to therapy. *Behavior Therapy, 25,* 51-66.

Birchwood, M., Mason, R., MacMillan, F. & Healy, J. (1993). Depression, demoralization and control over psychotic illness: A comparison of depressed and non-depressed patients with a chronic psychosis. *Psychological Medicine, 23,* 387-395.

Carpenter, W. T. (2009). Anticipating DSM-V: Should psychosis risk become a diagnostic class? *Schizophrenia Bulletin, 35,* 841-843.

Cougnard, A., Marcelis, M., Myin-Germey, I., De Graaf, R., Vollenbergh, W., Krabbendam, L., Lieb, R., Wittchen, H. U., Henquet, C., Spauwen, J. & van Os, J. (2007). Does normal developmental expression of psychosis combine with environmental risk to cause persistence of psychosis? A psychosis proneness–persistence model. *Psychological Medicine, 37,* 513-527.

Cummings, J. L. (1985). Organic Delusions: Phenomenology, anatomic correlations, and review. *British Journal of Psychiatry, 146,* 184-197.

Chapman, J. P., Chapman, L. J., Raulin, M. L. & Eckblad, M. (1994). Putatively Psychosis-prone Subjects 10 years later. *Journal of Abnormal Psychology, 87,* 399-407.

De Loore, E., Gunther, N., Drukker, M., Feron, F., Sabbe, B., Deboutte, D., van Os, J. & Myin-Germeys, I. (2008). Auditory hallucinations in adolescence: A longitudinal general population study. *Schizophrenia Research, 102,* 229-230.

Dhossche, D., Ferdinand, R., van der Ende, J., Hofstra, M. B. & Verhulst, F. (2002). Diagnostic outcome of self-reported hallucinations in a community sample of adolescents. *Psychological Medicine, 32,* 619-627.

Dominguez, M. G., Wichers, M., Lieb, R., Wittchen, H.-U. & van Os, J. (in press). Evidence that onset of clinical psychosis is an outcome of progressively more persistent subclinical psychotic experiences: An 8-year cohort study. *Schizophrenia Bulletin,* doi:10.1093/schbul/sbp022

Fonseca-Pedrero, E., Lemos-Giráldez, S., Muñiz, J., García-Cueto, E. & Campillo-Álvarez, A. (2008). Schizotypy in adolescence: The role of gender and age. *Journal of Nervous and Mental Disease, 196,* 161-165.

Fonseca-Pedrero, E., Lemos-Giráldez, E., Paino, M., Villazón-García, U., Sierra-Baigrie, S. & Muñiz, J. (2009). Experiencias psicóticas atenuadas en población adolescente [Attenuated psychotic experiences in adolescents]. *Papeles del Psicólogo, 30,* 63-73.

Fonseca-Pedrero, E., Paíno-Piñeiro, M., Lemos-Giráldez, S., Villazón-García, U. & Muñiz, J. (2009). Validation of the Schizotypal Personality Questionnaire-Brief Form in adolescents. *Schizophrenia Research, 111,* 53-60.

Fonseca-Pedrero, E., Muñiz, J., Lemos-Giráldez, S., Paino, M. & Villazón-García, U. (2010). *ESQUIZO-Q: Cuestionario Oviedo para la Evaluación de la Esquizotipia [ESQUIZO-Q: Oviedo Questionnaire for Schizotypy Assessment]*. Madrid: TEA ediciones.

Freeman, D. (2007). Suspicious minds: The psychology of persecutory delusions. *Clinical Psychology Review, 27,* 425-457.

Freeman, D. & Fowler, D. (2009). Routes to psychotic symptoms: Trauma, anxiety and psychosis-like experiences. *Psychiatry Research, 169,* 107-112.

Freeman, D., Garety, P. & Fowler, D. (2008). The puzzle of paranoia. In D. Freeman, R. Bentall & P. Garety (Eds.), *Persecutory delusions: Assessment, theory, and treatment* (pp. 121-142). Oxford: Oxford University Press.

Frith, C. D. (1992). *The cognitive neuropsychology of schizophrenia*. Hove, UK: Erlbaum.

Garety, P. A., Kuipers, E., Fowler, D., Freeman, D. & Bebbington, P. E. (2001). A cognitive model of the positive symptoms of psychosis. *Psychological Medicine, 31,* 189-195.

Gazzaniga, M. S., Ivry, R. B. & Mangun, G. R. (1998). *Cognitive neuroscience: The biology of mind*. New York: Norton.

Goldman-Rakic, P. S. (1991). Prefrontal cortical dysfunction in schizophrenia: The relevance of working memory. In B. J. Carroll & J. E. Barrett (Eds.), *Psychopathology and the brain* (pp. 1-23). New York: Raven Press.

Gooding, D. C., Tallent, K. A. & Matts, C. W. (2005). Clinical status of at-risk individuals 5 years later: Further validation of the psychometric high-risk strategy. *Journal of Abnormal Psychology, 114,* 170-175.

Häfner, H. (1992). Epidemiology of schizophrenia. In F. P. Ferrero, A. E. Haynal & N. Sartorius (Eds.), *Schizophrenia and affective psychoses: Nosology in contemporary psychiatry* (pp. 221-236). London: John Libbey.

Hanssen, M., Bak, M., Bijl, R., Vollebergh, W. & Van Os, J. (2005). The incidence and outcome of subclinical psychotic experiences in the general population. *British Journal of Clinical Psychology, 44,* 181-191.

Hanssen, M., Krabbendam, L., de Graaf, R., Vollebergh, W. & van Os, J. (2005). Role of distress in delusion formation. *British Journal of Psychiatry, 187 (Suppl. 48),* s55-s58.

Hemsley, D. R. (1994). A cognitive model for schizophrenia and its possible neural basis. *Acta Psychiatrica Scandinavica, 90 (Suppl. 284),* 80-86.

Henquet, C., Di Forte, M., Murray, R. M. & Van Os, J. (2008). The role of cannabis in inducing paranoia and psychosis. In D. Freeman, R. Bentall & P. Garety (Eds.), *Persecutory delusions: Assessment, theory, and treatment* (pp. 267-280). Oxford: Oxford University Press.

Horwood, J., Salvi, G., Thomas, K., Duffy, L., Gunnell, D., Hollis, C., Lewis, G., Menezes, P., Thompson, A., Wolke, D., Zammit, S. & Harrison, G. (2008). IQ and non-clinical psychotic symptoms in 12-year-olds: results from the ALSPAC birth cohort. *British Journal of Psychiatry, 193,* 185-191.

Karimi, Z., Windmann, S., Gunturkun, O. & Abraham, A. (2007). Insight problem solving in individuals with high versus low schizotypy. *Journal of Research in Personality, 41,* 473-480.

Kelleher, I., Harley, M., Lynch, F., Arseneault, L., Fitzpatrick, C. & Cannon, M. (2008). Associations between childhood trauma, bullying and psychotic symptoms among a school-based adolescent sample. *British Journal of Psychiatry, 193,* 378-382.

Kelly, B. D., O'Callaghan, E., Waddington, J. L., Feeney, L., Browne, S., Scully, P. J., et al. (2010). Schizophrenia and the city: A review of literature and prospective study of psychosis and urbanicity in Ireland. *Schizophrenia Research, 116,* 75-89.

Krabbendam, L., Myin-Germeys, I., Bak, M. & van Os, J. (2005). Explaining transitions over the hypothesized psychosis continuum. *Australian and New Zealand Journal of Psychiatry, 39,* 180-186.

Larkin, W. & Morrison, A. P. (Eds.). (2006). *Trauma and psychosis: New directions for theory and therapy.* London: Routledge.

Lemos-Giráldez, S., Vallina-Fernández, O., Fernández-Iglesias, P., Vallejo-Seco, G., Fonseca-Pedrero, E., Paíno-Piñeiro, M., Sierra-Baigrie, S., García-Pelayo, P., Pedrejón-Molino, C., Alonso-Bada, S., Gutiérrez-Pérez, A. & Ortega-Ferrández, J. A. (2009). Symptomatic and functional outcome in youth at ultra-high risk for psychosis: A longitudinal study. *Schizophrenia Research, 115,* 121-129.

Lenzenweger, M. F. (2006). Schizotaxia, schizotypy, and schizophrenia: Paul E. Meehl's blueprint for the experimental psychopathology and genetics of schizophrenia. *Journal of Abnormal Psychology, 115,* 195-200.

Linscott, R. J. & Van Os, J. (2010). Systematic reviews of categorical versus continuum models in psychosis: Evidence for discontinuous subpopulations underlying a psychometric continuum. Implications for DSM-V, DSM-VI, and DSM-VII. *Annual Review of Clinical Psychology, 6,* 391-419.

Maher, B. A. (1992). Models and methods for the study of reasoning in delusions. European *Review of Applied Psychology/Revue Europeenne de Psychologie Appliquee, 42,* 97-104.

Maher, B. A. & Spitzer, M. (1993). Delusions. In C. G. Costello (Ed.), *Symptoms of schizophrenia* (pp. 92-120). New York: Wiley.

McCreery, C. & Claridge, G. (2002). Healthy schizotypy: The case of out-of-the-body experiences. *Personality and Individual Differences, 32,* 141-154.

Meehl, P. E. (1990). Toward an integrated theory of schizotaxia, schizotypy, and schizophrenia. *Journal of Personality Disorders, 4,* 1-99.

Morgan, C. & Fisher, H. (2007). Environment and schizophrenia: Environmental factors in schizophrenia: Childhood trauma -a critical review. *Schizophrenia Bulletin, 33,* 3-10.

Morrison, A. P., Haddock, G. & Tarrier, N. (1995). Intrusive thoughts and auditory hallucinations: A cognitive approach. *Behavioural and Cognitive Psychotherapy, 23,* 265-280.

Morrison, A. P., Wells, A. & Nothard, S. (2000). Cognitive factors in predisposition to auditory and visual hallucinations. *British Journal of Clinical Psychology, 39,* 67-78.

Nelson, B., Yung, A., Bechdolf, A. & McGorry, P. D. (2008). The phenomenological critique and self-disturbance: Implications for ultra-high risk ("prodrome") research. *Schizophrenia Bulletin, 34,* 381-392.

Nelson, B. & Yung, A. R. (2009). Psychotic-like experiences as overdetermined phenomena: When do they increase risk for psychotic disorder? *Schizophrenia Research, 108,* 303-304.

Nuechterlein, K. H. & Dawson, M. E. (1984). Information processing and attentional functioning in the developmental course of schizophrenic disorders. *Schizophrenia Bulletin, 10,* 160-203.

Posner, M. (1982). Cumulative development of attentional theory. *American Psychologist, 37,* 168-179.

Poulton, R., Caspi, A., Moffitt, T. E., Cannon, M., Murray, R. & Harrington, H. (2000). Children's self-reported psychotic symptoms and adult schizophreniform disorder: a 15-year longitudinal study. *Archives of General Psychiatry, 57,* 1053-1058.

Sass, L. A. (2003). Self-disturbance in schizophrenia: Hyperreflexivity and diminished self-affection. In T. Kircher & A. David (Eds.), *The self in neuroscience and psychiatry* (pp. 242-271). Cambridge, UK: Cambridge University Press.

Sass, L. A. & Parnas, J. (2003). Schizophrenia, consciousness, and the self. *Schizophrenia Bulletin, 29,* 427-444.

Scott, J., Chant, D., Andrews, G. & McGrath, J. (2006). Psychotic-like experiences in the general community: The correlates of CIDI psychosis screen items in an Australian sample. *Psychological Medicine, 36,* 231-238.

Scott, J., Martin, G., Bor, W., Sawyer, M., Clark, J. & McGrath, J. (2009). The prevalence and correlates of hallucinations in Australian adolescents: Results from a national survey. *Schizophrenia Research, 109,* 179-185.

Scott, J., Martin, G., Welham, J., Bor, W., Najman, J. & O'Callaghan, M. (2009). Psychopathology during childhood and adolescence predicts delusional-like experiences in adults: A 21-year birth cohort study. *American Journal of Psychiatry, 166,* 567-574.

Scott, J., Martin, G., Welham, J., Bor, W., Najman, J., O'Callaghan, M., Williams, G., Aird, R. & McGrath, J. (2009). Psychopathology during childhood and adolescence predicts delusional-like experiences in adults: A 21-year birth cohort study. *American Journal of Psychiatry, 166,* 567-574.

Scott, J., Welham, J., Martin, G., Bor, W., Najman, J., O' Callaghan, M., Williams, G., Aird, R. & McGrath, J. (2008). Demographic correlates of psychotic-like experiences in young Australian adults. *Acta Psychiatrica Scandinavica, 118,* 230-237.

Schiffman, J., Nakamura, B., Earleywine, M. & LaBrie, J. (2005). Symptoms of schizoypy precede cannabis use. *Psychiatry Research, 134,* 1429-1435.

Smith, B., Fowler, D. G., Freeman, D., Bebbington, P. E., Bashforth, A., Garety, P., Dunn, G. & Kuipers, E. (2006). Emotion and psychosis: Links between depression, self-esteem, negative schematic beliefs and delusions and hallucinations. *Schizophrenia Research, 86,* 181-188.

Spauwen, J., Krabbendam, L., Lieb, R., Wittchen, H. U. & van Os, J. (2006). Evidence that the outcome of developmental expression of psychosis is worse for adolescents growing up in an urban environment. *Psychological Medicine, 36,* 407-415.

Tien, A. Y. (1991). Distributions of hallucinations in the population. *Social Psychiatry and Psychiatric Epidemiology, 26,* 287-292.

van Os, J., Hanssen, M., Bak, M., Bijl, R. V. & Vollebergh, W. (2003). Do urbanicity and familial liability coparticipate in causing psychosis? *American Journal of Psychiatry, 160,* 477-482.

van Os, J., Hanssen, M., Bijl, R. V. & Ravelli, A. (2000). Strauss (1969) revisited: A psychosis continuum in the general population? *Schizophrenia Research, 45,* 11-20.

van Os, J., Linscott, R. J., Myin-Germeys, I., Delespaul, P. & Krabbendam, L. (2009). A systematic review and meta-analysis of the psychosis continuum: Evidence for a psychosis proneness-persistence-impairment model of psychotic disorder. *Psychological Medicine, 39,* 179-195.

van Os, J. & Poulton, R. (2009). Environmental vulnerability and genetic-environmental interactions. In H. J. Jackson & P. D. McGorry (Eds.), *The recognition and management of early psychosis: A preventive approach (2nd.ed.)* (pp. 47-59). Cambridge, UK: Cambridge University Press.

Verdoux, H. & van Os, J. (2002). Psychotic symptoms in non-clinical populations and the continuum of psychosis. *Schizophrenia Research, 54,* 59-65.

Verdoux, H., van Os, J. & Maurice-Tison, S. (1999). Increased occurrence of depression in psychosis-prone subjects: A follow-up study in primary care Settings. *Comprehensive Psychiatry, 40,* 462-468.

Weiser, M. & Noy, S. (2005). Interpreting the association between cannabis use and increased risk for schizophrenia. *Dialogues in Clinical Neuroscience, 7,* 81-85.

Welham, J., Scott, J., Williams, G., Najman, J., Bor, W., O'Callaghan, M. & McGrath, J. (2009). Emotional and behavioural antecedents of young adults who screen positive for non-affective psychosis: a 21-year birth cohort study. *Psychological Medicine, 39,* 625-634.

Wigman, J. T. W., Vollebergh, W. A. M., Raaijmakers, Q. A. W., Iedema, J., van Dorsselaer, S., Ormel, J., Verhulst, F. C. & van Os, J. (in press). The structure of the extended psychosis phenotype in early adolescence--A cross-sample replication. *Schizophrenia Bulletin*, doi: 10.1093/schbul/sbp154

Woods, S. W., Addington, J., Cadenhead, K. S., Cannon, T. D., Cornblatt, B. A., Heinssen, R., Perkins, D. O., Seidman, L. J., Tsuang, M. T., Walker, E. F. & McGlashan, T. H. (2009). Validity of the prodromal risk syndrome for first psychosis: Findings from the North American prodrome longitudinal study. *Schizophrenia Bulletin, 35,* 894-908.

Yoshizumi, T., Murase, S., Honjo, S., Kanedo, H. & Murakami, T. (2004). Hallucinatory experiences in a comunity sample of Japanese children. *Journal of American Academy of Child and Adolescent Psychiatry, 43,* 1030-1036.

Young, H. F., Bentall, R. P., Slade, P. D. & Dewey, M. E. (1986). Disposition towards hallucination, gender and IQ scores. *Personality and Individual Differences, 7,* 247-249.

Yung, A. R., Yuen, H. P., Berger, G., Francey, S., Hung, T., Nelson, B., et al. (2007). Declining transition rate in ultra high risk (prodromal) services: Dilution or reduction of risk? *Schizophrenia Bulletin, 33,* 673-681.

Yung, A. R., Nelson, B., Baker, K., Buckby, J. A., Baksheev, G. & Cosgrave, E. M. (2009). Psychotic-like experiences in a community sample of adolescents: Implications for the continuum model of psychosis and prediction of schizophrenia. *Australian and New Zealand Journal of Psychiatry, 43,* 118-128.

In: Hallucinations: Types, Stages and Treatments
Editor: Meredith S. Payne, pp. 147-161
ISBN: 978-1-61728-275-1
© 2011 Nova Science Publishers, Inc.

Chapter 8

Nonpharmacological Inhibition of Cerebral Dopaminergic Activity May Be an Option for Medication-Resistant Hallucinations

Nikolai A. Shevchuk
BioTest LLC, Novosibirsk, Russia

Abstract

Some percentage of patients experience hallucinations that are not responsive to different classes of neuroleptic drugs and to electroconvulsive therapy. Interestingly, some nonpharmacological treatments can inhibit dopaminergic activity in the brain and produce physiological effects that are similar to those of neuroleptic medication, suggesting that these approaches may potentially be useful as a therapeutic option for medication-resistant hallucinations. Two examples are temporary hyperthermia and low-protein diets.

A temporary increase in core body temperature via external heating, such as immersion in hot water (39-40 degrees Celsius), can increase the plasma and brain level of serotonin and the plasma level of prolactin. Hyperthermia typically induces fatigue and can cause lethargy and loss of motivation. All of these changes are consistent with increased serotonergic and reduced dopaminergic activity in the brain. It is also noteworthy that cerebral serotonergic neurons, for the most part, have inhibitory projections to dopaminergic neurons.

Low-protein diets lower the plasma levels of tyrosine and phenylalanine, which are metabolic precursors of cerebral dopamine. Experiments on laboratory rats have shown that low-protein diets can lower the total concentration of dopamine in the striatum and reduce the density of dopamine D2 receptors in this brain region. Low protein diets are also known to impair the coping ability of laboratory animals in experimental models of depression such as Porsolt swim test. These changes are consistent with reduced dopaminergic activity in the brain and are similar to the effects of neuroleptic drugs. It should be noted that neuroleptics inhibit most dopamine receptors and tend to reduce dopaminergic transmission overall, although these drugs typically cause a compensatory increase in the density of D2 receptors and a temporary increase in the level of extracellular dopamine due to inhibition of presynaptic D2 receptors.

The two aforementioned treatments cannot be used on a permanent basis, but each of them can be used intermittently, for example, 30-minutes of whole-body hyperthermia per day or alternation of one week of very-low-protein diet with two weeks of a balanced diet. Although the proposed treatments are temporary, they may produce lasting changes in the dopaminergic system due to neural plasticity. Clinical effectiveness of these approaches is currently unknown. The dietary approach is likely to be safe to use in combination with pharmacotherapy, whereas hyperthermic treatments are known to be dangerous for patients taking neuroleptics.

Introduction

Hallucinations, particularly auditory hallucinations (the person is "hearing voices," often unpleasant and derogatory voices), are among the most typical symptoms of a psychotic episode as defined in the Diagnostic and Statistical Manual of Mental Disorders [1]. Hallucinations can also occur during a manic episode [1] and in some organic brain disorders such as Parkinson's disease [2]. In the context of the diagnosis of schizophrenia, hallucinations belong to the category of "positive symptoms," as do bizarre delusions and disorganization of thought/speech [3]. The adjective "positive" here means that these symptoms "add something new," so to speak, to the symptomatology of a patient, while the so-called "negative symptoms," namely, emotional blunting, social withdrawal, poverty of thought, and demotivation, "subtract," as it were, from existing personal qualities of a patient. Aside from the positive and negative symptoms, there is another category, namely, "cognitive symptoms" of schizophrenia, which include deficits in attention and short-term memory. Patients diagnosed with schizophrenia do not always experience hallucinations; however, the existing biological theories of hallucinations overlap to a large extent with the existing theories of schizophrenia [4]. Etiology of schizophrenia is believed to involve an unknown combination of genetic and environmental factors [5]. Several factors of small effect may collectively contribute to the development of the illness, while no single factor has a strong causal association with schizophrenia [5]. Particularly, no single gene has been shown to cause schizophrenia so far, while large groups of genes may be associated more strongly with this disorder [6]. It is noteworthy that brain imaging studies found some abnormalities in the brain structure of schizophrenic patients, but these deviations are relatively small, on average, and fall within the normal range [5]. Therefore, brain imaging, genetic analyses, and other laboratory tests cannot be used to diagnose schizophrenia at the time of this writing and this disorder is currently diagnosed using a special questionnaire and a clinical interview.

Hallucinations can also be caused by detectable physical changes in the brain, such as those that occur during Parkinson's disease, Alzheimer's or other neurodegenerative diseases. The former disorder is characterized by a progressive loss of dopaminergic neurons that project to the striatum and some patients with Parkinson's present with hallucinations [2].

Several theories regarding pathophysiology of hallucinations have been proposed in the last half century [4]. The "dopamine hypothesis of psychosis" is one of the few theories that have been widely applied to the development of therapeutic agents during that past two decades. This theory derives from a serendipitous finding that drugs which block dopamine

D2 receptors can reduce hallucinations and other psychotic symptoms in schizophrenic patients [7]. Conversely, drugs that increase extracellular level of dopamine in the brain such as cocaine and amphetamine, when administered at high doses, can cause positive symptoms of schizophrenia (e.g. delusions and hallucinations) in healthy people [8]. According to the dopamine hypothesis, schizophrenia may be associated with increased sensitivity of dopamine D2 receptors in the striatum [8]. Therefore, pharmacological antagonists of D2 receptors would be expected to reduce psychotic symptoms. Traditional antipsychotic drugs such as haloperidol and chlorpromazine are believed to exert their action through this mechanism and these pharmacological agents can significantly reduce positive symptoms (including hallucinations) in up to 60% of schizophrenic patients without causing significant sedation [5,9]. Serious concerns have been raised about the side effects of chronic administration of the traditional antipsychotics, which may include motor abnormalities such as akathisia, bradykinesia, tremor, tardive dyskenisia and muscle rigidity (so-called extrapyramidal symptoms) as well as neuroleptic malignant syndrome (hyperthermia, delirium, unstable vital signs, rigidity) [9]. The motor side effects are thought to result from the blockade of dopamine D2 receptors in the basal ganglia (located in the dorsal striatum) which are involved in the regulation of the motor function. The peculiarity of extrapyramidal symptoms is that they often persist even after withdrawal from antipsychotic drugs [9].

The dopamine theory of psychosis was updated in the last two decades in order to explain the role of serotonin 5-HT2A receptors in the pathophysiology of psychosis as well as the clinical effectiveness of the newer generation of "atypical" antipsychotics, which have a relatively low affinity for dopamine D2 receptors and a stronger inhibitory effect on 5-HT2A receptors [8,9]. It was found some time ago that many hallucinogens (e.g., mescaline and lysergic acid diethylamide) stimulate serotonin 5-HT2A receptors in the brain, and their psychotogenic effects can be blocked by 5-HT2A antagonists [10]. Unfortunately, selective 5-HT2A antagonists do not reduce hallucinations in schizophrenia and neurodegenerative disorders and it is currently believed that clinically effective antipsychotic drugs must have a significant inhibitory effect on 5-HT2A receptors and at the same time exert a moderate-to-weak inhibitory effect on dopamine D2 receptors [5,10]. This sort of antipsychotic agents, which exert dual action by inhibiting dopamine D2 and serotonin 5-HT2A receptors, are expected to cause a lower incidence of dopamine-related side effects compared to the typical antipsychotics such as haloperidol. The atypical antipsychotic drugs such as clozapine, olanzapine and risperidone, which fit the above pharmacodynamic criteria, indeed have a significantly lower risk of extrapyramidal symptoms at clinically effective doses [5,9].

Clozapine seems to stand out among other atypical antipsychotics with respect to its high clinical effectiveness: a high percentage of patients who do not respond to either traditional or atypical antipsychotics seem to benefit from clozapine and the mechanism of this effect is unknown [5,9]. Additionally, clozapine can improve negative symptoms in some patients, while most neuroleptics (both traditional and atypical) have little or no effect on negative symptoms of schizophrenia [5]. At present, clozapine is the only proven treatment for hallucinations in patients with Parkinson's disease [11]. Incidentally, the affinity of clozapine for dopamine D2 receptors is approximately 10-fold lower than that of haloperidol and clozapine's occupancy of striatal D2 receptors is some 2 to 3 times lower than that of haloperidol at clinically effective doses [10,12]. It has been hypothesized that the anomalous effectiveness of clozapine may have to do with its simultaneous inhibition of a broad range of dopaminergic (D1, D2, D3, D4), serotonergic (5-HT2A, 5-HT2C, possibly 5-HT3 and 5-HT6, plus partial agonism of 5-HT1A) receptors plus its interaction with some adrenergic, cholinergic and histamine receptors [13].

The latest generation of atypical antipsychotics is represented by aripiprazole, which is a partial agonist of the dopamine D2 receptor and can inhibit its function when the receptor is in its active conformation, but will stimulate the receptor in the inactive conformation [3]. These dual properties of aripiprazole are expected to improve both positive and some negative symptoms of schizophrenia, with low risk of dopaminergic side effects [3]. Recent systematic reviews suggest that aripiprazole is not more clinically effective than typical antipsychotics, but causes fewer extrapyramidal symptoms and overall seems to be tolerated better than the typical antipsychotics, however the risk of dizziness and nausea is higher with aripiprazole [14]. It should be pointed out that the risk of extrapyramidal symptoms and neuroleptic malignant syndrome is not eliminated completely with the atypical antipsychotic drugs and these agents can cause adverse effects that are seldom observed with the traditional neuroleptics: clozapine can cause hematotoxicity (agranulocytosis), while other atypical antipsychotics (as well as clozapine) can cause rapid weight gain and type II diabetes [9]. As mentioned above, most of the traditional and atypical antipsychotics are effective against positive symptoms, but have little or no effect on negative and cognitive symptoms of schizophrenia, which is one of the shortcomings of the dopamine hypothesis [15]. A large percentage of schizophrenic patients (up to 40%) do not respond to treatment with most known antipsychotics [16]. Another drawback of the dopamine hypothesis is that genetic studies of schizophrenic patients failed to identify any genes that are specifically related to dopamine or D2 receptors with the exception of the gene encoding catechol-o-methyl transferase (COMT), an enzyme that is not specific to dopamine and is involved in degradation of other catecholamines, such as adrenaline and noradrenaline [6,17]. The aforementioned genetic studies identified a couple dozen genes that may be associated with schizophrenia and many of these genes have to do with GABAergic and glutamatergic systems in the brain, which is the subject of the latest major theory of schizophrenia, as discussed next [6,17].

The newer perspective on the pathophysiology of schizophrenia is reflected in the n-methyl-d-aspartate (NMDA) receptor hypofunction theory of schizophrenia. This hypothesis was formulated based on the observation that NMDA receptor antagonists such as ketamine and phencyclidine (PCP) can cause both positive (hallucinations) and negative symptoms of schizophrenia in healthy subjects [15]. In contrast, dopaminergic drugs such as amphetamine and cocaine can reproduce only positive symptoms (and few or no negative symptoms) in humans and laboratory animals, as was mentioned above [15]. NMDA receptors are glutamate receptors located mostly postsynaptically and they are thought to play a major role in learning and memory because they are involved in mechanisms of long-term potentiation. The possible involvement of NMDA receptors in schizophrenia was puzzling at first because the behavioral symptoms induced by NMDA antagonists seemed at odds with the known function of these receptors [17]. It was later found that NMDA receptors mediate excitatory postsynaptic potentials on dendrites of inhibitory GABAergic neurons known as fast-spiking interneurons [17]. Lisman and colleagues have recently proposed a circuit-based model according to which, the fast-spiking interneurons have inhibitory projections onto pyramidal cells (glutamatergic neurons with excitatory output), which are mostly located in the cortex and hippocampus [17]. The inhibitory fast-spiking interneurons are thought to be involved in the homeostatic regulation of the activity pyramidal cells via a negative feedback loop: the pyramidal cells have projections to the fast-spiking interneurons and these synapses (many of them contain NMDA receptors) may serve as "sensors" of the level of activity of pyramidal cells [17]. Inhibition of NMDA receptors by PCP in this system would be expected to destabilize the feedback regulation and cause excessive activity of pyramidal cells (via disinhibition), possibly leading to hallucinations and other psychotic symptoms. Experiments on laboratory animals indeed show that administration of PCP or ketamine can increase disorganized spiking activity of glutamatergic neurons projecting to the prefrontal cortex and this was determined both by measuring the glutamate efflux and by electrophysiological methods [18]. NMDA receptors are known to enhance glutamatergic transmission (via long-term potentiation) and their main ligand is glutamate, therefore it would seem that blockade of NMDA receptors should logically reduce glutamate signaling [19], but experimental data suggest that NMDA antagonists actually cause a hyperglutamatergic state at least in discrete regions of the brain [20]. Deficiencies in the signaling/metabolism of GABA (gamma-aminobutyric acid) in the fast-spiking interneurons would also be expected to contribute to psychotic symptoms according to the above model [17], and genetic linkage studies of schizophrenia have indeed identified a number of genes relevant to the GABAergic system [6].

There may also be a connection between the theorized dysregulation of the glutamate system on the one hand and the dopaminergic abnormalities in the striatum that form the basis of the dopamine hypothesis on the other hand [17]. In particular, some studies have shown that NMDA antagonists (hallucinogens such as ketamine and PCP) can increase extracellular dopamine in the striatum and there may exist another feedback loop between hippocampal pyramidal cells and dopaminergic neurons of the ventral tegmental area [21]. The readers can find an excellent review of this topic in a recent article by Lisman *et al* [17].

Various therapeutic approaches aimed at enhancing NMDA receptor function have been tested in clinical studies and the data show that these treatments can significantly reduce negative symptoms and improve cognitive symptoms in schizophrenic patients, but, unfortunately, the effect on positive symptoms is either modest or non-existent [5,19]. Since direct glutamate agonists would be excitotoxic, the above strategies are based on stimulation of NMDA receptors via an obligatory co-activator site on these receptors, which is known as a "glycine modulatory site" [19]. Activation of the NMDA receptor requires three events to occur simultaneously: 1) binding of a glutamate molecule, 2) binding of a molecule of glycine or D-serine to the glycine modulatory site, and 3) depolarization of the postsynaptic membrane [22]. Glycine reuptake inhibitors and glycine agonists such as glycine itself, d-serine, and d-cycloserine have all been shown to be effective for negative and some cognitive symptoms of schizophrenia as mentioned above, and may be beneficial as a supplementary treatment [22].

Until recently, it's been widely believed that D2 receptor inhibitory activity is absolutely mandatory for a neuroleptic drug to be clinically effective [7]. An intriguing development several years ago was the discovery of a prospective antipsychotic agent (LY404039) that has no activity at any known dopamine receptors [23]. This compound is a selective agonist of type II metabotropic glutamate receptors (mGluR2 and mGluR3) and was originally developed as a candidate antianxiety agent, since it can reduce synaptic release of glutamate. The finding that a gene called GRM3, which encodes mGluR3, is linked to schizophrenia, as well as animal studies, which showed that LY404039 can reverse many of the behavioral effects of PCP in a mouse model of schizophrenia, prompted Patil and colleagues to conduct a clinical study of an oral prodrug (LY2140023) in schizophrenic patients [23]. That study showed that this drug can reduce positive symptoms in patients almost as effectively as olanzapine (an atypical antipsychotic), but can also improve negative symptoms. The preliminary data suggest that LY2140023 does not produce extrapyramidal symptoms, weight gain or hyperprolactinemia, which can be caused by typical and atypical antipsychotics [23]. The mechanism of action of LY404039 may seem to contradict the NMDA receptor hypofunction hypothesis of schizophrenia, since the drug tends to downregulate synaptic release of glutamate (the main agonist of NMDA receptors). Nonetheless, several studies have shown that administration of NMDA antagonists (as a model of schizophrenia) appears to cause a hyperglutamatergic state in some brain regions as was already mentioned above [21], and therefore attenuation of glutamate efflux via stimulation of mGluR2/3 would be expected to reduce psychotic symptoms [24-26]. In particular, studies in laboratory animals have shown that mGluR2/3 agonists can reduce cortical glutamate efflux caused by PCP or 5-HT2A agonists (hallucinogens) as well as inhibit dopamine release in the nucleus accumbens (ventral striatum) [24,25]. Additionally, one study showed that mGluR2/3 agonists can enhance NMDA receptor-associated postsynaptic currents in the prefrontal cortex, suggesting that these pharmacological agents can enhance NMDA receptor function in some brain regions [26]. In summary, both stimulation of mGlu2/3 receptors and enhancement of NMDA receptor function by means of glycine modulatory site agonists are novel and promising approaches to the treatment of schizophrenia and further research is necessary. The manufacturer of LY2140023, Eli Lilly, Inc. announced in April 2009 that the second trial of this compound in schizophrenia failed to show clinical benefits that are greater than the placebo effect. Further research will be needed. To summarize, pharmacological agents that act on the dopamine D2 receptors are currently the only proven type of neuroleptic drugs [5].

It is worth mentioning that there are nonpharmacological treatments for hallucinations, such as electroconvulsive therapy, repetitive transcranial magnetic stimulation (rTMS), and psychotherapy. Recent systematic reviews suggest that electroconvulsive therapy and rTMS can be beneficial [27], while cognitive-behavioral therapy is not effective against positive symptoms of schizophrenia (delusions, hallucinations and thought disorder) [28]. Among other possible nonpharmacological treatments, dietary interventions are somewhat similar in their mode of action to the pharmacological approach and, in theory, a specially designed diet could be beneficial in psychosis. At present, dietary interventions that have a proven neuroleptic effect are unknown.

This article discusses a dietary intervention and a physical treatment that may produce some of the physiological effects of neuroleptic agents that were discussed above. Hyperthermia (increased core body temperature) produces some biological effects that are similar to those of neuroleptic drugs, such as loss of motivation and hyperprolactinemia. Additionally, literature suggests that radical dietary changes can be used successfully for the treatment of some brain disorders: for example, a ketogenic diet (high-fat, protein-normal, low-carbohydrate) has been shown to be beneficial for patients with treatment-refractory epilepsy [29,30]. Recent studies suggest that a restrictive elimination diet can be effective in the treatment of attention deficit hyperactivity disorder (ADHD) [31]. Interestingly, several studies have shown that low-protein diets (and, to a lesser extent, low-fat diets) can affect the level of dopamine, serotonin, glycine, the density of dopamine D2 receptors and dopamine transporter (DAT), as well as synaptic release of glutamate in the brain as discussed in more detail below. Therefore, low-protein or protein-free diets may have psychoactive properties that may be useful for the treatment of hallucinations. The arguments presented below attempt to show that repeated hyperthermia and a temporary protein-free diet produce effects that are similar to those of neuroleptic drugs and therefore these nonpharmacological treatments could be beneficial for patients who do not respond to existing types of neuroleptic medication. This is because patients respond differently to different classes of neuroleptic drugs and even to different drugs within the same class.

Rationale for a Temporary Protein-Free Diet

a) Some studies showed that low-protein diets can increase the plasma and brain levels of glycine without changing the levels of glutamate [32-35]. This can stimulate the activity of n-methyl-d-aspartate (NMDA) receptors and may have a therapeutic effect on negative symptoms of schizophrenia in accordance with the NMDA hypofunction hypothesis of schizophrenia [19].

b) One report showed that a low-protein diet can reduce the density of dopamine D2 receptors in the striatum of rats [36] and also reduce the total tissue level of dopamine in this brain region and in the ventral tegmental area [79]. The sensitivity of D2 receptors was not changed in that experiment. Restriction of dietary protein in humans can reduce the level of homovanillic acid, a major metabolite of dopamine, in the cerebrospinal fluid, which can be interpreted as reduced dopaminergic activity in the brain [37]. Additionally, a low-protein diet was shown to worsen coping behavior in an animal model of depression, the Porsolt swim test [38]. These alterations are suggestive of reduced dopaminergic activity in the brain and bear a resemblance to the effects of neuroleptic drugs. Most antipsychotic drugs inhibit activity of many dopamine receptors (D1, D2, D3, and D4) but their neuroleptic effect is attributed to the antagonism of cerebral dopamine D2 receptor. Neuroleptics also promote behavioral despair (worsen coping behavior) in the animal models of depression [39]. Neuroleptic drugs are also known to appreciably lower mood in human subjects within hours [40,41]. One possible problem with the argument outlined above is that neuroleptic drugs tend to increase the density of dopamine D2 receptors [42,43], and they can elevate extracellular dopamine in the relevant brain regions by inhibiting presynaptic D2 receptors [44,45]. Nevertheless, in general, neuroleptics downregulate cerebral dopamine activity via inhibition of postsynaptic dopamine receptors [46].

c) In primates, reduction of dietary protein intake can decrease the synthesis and turnover of serotonin in the brain [47]. The inhibition of both dopaminergic and serotonergic transmission in the brain by a low-protein diet may be similar to the effects of clozapine. This drug inhibits several serotonin receptors (5-HT2A, 5-HT2C, and possibly 5-HT3 and 5-HT6 [13,48-52]) and dopamine receptors (D1, D3, and D4) in addition to its moderate inhibition of D2 receptor function [13,53-56].

d) Manipulations of dietary fat have been reported to change the density of D2 receptors as well as the density of the dopamine transporter in the striatum in laboratory animals [57,58]. This observation suggests that a low-fat diet may affect the activity of the dopamine system in the brain.

e) Low-protein, low-fat, high-carbohydrate diets are rather common among mammals. Although the closest genetic relatives of humans among primates are omnivores, there are some primate species that are frugivores [59,60].

A good example of a low-protein diet is the fruit-and-vegetable diet. It contains very low amounts of fat and protein and can be considered an ancestral diet of primates [59,60]. The quality of protein in this diet is low too [61-63]. For this reason, the fruit-and-vegetable diet can be considered a "protein-free diet." For the purposes of the proposed experiment, this diet should exclude protein-rich plant foods such as nuts, grains, and legumes. This author's unpublished personal observations suggest that pungent vegetables such as garlic, onion, and horseradish may increase irritability in the context of this diet and may have to be excluded too. Up to 90% of the fruits and vegetables in this diet can be cooked at moderate temperature (by boiling or steaming). All food additives, salad dressings, and other seasonings will be excluded from the fruit-and-vegetable diet in order to facilitate interpretation of the psychotropic effects of this approach.

This author (a healthy subject) has tested the fruit-and-vegetable diet extensively on himself, but since he has never been diagnosed with a psychotic disorder, it is unknown if this approach can be effective as a neuroleptic treatment. In principle, it appears that the dietary and pharmacological approaches are not mutually exclusive and could be combined if necessary. It must be noted that the high-carbohydrate diet such as the one described above can be problematic for patients with diabetes.

Rationale for Repeated Hyperthermia

It is possible that intermittent hyperthermia has an antipsychotic effect because this approach is expected to have some neurobiological effects that are similar to those of neuroleptic drugs. It should be mentioned that hyperthermia carries a risk of serious side effects, especially when combined with neuroleptic medication. The prospective participants in this kind of clinical trial should consult with their doctor about the safety of this approach, especially participants who have a chronic medical condition and/or take any medication.

i. The dopamine system in the brain serves many functions including regulation of mood. Dopamine reuptake inhibitors such as cocaine and amphetamine can quickly elevate mood [64,65], while dopamine antagonists such as neuroleptic drugs can lower mood within hours [40,41]). Exposure to heat can quickly lower mood [66,67] possibly because this treatment inhibits dopamine activity in the brain as explained below. The mood recovers within about 60 minutes after exposure to heat is discontinued [66,67].

ii. Hyperthermia can increase the level of serotonin and serotonergic activity in the brain judging by the elevation of plasma prolactin in humans [68] and direct measurements in the brains of rodents [69,70]. The plasma concentration of prolactin is negatively regulated by dopaminergic neurons and positively regulated by serotonergic neurons [71,72]. Serotonergic neurons largely inhibit the activity of dopaminergic neurons in the mesolimbic pathway [73]. Therefore, it is possible that hyperthermia inhibits cerebral dopamine activity. Inhibition of dopaminergic activity in the brain may be beneficial during hallucinations because the widely accepted theory of psychosis (dopamine hypothesis of schizophrenia) suggests that hallucinations and other psychotic symptoms can be caused by hyperfunction of the dopaminergic system.

iii. As mentioned above, neuroleptic drugs can lower mood [40,41] and tend to inhibit dopaminergic activity in the brain; these drugs can also raise the level of prolactin in blood plasma [71,72]. It is noteworthy that antipsychotic drugs can affect thermoregulation: one of the rare side effects of these drugs is neuroleptic malignant syndrome, which often includes the symptom of dangerously high body temperature (hyperthermia).

iv. In the past, antipsychotic drugs were often referred to as "major tranquilizers." This name implies that these drugs can tranquilize the most agitated and violent patients. Hyperthermia may also be effective as a "major tranquilizer" because high core body temperature can cause disabling fatigue and loss of motivation [74,75].

Practical aspects of using hyperthermia warrant some elaboration. Hyperthermia does not have to be maintained constantly and a temporary hyperthermia that is repeated daily (let's say, 30 minutes per day) may be effective. A convenient way to increase core body temperature is a hot bath or immersion in hot water up to the neck. This author's unpublished observations suggest that hyperthermia can induce temporary disabling fatigue if core body temperature reaches 39°C. One possible problem with hot baths is that if the temperature is relatively high (42-43°C), then this treatment can inhibit the function of T lymphocytes [76,77], i.e. it may negatively affect the immune system (blood carrying T lymphocytes passes through the overheated epidermis). Another potential problem is skin irritation if the water is too hot. Thus, the high temperature of water can induce hyperthermia relatively quickly (within 30 minutes), but may cause immunosuppression and skin irritation if it is used on a daily basis. Thus, a slower protocol may be safer. For example, water temperature can be set to 39.5°C in a bath and vigorous (automatic) stirring of water may accelerate body heating. The author (a healthy subject) did some self-experimentation with hyperthermia, but since he does not have a history of hallucinations (or psychotic disorders in general), it is currently unknown if this approach can be effective in psychosis. As mentioned above, the hyperthermia treatment cannot be combined with neuroleptic medication because this combination is unsafe [75].

Testing

An intermittent fruit-and-vegetable diet can be tested in a clinical trial with schizophrenic patients with controls who take a proven neuroleptic treatment such as olanzapine. The effectiveness of these two treatments can be compared using a symptom rating scale such as PANSS. Sample size requirements can be calculated using PASS software [78] (equivalency study design). The possible intermittent schedule of the diet can be as follows: one week of the protein-free diet, followed by two weeks of a balanced diet, then the cycle repeats and ends with one week of the protein-free diet during week 7. Although the protein-free diet is used only intermittently, it may have lasting effects on the dopaminergic system due to neuronal plasticity.

Sessions of hyperthermia (30 minutes, 39°C core body temperature) once or twice a day can be compared to a proven neuroleptic treatment as described in the previous paragraph, except that hyperthermic treatments would be performed every day for 7 weeks.

Conclusion

At present, clinical effectiveness of the repeated hyperthermia and temporary protein-free diet is unknown. The theoretical evidence presented above suggests that these treatments may be effective against hallucinations and further research will be needed to test these ideas.

Acknowledgments

No extramural funding was used for preparation of this manuscript and the author declares that he has no conflicts of interest with respect to the contents of this publication.

References

[1] American Psychiatric Association: *Diagnostic and Statistical Manual of Mental Disorders*, 4th ed., text revision.; 2000.
[2] Goetz, CG; Fan, W; Leurgans, S. Antipsychotic medication treatment for mild hallucinations in Parkinson's disease: Positive impact on long-term worsening. *Mov Disord*, 2008 vol. 23, 1541-1545.
[3] Hirose, T; Kikuchi, T. Aripiprazole, a novel antipsychotic agent: dopamine D2 receptor partial agonist. *J Med Invest*, 2005, vol. 52, 284-290.
[4] Ertugrul, A; Rezaki, M. The neurobiology of hallucinations. *Turk Psikiyatri Derg*, 2005, vol. 16, 268-275.
[5] Tandon, R; Keshavan, MS; Nasrallah, HA. Schizophrenia, "Just the Facts": what we know in 2008 part 1: overview. *Schizophr Res*, 2008, vol. 100, 4-19.
[6] Sullivan, PF. Schizophrenia genetics: the search for a hard lead. *Curr Opin Psychiatry*, 2008, vol. 21, 157-160.
[7] Weinberger, DR. Schizophrenia drug says goodbye to dopamine. *Nat Med*, 2007, vol. 13, 1018-1019.
[8] Meisenzahl, EM; Schmitt, GJ; Scheuerecker, J; Moller, HJ. The role of dopamine for the pathophysiology of schizophrenia. *Int Rev Psychiatry*, 2007, vol. 19, 337-345.
[9] Gardner, DM; Baldessarini, RJ; Waraich, P. Modern antipsychotic drugs: a critical overview. *CMAJ*, 2005, vol. 172, 1703-1711.
[10] Meltzer, HY; Li, Z; Kaneda, Y; Ichikawa, J. Serotonin receptors: their key role in drugs to treat schizophrenia. *Prog Neuropsychopharmacol Biol Psychiatry*, 2003, vol. 27, 1159-1172.

[11] Diederich, NJ; Fenelon, G; Stebbins, G; Goetz, CG. Hallucinations in Parkinson disease. *Nat Rev Neurol*, 2009, vol. 5, 331-342.

[12] Millan, MJ. Improving the treatment of schizophrenia: focus on serotonin (5-HT)(1A) receptors. *J Pharmacol Exp Ther*, 2000, vol. 295, 853-861.

[13] Theisen, FM; Haberhausen, M; Firnges, MA; Gregory, P; Reinders, JH; Remschmidt, H; Hebebrand, J; Antel, J. No evidence for binding of clozapine, olanzapine and/or haloperidol to selected receptors involved in body weight regulation. *Pharmacogenomics J*, 2007, vol. 7, 275-281.

[14] Bhattacharjee, J; El-Sayeh, HG. Aripiprazole versus typical antipsychotic drugs for schizophrenia. *Cochrane Database Syst Rev*, 2008, CD006617.

[15] Coyle, JT. Glutamate and schizophrenia: beyond the dopamine hypothesis. *Cell Mol Neurobiol*, 2006, vol. 26, 365-384.

[16] Solanki, RK; Singh, P; Munshi, D. Current perspectives in the treatment of resistant schizophrenia. *Indian J Psychiatry*, 2009, vol. 51, 254-260.

[17] Lisman, JE; Coyle, JT; Green, RW; Javitt, DC; Benes, FM; Heckers, S; Grace, AA. Circuit-based framework for understanding neurotransmitter and risk gene interactions in schizophrenia. *Trends Neurosci*, 2008, vol. 31, 234-242.

[18] Jackson, ME; Homayoun, H; Moghaddam, B. NMDA receptor hypofunction produces concomitant firing rate potentiation and burst activity reduction in the prefrontal cortex. *Proc Natl Acad Sci*, U S A, 2004 vol. 101, 8467-8472.

[19] Shim, SS; Hammonds, MD; Kee, BS. Potentiation of the NMDA receptor in the treatment of schizophrenia: focused on the glycine site. *Eur Arch Psychiatry Clin Neurosci*, 2008 vol. 258, 16-27.

[20] Moghaddam, B; Adams, B; Verma, A; Daly, D. Activation of glutamatergic neurotransmission by ketamine: a novel step in the pathway from NMDA receptor blockade to dopaminergic and cognitive disruptions associated with the prefrontal cortex. *J Neurosci*, 1997, vol. 17, 2921-2927.

[21] Vollenweider, FX; Vontobel, P; Oye, I; Hell, D; Leenders, KL. Effects of (S)-ketamine on striatal dopamine: a [11C]raclopride PET study of a model psychosis in humans. *J Psychiatr Res*, 2000, vol. 34, 35-43.

[22] Stahl, SM. Novel therapeutics for schizophrenia: targeting glycine modulation of NMDA glutamate receptors. *CNS Spectr*, 2007, vol. 12, 423-427.

[23] Patil, ST; Zhang, L; Martenyi, F; Lowe, SL; Jackson, KA; Andreev, BV; Avedisova, AS; Bardenstein, LM; Gurovich, IY; Morozova, MA; Mosolov, SN; Neznanov, NG; Reznik, AM; Smulevich, AB; Tochilov, VA; Johnson, BG; Monn, JA; Schoepp, DD. Activation of mGlu2/3 receptors as a new approach to treat schizophrenia: a randomized Phase 2 clinical trial. *Nat Med*, 2007, vol. 13, 1102-1107.

[24] Hu, G; Duffy, P; Swanson, C; Ghasemzadeh, MB; Kalivas, PW. The regulation of dopamine transmission by metabotropic glutamate receptors. *J Pharmacol Exp Ther*, 1999, vol. 289, 412-416.

[25] Marek, GJ; Wright, RA; Schoepp, DD; Monn, JA; Aghajanian, GK. Physiological antagonism between 5-hydroxytryptamine(2A) and group II metabotropic glutamate receptors in prefrontal cortex. *J Pharmacol Exp Ther*, 2000, vol. 292, 76-87.

[26] Tyszkiewicz, JP; Gu, Z; Wang, X; Cai, X; Yan, Z. Group II metabotropic glutamate receptors enhance NMDA receptor currents via a protein kinase C-dependent

mechanism in pyramidal neurones of rat prefrontal cortex. *J Physiol*, 2004 vol. 554, 765-777.

[27] Matheson, SL; Green, MJ; Loo, C; Carr, VJ. Quality assessment and comparison of evidence for electroconvulsive therapy and repetitive transcranial magnetic stimulation for schizophrenia: *A systematic meta-review*. Schizophr Res, 2010.

[28] Lynch, D; Laws, KR; McKenna, PJ. Cognitive behavioural therapy for major psychiatric disorder: does it really work? A meta-analytical review of well-controlled trials. *Psychol Med*, 2010, vol. 40, 9-24.

[29] Freitas, A; da Paz, JA; Casella, EB; Marques-Dias, MJ. Ketogenic diet for the treatment of refractory epilepsy: a 10 year experience in children. *Arq Neuropsiquiatr*, 2007, vol. 65, 381-384.

[30] Papandreou, D; Pavlou, E; Kalimeri, E; Mavromichalis, I. The ketogenic diet in children with epilepsy. *Br J Nutr*, 2006, vol. 95, 5-13.

[31] Pelsser, LM; Frankena, K; Toorman, J; Savelkoul, HF; Pereira, RR; Buitelaar, JK. A randomised controlled trial into the effects of food on ADHD. *Eur Child Adolesc Psychiatry*, 2008.

[32] Pao, SK; Dickerson, JW. Effect of a low protein diet and isoenergetic amounts of a high protein diet in the weanling rat on the free amino acids of the brain. *Nutr Metab*, 1975, vol. 18, 204-216.

[33] Fernstrom, JD; Wurtman, RJ; Hammarstrom-Wiklund, B; Rand, WM; Munro, HN; Davidson, CS. Diurnal variations in plasma concentrations of tryptophan, tryosine, and other neutral amino acids: effect of dietary protein intake. *Am J Clin Nutr*, 1979 vol. 32, 1912-1922.

[34] Fujita, Y; Yamamoto, T; Rikimaru, T; Inoue, G. Effect of low protein diets on free amino acids in plasma of young men: effect of wheat gluten diet. *J Nutr Sci Vitaminol*, (Tokyo), 1979, vol. 25, 427-439.

[35] Suzic, S; Radunovic, L; Jankovic, V; Segovic, R. Effects of protein-free diet in amino acid homeostasis of rat blood plasma and gut contents. *FEBS Lett*, 1987, vol. 216, 287-290.

[36] Hamdi, A; Onaivi, ES; Prasad, C. A low protein-high carbohydrate diet decreases D2 dopamine receptor density in rat brain. *Life Sci*, 1992, vol. 50, 1529-1534.

[37] Hirata, H; Asanuma, M; Kondo, Y; Ogawa, N. Influence of protein-restricted diet on motor response fluctuations in Parkinson's disease. *Rinsho Shinkeigaku*, 1992, vol. 32, 973-978.

[38] Lieberman, HR; Yeghiayan, SK; Maher, TJ. A low-protein diet alters rat behavior and neurotransmission in normothermic and hyperthermic environments. *Brain Res Bull*, 2005, vol. 66, 149-154.

[39] Iversen, L; Iversen, S; Bloom, FE. *Introduction to Neuropsychopharmacology*. USA: Oxford University Press; 2008.

[40] Mizrahi, R; Rusjan, P; Agid, O; Graff, A; Mamo, DC; Zipursky, RB; Kapur, S. Adverse subjective experience with antipsychotics and its relationship to striatal and extrastriatal D2 receptors: a PET study in schizophrenia. *Am J Psychiatry*, 2007, vol. 164, 630-637.

[41] Saeedi, H; Remington, G; Christensen, BK. Impact of haloperidol, a dopamine D2 antagonist, on cognition and mood. *Schizophr Res*, 2006, vol. 85, 222-231.

[42] See, RE; Lynch, AM; Sorg, BA. Subchronic administration of clozapine, but not haloperidol or metoclopramide, decreases dopamine D2 receptor messenger RNA

levels in the nucleus accumbens and caudate-putamen in rats. *Neuroscience*, 1996, vol. 72, 99-104.

[43] Lee, T; Tang, SW. Loxapine and clozapine decrease serotonin (S2) but do not elevate dopamine (D2) receptor numbers in the rat brain. *Psychiatry Res*, 1984, vol. 12, 277-285.

[44] Volonte, M; Ceci, A; Borsini, F. Effect of haloperidol and clozapine on (+)SKF 10,047-induced dopamine release: role of 5-HT3 receptors. *Eur J Pharmacol*, 1992, vol. 213, 163-164.

[45] Westerink, BH; de Vries, JB. On the mechanism of neuroleptic induced increase in striatal dopamine release: brain dialysis provides direct evidence for mediation by autoreceptors localized on nerve terminals. *Neurosci Lett*, 1989, vol. 99, 197-202.

[46] Wise, RA. Dopamine, learning and motivation. *Nat Rev Neurosci*, 2004, vol. 5, 483-494.

[47] Grimes, MA; Cameron, JL; Fernstrom, JD. Cerebrospinal fluid concentrations of tryptophan and 5-hydroxyindoleacetic acid in Macaca mulatta: diurnal variations and response to chronic changes in dietary protein intake. *Neurochem Res*, 2000, vol. 25, 413-422.

[48] Cussac, D; Newman-Tancredi, A; Nicolas, JP; Boutin, JA; Millan, MJ. Antagonist properties of the novel antipsychotic, S16924, at cloned, human serotonin 5-HT2C receptors: a parallel phosphatidylinositol and calcium accumulation comparison with clozapine and haloperidol. Naunyn Schmiedebergs *Arch Pharmacol*, 2000, vol. 361, 549-554.

[49] Kuoppamaki, M; Palvimaki, EP; Hietala, J; Syvalahti, E. Differential regulation of rat 5-HT2A and 5-HT2C receptors after chronic treatment with clozapine, chlorpromazine and three putative atypical antipsychotic drugs. *Neuropsychopharmacology*, 1995, vol. 13, 139-150.

[50] Gobbi, G; Janiri, L. Clozapine blocks dopamine, 5-HT2 and 5-HT3 responses in the medial prefrontal cortex: an in vivo microiontophoretic study. Eur *Neuropsychopharmacol*, 1999, vol. 10, 43-49.

[51] Hermann, B; Wetzel, CH; Pestel, E; Zieglgansberger, W; Holsboer, F; Rupprecht, R. Functional antagonistic properties of clozapine at the 5-HT3 receptor. *Biochem Biophys Res Commun*, 1996, vol. 225, 957-960.

[52] Frederick, JA; Meador-Woodruff, JH. Effects of clozapine and haloperidol on 5-HT6 receptor mRNA levels in rat brain. *Schizophr Res*, 1999, vol. 38, 7-12.

[53] Tauscher, J; Hussain, T; Agid, O; Verhoeff, NP; Wilson, AA; Houle, S; Remington, G; Zipursky, RB; Kapur, S. Equivalent occupancy of dopamine D1 and D2 receptors with clozapine: differentiation from other atypical antipsychotics. *Am J Psychiatry*, 2004, vol. 161, 1620-1625.

[54] Burstein, ES; Ma, J; Wong, S; Gao, Y; Pham, E; Knapp, AE; Nash, NR; Olsson, R; Davis, RE; Hacksell, U; Weiner, DM; Brann, MR. Intrinsic efficacy of antipsychotics at human D2, D3, and D4 dopamine receptors: identification of the clozapine metabolite N-desmethylclozapine as a D2/D3 partial agonist. *J Pharmacol Exp Ther*, 2005, vol. 315, 1278-1287.

[55] Cussac, D; Pasteau, V; Millan, MJ. Characterisation of Gs activation by dopamine D1 receptors using an antibody capture assay: antagonist properties of clozapine. *Eur J Pharmacol*, 2004, vol. 485, 111-117.

[56] Lanig, H; Utz, W; Gmeiner, P. Comparative molecular field analysis of dopamine D4 receptor antagonists including 3-[4-(4-chlorophenyl)piperazin-1-ylmethyl]pyrazolo[1,5-a]pyridine (FAUC 113), 3-[4-(4-chlorophenyl)piperazin-1-ylmethyl]-1H-pyrrolo-[2,3-b]pyridine (L-745,870), and clozapine. *J Med Chem*, 2001, vol. 44, 1151-1157.

[57] South, T; Huang, XF. High-fat diet exposure increases dopamine D2 receptor and decreases dopamine transporter receptor binding density in the nucleus accumbens and caudate putamen of mice. *Neurochem Res*, 2008, vol. 33, 598-605.

[58] Huang, XF; Zavitsanou, K; Huang, X; Yu, Y; Wang, H; Chen, F; Lawrence, AJ; Deng, C. Dopamine transporter and D2 receptor binding densities in mice prone or resistant to chronic high fat diet-induced obesity. *Behav Brain Res*, 2006, vol. 175, 415-419.

[59] Milton, K. The critical role played by animal source foods in human (Homo) evolution. *J Nutr*, 2003, vol. 133, 3886S-3892S.

[60] Ulijaszek, SJ. Human eating behaviour in an evolutionary ecological context. *Proc Nutr Soc*, 2002, vol. 61, 517-526.

[61] Volkova, LD; Nam, OI; Chernikov, MP; Smetanina, LB; Dakhundaridze, VV. Determination of the biological value of beef and rice proteins and their combinations. *Vopr Pitan*, 1988, 55-59.

[62] Shiell, AW; Campbell-Brown, M; Haselden, S; Robinson, S; Godfrey, KM; Barker, DJ. High-meat, low-carbohydrate diet in pregnancy: relation to adult blood pressure in the offspring. *Hypertension*, 2001, vol. 38, 1282-1288.

[63] Watts, JH; Booker, LK; Mc, AJ; Williams, EG; Wright, WG; Jones, F, Jr. Biological availability of essential amino acids to human subjects. I. Whole egg, pork muscle and peanut butter. *J Nutr*, 1959, vol. 67, 483-496.

[64] Di Chiara, G; Bassareo, V; Fenu, S; De Luca, MA; Spina, L; Cadoni, C; Acquas, E; Carboni, E; Valentini, V; Lecca, D. Dopamine and drug addiction: the nucleus accumbens shell connection. *Neuropharmacology*, 2004, vol. 47, 227-241.

[65] Ikemoto, S. Involvement of the olfactory tubercle in cocaine reward: intracranial self-administration studies. *J Neurosci*, 2003, vol. 23, 9305-9311.

[66] McMorris, T; Swain, J; Smith, M; Corbett, J; Delves, S; Sale, C; Harris, RC; Potter, J. Heat stress, plasma concentrations of adrenaline, noradrenaline, 5-hydroxytryptamine and cortisol, mood state and cognitive performance. *Int J Psychophysiol*, 2006, vol. 61, 204-215.

[67] Yamamoto, S; Iwamoto, M; Inoue, M; Harada, N. Evaluation of the effect of heat exposure on the autonomic nervous system by heart rate variability and urinary catecholamines. *J Occup Health*, 2007, vol. 49, 199-204.

[68] Koska, J; Rovensky, J; Zimanova, T; Vigas, M. Growth hormone and prolactin responses during partial and whole body warm-water immersions. *Acta Physiol Scand,*, 2003, vol. 178, 19-23.

[69] Dey, S; Dey, PK; Sharma, HS. Regional metabolism of 5-hydroxytryptamine in brain under acute and chronic heat stress. *Indian J Physiol Pharmacol*, 1993, vol. 37, 8-12.

[70] Sharma, HS; Dey, PK. Influence of long-term acute heat exposure on regional blood-brain barrier permeability, cerebral blood flow and 5-HT level in conscious normotensive young rats. *Brain Res*, 1987, vol. 424, 153-162.

[71] Emiliano, AB; Fudge, JL. From galactorrhea to osteopenia: rethinking serotonin-prolactin interactions. *Neuropsychopharmacology*, 2004, vol. 29, 833-846.

[72] Freeman, ME; Kanyicska, B; Lerant, A; Nagy, G. Prolactin: structure, function, and regulation of secretion. *Physiol Rev*, 2000, vol. 80, 1523-1631.
[73] Guiard, BP; El Mansari, M; Merali, Z; Blier, P. Functional interactions between dopamine, serotonin and norepinephrine neurons: an in-vivo electrophysiological study in rats with monoaminergic lesions. *Int J Neuropsychopharmacol*, 2008, vol. 11, 625-639.
[74] Glazer, JL. Management of heatstroke and heat exhaustion. *Am Fam Physician*, 2005, vol. 71, 2133-2140.
[75] Wexler, RK. Evaluation and treatment of heat-related illnesses. *Am Fam Physician*, 2002, vol. 65, 2307-2314.
[76] Dieing, A; Ahlers, O; Kerner, T; Wust, P; Felix, R; Loffel, J; Riess, H; Hildebrandt, B. Whole body hyperthermia induces apoptosis in subpopulations of blood lymphocytes. *Immunobiology*, 2003 vol. 207, 265-273.
[77] Shen, RN; Lu, L; Young, P; Shidnia, H; Hornback, NB; Broxmeyer, HE. Influence of elevated temperature on natural killer cell activity, lymphokine-activated killer cell activity and lectin-dependent cytotoxicity of human umbilical cord blood and adult blood cells. *Int J Radiat Oncol Biol Phys*, 1994, vol. 29, 821-826.
[78] Power Analysis and Sample Size software, NCSS [online].2008 [cited 2010-02-16] Available from: URL: http://www.ncss.com/pass.html.
[79] Farooqui, SM; Brock, JW; Onaivi, ES; Hamdi, A; Prasad, C. Differential modulation of dopaminergic systems in the rat brain by dietary protein. *Neurochem Res*, 1994 vol. 19, 167-176.

In: Hallucinations: Types, Stages and Treatments
Editor: Meredith S. Payne, pp. 163-178
ISBN: 978-1-61728-275-1
© 2011 Nova Science Publishers, Inc.

Chapter 9

Hallucinations and Suicide Risk: Future Directions for Research and Clinical Implications

Maurizio Pompili[a,b], Gianluca Serafini,[a] Marco Innamorati[c], S. Diletta Del Bono,[a] Eleonora Piacentini,[a] David Lester[d] and Roberto Tatarelli[a]

[a]Department of Neurosciences, Mental Health and Sensory Functions, Suicide Prevention Center, Sant'Andrea Hospital, Sapienza University of Rome, Italy
[b]McLean Hospital – Harvard Medical School, USA
[c]Università Europea di Roma, Italy
[d]The Richard Stockton College of New Jersey, USA

Introduction

Suicide has taken lives around the world and across the centuries, and it accounts for about one million deaths annually, with devastating socioeconomic costs and consequences (Mann, 2003). It's one of the world's largest public health problems and has multiple causes in which, according to a stress-diathesis model, both genetic make up and acquired susceptibility contribute to a person's predisposition to suicidal acts in stressful situations (Mann, 2003; Wasserman, 2001). Suicide is a complex phenomenon resulting from various factors, including psychiatric, biological and environmental factors. Mental disorders (particularly depression and schizophrenia) are associated with suicide, and over 90% of suicide attempters and 60% of completed suicides have mood disorders (Beautrais et al., 1996; Shaffer et al., 1996), and between 70-95% of suicide victims have some form of diagnosable mental illness (Conwell et al., 2002; Conwell et al., 2002; American Psychiatric Association, 2003). Depression and schizophrenia, no doubt, both play a critical role in suicidal behaviour. Suicide is the leading cause of death among people with schizophrenia (Allebeck and Wistedt, 1986; Caldwell and Gottesman, 1990; Pompili et al, 2007; Pompili et al, 2008; Roy and Pompili, 2009), and people with schizophrenia have an 8.5-fold greater risk for suicide than those in the general population (Harris and Barraclough, 1997).

Nearly half of schizophrenic individuals report suicidal ideation at some point during their lives, while 20-50% have a history of suicide attempts (Breier and Pickar, 1991; Roy, 1986) and 4-13% of them eventually take their own lives (Allebeck, 1989; Drake et al., 1985; Inskip et al., 1998; Meltzer and Okayli, 1995; Miles, 1977; American Psychiatric Association, 2003).

Schizophrenia often leads to decreased social support (Drake et al., 1985; Caldwell and Gottesman, 1992; Pinikahana et al., 2003; Siris, 2001; Raymont, 2001), lower levels of occupational and daily functioning, decreased insight, and maladaptive coping skills (Raymont, 2001; Modestin et al., 1992). Additionally, people with schizophrenia have two or more of the following indicators: (a) delusions, (b) hallucinations, (c) disorganized speech, (d) grossly disorganized behavior, and (e) negative symptoms (American Psychiatric Association, 1994).

Hallucinations may be auditory, visual or tactile and may include highly idiosyncratic content (e.g., threats, suggestions, affirmations) (American Psychiatric Association, 1994; World Health Organization, 1973). Command hallucinations are a particular subtype of auditory hallucination in which the patient is instructed to "act, making a gesture or grimace to committing suicidal or homicidal acts" (Hellerstein, Frosch, & Koenigsberg, 1987, p. 219). Patients with schizophrenia may hear voices that instruct them to engage in suicidal acts or to proceed with violent acts toward others.

Command hallucinations in schizophrenic individuals may be common but often ignored by psychiatrists (Rogers, 1988). The prevalence of this symptom is reported to vary from 18-50% (Harkavy-Friedman, et al, 2003), and several studies have reported rates between 30-50% (Zisook et al., 1995; McNiel et al., 2000; Kasper et al., 1996; Rogers et al., 1990). The presence of hallucinations, especially command hallucinations, in schizophrenic patients may increase the risk of suicide.

This chapter investigates whether hallucinations may impact on suicidal behaviour in schizophrenia. We review the literature, citing the most relevant studies about the association between hallucinations and suicidal behaviour. We also report the most common indicators of treatment adherence and treatment options in people with schizophrenia having hallucinations, and we emphasize research in this field and provide clinical implications for future research.

Auditory Hallucinations

Auditory hallucinations are often related to anxiety, presumably having adaptive properties for patients such as decreasing anxiety (Slade, 1976)). This model may partially explain how some patients, particularly those who are socially isolated, appear so convinced by their experience of voices.

Excessive dopamine is the most plausible neurobiological explanation for the occurrence of command hallucinations in schizophrenia. This theory is confirmed by the fact that antipsychotic medications blocking D2 receptors in the brain decrease dopamine production (Nasrallah and Smeltzer, 2002), while other drugs (amphetamines, L-dopa, etc.) increase dopamine production and may induce hallucinations in people with no diagnosable disorder (Lakeman, 2001). In addition, stress-producing excessive dopamine in the mesolimbic system may touch off psychotic symptoms (O'Connor, 1994; O'Connor, 1991).

Other theories have proposed that auditory hallucinations may reflect a degree of "sub-vocal" speech mistakenly attributed to external sources (Nelson, 1997). It has been found that several activities, such as reading, watching television, and listening to the radio, may distract patients experiencing auditory hallucinations, and listening to "white noise" may exacerbate symptoms (Delespaul et al, 2002). However, it is poorly understood whether such activities decrease the intensity of hallucinations as a result of the suppression of sub-vocal speech or because the patient is focusing on a divergent task.

Cognitive models have also suggested hypotheses regarding the formation and maintenance of auditory hallucinations (Beck and Rector, 2003; Byrne et al., 2003; Chadwick and Birchwood, 1994). For these theories, hallucinations represent a combination of several factors: hyperactive cognitions, predispositions for imagining, disinhibitions of normal constraints on imagining, biases toward externalization, and deficits in reality testing and reasoning (Beck and Rector, 2003). According to this model, hallucinations may be paradoxically accentuated when patients attempt to suppress them.

Command Hallucinations and Suicidal Behaviour

Several investigators have speculated about the relationship between hallucinations and suicide. Researchers have investigated the association between hallucinations, especially command hallucinations, and suicide attempts, completed suicide and self-harming behavior.

Command hallucinations happen when patients hear voices explicitly instructing them to engage in specific acts (Hellerstein, et al., 1987). They occur in 18–50% of the schizophrenia-spectrum disorder population (Harkavy-Friedman et al., 2003; Zisook, Byrd, Kuck, & Jeste, 1995). Often these command hallucinations are suicidal in nature, thereby placing individuals who are vulnerable to suicide at even greater risk.

Considering that aggression and impulsivity have been found to be relevant factors involved in suicide, command hallucinations have been studied in relationship both to violence and to suicidal behaviour; (Conner et al, 2004). However, there are few empirical studies in this area, and the findings conflict as to the legitimacy of command hallucinations as a consistent risk factor either in suicide or violence toward others (see Table 1).

Several authors have reported that command hallucinations may cause patients with schizophrenia to complete suicide (Barraclough, Bunch, Nelson, & Sainsbury, 1974; Planansky & Johnston, 1973). However, initial studies found no association between command hallucinations and suicidal behaviour. Breier and Astrachan (1984) compared 20 patients with schizophrenia who committed suicide to three other patient groups and found that none of the suicides had experienced command hallucinations. Similarly, Cotton et al. (1985) interviewed 20 therapists whose schizophrenic patients had committed suicide and found that all their patients had been relatively non-psychotic at the time of the suicide.

Table 1. Studies about the association between command hallucinations and suicidal risk or violent behavior

Study	Design	Sample Size	Conclusions
Breier and Astrachan (1984)	Four group comparison: 1) patients with schizophrenia who committed suicide, 2) patients without schizophrenia who committed suicide, 3) randomly selected patients with schizophrenia who did not commit suicide, and 4) sex-matched group of patients with schizophrenia who did not commit suicide	Total n for all four groups = 139	None of the 20 patients with schizophrenia who committed suicide were found to have hallucinatory suicidal commands
Hellerstein et al., (1987) *	Between-groups comparison based on retrospective records. Studied the following four types of inpatients: 1) those with auditory hallucinations, 2) those without auditory hallucinations, 3) those with command hallucinations, and 4) those with non-command hallucinations	Total n = 789; auditory hallucination group = 151; non-hallucination group = 638; command hallucination group = 58; non-command group = 93	No significant differences were found between the command hallucination groups with regard to suicidal or assaultive acts
Zisook et al., (1995) *	Retrospective clinical record and secondary source review. Studied only patients with schizophrenia who had documented auditory hallucinations	106 patients with schizophrenia	Patients with command hallucinations did not significantly differ from patients without command hallucinations in the number of prior suicide attempts or histories of violent/ impulsive acts
Rudnick (1999) *	Literature review of research published between 1966 and 1997	Focused on the 11 controlled studies from among 34 studies relating to command hallucinations and dangerous behavior	All controlled studies related to suicide and command hallucinations found no significant relationship. Six of seven controlled studies pertaining to violence and command hallucinations suggested the non-existence of a significant relationship.

Table 1. (Continued)

Study	Design	Sample Size	Conclusions
Harkavy-Friedman et al., (2003) *	Between-group comparison of inpatients with schizophrenia who reported command auditory hallucinations with inpatients with schizophrenia who did not	Total sample =100; patients with command auditory hallucinations = 22; group without = 78	The rate of suicide attempts did not differ significantly between the groups of patients with and without command auditory hallucinations
Rogers et al., (2002) *	Between-groups comparison of forensic patients with mixed diagnoses based on clinical or legal records. Separated groups based on the presence/absence of lifetime histories of command hallucinations	Command hallucinators = 54, non-command hallucinators = 56	Violent command hallucinations and inpatient violence were not significantly related Self-harm command hallucinations significantly predicted self-harming behavior on the unit
Nordentoft et al., (2002) +	Randomized controlled trial, placing patients with first-episode schizophrenia-spectrum disorders into integrated treatment or treatment as usual conditions	Total n = 341; 173 given integrated treatment	The presence of hallucinations and prior suicide attempts were the only two significant predictors (when using multivariate analyses) of attempted suicide during study follow-up period
McNiel et al., (2000) *	Between-group comparison of inpatients with mixed diagnoses. Groups were divided into those who had or had not experienced command hallucinations to hurt others	Total n = 103; violent command hallucinators = 31; non-violent group = 72	Patients with violent command hallucinations were more likely to report being violent
Cheung et al., (1997) *	Between-group comparison of violent patients with chronic schizophrenia to matched controls with schizophrenia	Violent group = 31; matched control group = 31	No association was found between command hallucinations and any violent behavior on the unit
Hawton et al., (2005)	Systematic review of prospective cohort study; retrospective cohort study; nested case–control study; case–control study, with similar patient groups; case–control study in which the status of the controls was unclear or different.		Reduced risk was associated with hallucinations (OR¼0.50,95% CI 0.35^0.71), previous depressive disorders (OR¼3.03, 95% CI 2.06-4.46), previous suicide attempts (OR¼4.09,95% CI 2.79-6.01), drug misuse (OR¼3.21,95%

Table 1. (Continued)

Study	Design	Sample Size	Conclusions
			CI1.99-5.17), agitation or motor restlessness (OR¼2.61, 95% CI1.54-4.41), fear of mental disintegration (OR¼12.1,95% CI1.89-81.3), poor adherence to treatment (OR¼3.75,95% CI 2.20-6.37) and recent loss (OR¼4.03,95%CI1.37-11.8) were robustly associated with increased risk of suicide
Tarrier et al., (2007)	Cross sectional study	Data from the SoCRATES Trial of cognitive-behaviour therapy in recent onset schizophrenia. 306 patients of which 80% were first episode and 20% second episode patients.	A logistic regression analysis revealed that emotional withdrawal, but not blunted affect, was significant and negatively associated, and depression positively associated, with suicide behaviour. Restricted emotions were associated with reduced suicide risk.
Preti et al. (2010)	Cross sectional study	1,547 patients admitted over a 12-day index period during the year 2004 to 130 public and 36 private psychiatric facilities in Italy	Disordered eating behavior, depressive symptoms, substance abuse, and non-prescribed medication abuse were positively related to attempted suicide, as were any traumatic events in the week prior to admission. Symptoms of psychosis (hallucinations/delusions) and lack of self-care were negatively associated with suicide attempt admission.

+Command auditory hallucinations were not explicitly addressed in these studies.
*Command auditory hallucinations served as a primary variable of interest in these reports.
Source: Adapted from Montross LP, Zisook S, Kasckow J. Command Hallucinations and Suicide Risk. In: Suicide in Schizophrenia. Tatarelli R, Pompili M, Girardi P (Eds): 2007, Nova Science Publishers, Inc.

Hellerstein et al. (1987) conducted one of the first controlled studies investigating the relevance of command hallucinations in suicidal behaviour or violence. Comparing patients with and without command hallucinations yielded no significant differences in rates of suicidal or assaultive acts. More broadly, patients with hallucinations (regardless of type) were just as likely to report suicidal ideation as those not experiencing hallucinations.

Cheng et al. (1990) conducted a study in 74 chinese schizophrenics who committed suicide and 74 case-control subjects. When comparing these two groups, no sociodemographic variables significantly differentiated between those who committed suicide and those who did not. The patients who had committed suicide were found to have more severe courses of illness, histories of major depressive episodes, past suicide attempts, hospitalizations for reasons other than schizophrenia and documented suicidal ideation during clinical consultations. Patients who committed suicide were also more likely to exhibit violent acts prior to their last admission, and the presence of violent acts increased the risk for suicide 10-fold among people with schizophrenia. However, it was unclear whether the acts of violence were in response to internal directives.

Cheung et al. (1997) found similar results in a study of 62 patients with chronic schizophrenia, the majority of whom had been defined as violent. They found that 74% of the schizophrenic patients had auditory hallucinations, usually command in nature. There was no association between command hallucinations and violent behavior in the long-term unit.

These findings were supported in a literature review by Rudnick (1999) who found a lack of a relationship between command hallucinations and violence toward self or others and by Zisook et al. (1995) who reported that patients with command hallucinations and those without command hallucinations did not differ in number of prior suicide attempts or in a history of violent/impulsive acts.

McNiel et al. (2000) completed a more targeted study on the relationship between command hallucinations and violence among 103 psychiatric inpatients. The participants had various diagnoses such as schizophrenia (20% of the sample), bipolar disorder, and substance-related disorders. Patients with command hallucinations were 2.5 times more likely to be violent in the two months prior to hospitalization. When controlling for the severity of symptoms, command hallucinations no longer made a significant contribution to the determination of violence. However, they found that 30% of patients heard voices telling them to harm others during the last year, and 22% stated they complied with those commands.

Rogers et al. (2002) compared 56 forensic patients with a lifetime history of command hallucinations to 54 non-command hallucinators, all of whom were being treated in a medium-security hospital between the years of 1995-1999 and found no relationship between violent command hallucinations and inpatient violence. However, the presence of self-injurious command hallucinations was a significant predictor of self-harming behavior. The authors reported that violent incidents were not predicted by gender, paranoid delusions, previous violent sentence, or a history of alcohol/drug abuse. On the other hand, Harkavy-Friedman et al. (2003) sampled 100 inpatients with schizophrenia or schizoaffective disorder, divided between those who had experienced command auditory hallucinations (n = 22) and those who had not (n = 78). The rate of suicide attempts did not differ significantly between the two groups.

Nordentoft et al. (2002) carried out a randomized controlled trial of integrated treatment in 341 patients with a first episode of schizophrenia-spectrum disorders, randomized into a first group (assertive community treatment, antipsychotic medication, psychoeducational family treatment, and social skills training) and a second group (treatment as usual). Hallucinations were one of only two significant variables predicting attempted suicide. However, this study had several limitations. First, it was not known whether these hallucinations were command in nature, and the content of such hallucinations was not specified (e.g., violent toward self, violent toward others, or benign). Finally, the study was not designed to measure the role of command hallucinations *per se*.

Hawton et al. (2005) tried to identify risk factors for suicide in schizophrenia and systematically reviewed the international literature on case-control and cohort studies of patients with schizophrenia or related conditions. They investigated delusions and hallucinations separately and found that, overall, hallucinations were associated with a reduced suicide risk (OR=0.50,95% CI 0.35-0.71). However, the finding for the three studies on command hallucinations showed significant heterogeneity (P=0.006), and the authors stated that although there was no overall association with suicide risk, although conclusion this was based on relatively few data.

Tarrier et al. (2007) carried out a logistic regression analysis on 278 recent onset schizophrenic patients, measuring suicide behaviour as the dependent variable and negative symptoms, delusions, hallucinations, depression, gender, episode, ethnicity, education, age, duration of untreated psychosis and substance use as independent variables. They found no association between hallucinations and suicide risk.

More recently, Preti et al. (2010) examined 1,547 patients admitted over a 12-day index period during 2004 to 130 public and 36 private psychiatric facilities in Italy and reported that, while symptoms of depression and substance abuse were the most important features linked to admission after attempted suicide, symptoms of psychosis (hallucinations/delusions) and lack of self-care were negatively associated with admission and did not appear to be precipitating factors for a suicide attempt in the week prior to admission. The authors stated that this negative association between hallucinations/delusions and suicide risk may possibly be explained by the fact that their disruptive impact leads patients to hospitals before more severe consequences can occur.

The findings of the majority of the studies examining the role of command hallucinations in both suicidal and violent behavior suggest that the nature of this association appears unclear. Some researchers find a connection, whereas other find no empirical evidence of a relationship between command hallucinations and various forms of violence. However, several studies agree on the fact that the rates of occurrence for command hallucinations is high, the symptoms are underreported, and command hallucinations may have clinical implications for predicting violence.

Finally, studies of the association between command hallucinations and suicide have resulted in contradictory results, and the majority of studies focusing on the role of command hallucinations and violence toward others are also mixed. Thus, it seems to be difficult to establish the prognostic significance of command hallucinations.

Methodological Problems

These conflicting research findings are probably the result of the methodological problems inherent in this type of research: underreporting of the symptoms (Rogers, Gillis, Turner, & Frise-Smith, 1990; Zisook, et al., 1995), small sample sizes (Caldwell & Gottesman, 1992), and a lack of standardization in defining suicidal behavior and the presence of hallucinations. Specifically, the type of hallucination has not always been clearly stated in the studies, leaving readers unclear about whether patients were experiencing violent, suicidal, or benign command hallucinations. Research also faces the problem of knowing whether patients were actively hallucinating during the behavior being studied (suicidal or violent behavior) (Buckley et al., 2004). Furthermore, researchers in the past have sampled diagnostically heterogeneous groups, mixing schizophrenia with bipolar disorders, personality disorders and severe mood disorders (McNiel, Eisner, & Binder, 2000; P. Rogers, et al., 2002; Rudnick, 1999). These results have then been compared, perhaps unfairly, to studies that sampled only people with schizophrenia (Cheung, Schweitzer, Crowley, & Tuckwell, 1997; Erkwoh, Willmes, Eming-Erdmann, & Kunert, 2002; Rudnick, 1999).

It's also important to note that command hallucinations are often underreported. Rogers et al. (1990) found numerous patients in their forensic sample who either denied or omitted to mention the presence of command hallucinations to treating clinicians, thereby allowing for nearly 50% of the patients experiencing these phenomena to go undetected. Zisook et al. (1995) also reported approximately one-third of command hallucination cases in their study went undocumented by clinicians.

Many researchers continue to believe that, although the association between command hallucinations and violence is unclear, it is important that people with schizophrenia continue to be monitored. Clinicians should recognize any signs that may predict command hallucinations, particularly in patients with risk factors for suicide. Command hallucinations occur more frequently than is often recognized and hold potentially vital clinical significance. In order to prevent suicide, direct screening for command hallucinations should be incorporated into any suicide assessment.

The Association between Command Hallucinations and Suicidal Behaviour: The Role of Compliance

Determining how or why patients comply with command hallucinations has been of interest for researchers and for clinicians. The majority of studies indicate that high numbers of patients comply with the command hallucinations experienced. Rogers et al. (1990) reported that 80% of 25 patients with command hallucinations in the last 30 days had obeyed with them (56% of them with "unquestioning obedience"). Kasper et al. (1996) found in 86 psychotic inpatients that 84% of those experiencing command hallucinations had recently complied. Forty-eight percent of those in the command hallucination group heard messages pertaining to self-harm within the past month, and 92% of those patients obeyed such commands.

Three basic elements have been reported as increasing command hallucination compliance: voice familiarity, perceived type of voice and subsequent emotional reaction, and the presence of corresponding delusional beliefs.

About the first aspect, it is presumably that, when a voice is identifiable by the patient and appears as familiar, the likelihood of obeying it increases (Junginger, 1990; Erkwoh, et al., 2002; Junginger and McGuire, 2001; Kasper et al., 1996; Rudnick, 1999).

About the second point, it is possible that the tone, perceived intention, and resulting affect may promote compliance. Rogers et al. (1990) stated that aggressive attitudes were more common in a group of forensic inpatients with command hallucinations compared to a group with non-command hallucination. Erkwoh et al. (2002) found that in a sample of 31 patients with schizophrenia or schizoaffective disorder, compliers were significantly more likely to have post-hallucinatory affect that included fear, despair, anger, and restlessness. Patients who complied with command hallucinations were also more likely to view the voice as "real" and to be alone when the voices were heard. Cheung et al. (1997) found that violent people with schizophrenia were more likely to report that command auditory hallucinations made them feel sad, angry, anxious and violated. The non-violent group of matched patients described the voices as gentle, comforting, loving, kind and helpful.

Delusional beliefs may affect compliance since delusions may support or reinforce command hallucinations (Junginger, 1990; Junginger and McGuire, 2001; Kasper et al., 1996). Junginger (1990) reported that, in 51 psychiatric patients with mixed diagnoses, delusions provided evidence for subsequent compliance with commands. Cheung et al. (1997) compared violent and non-violent patients with schizophrenia and found that the presence of persecutory delusional beliefs occurred more often in the violent group. The delusions justified harm directed toward others although the auditory hallucinations experienced by the two groups were similar with regard to frequency, duration, volume, or perceived reality.

Therefore, not only is it crucial to detect the presence of command hallucinations among people with schizophrenia, but it is critical to detect which patients are most likely to comply with such commands.

Treatment Interventions

Pharmacological interventions. The efficacy of antipsychotic medication for the positive symptoms of schizophrenia, including hallucinations, is well established (American Psychiatric Association, 1997; Davis et al., 2003; Leucht et al., 2003; Marder et al., 2002; Miller et al., 2004; Miller et al., 1999; Frances et al., 1996). However, there is poor data on whether patients with command hallucinations respond differently to medication than patients without command hallucinations, or whether patients with command hallucinations respond differently to patients with other types of hallucination.

Atypical antipsychotics such as clozapine, risperidone, olanzapine, quetiapine, ziprasidone and aripiprazole, compared to typical antipsychotic medications, have been found to have at least equal efficacy for positive symptoms; greater efficacy for negative, cognitive and affective symptoms; and reduced risk of extrapyramidal symptoms and tardive dyskinesia. However, the newer generation antipsychotic medications are considered first-line treatments for patients with schizophrenia and schizoaffective disorder. It is not clear if any of the newer atypical antipsychotics are more effective than others, but each has specific side-effect profiles. Therefore, the decision of which of the newer generation antipsychotic medications is best suited for an individual should be based on the unique clinical characteristics of the patient and side-effect profile of each agent (Marder et al., 2002; Miller et al., 2004).

Clozapine appears to be the most effective agent presently available for treating refractory patients (Chakos et al., 2001; Essock et al., 2000; Kane et al., 2001; Meltzer, 2004) and, of particular relevance to this chapter, it may be more effective in reducing hostility and aggression (Kane et al., 2001; Citrone et al., 2001) as well as reducing mortality from suicide in patients with schizophrenia (Meltzer, 2004; Meltzer and Okayli, 1995; Meltzer, Alphs, Green, Altamura, Anand, Bertoldi, Bourgeois, Chouinard, Islam, Kane, Krishnan, Lindenmayer, Potkin, and International Suicide Prevention Trial Study Group, 2003). Thus, in patients with schizophrenia and schizoaffective disorder with command hallucinations to harm themselves, clozapine should be seriously considered in non-responding and partially-responding patients to a trial of one of the other atypical antipsychotics rather than waiting for two or three failed trials as is customarily done for non-responders in other clinical situations (Marder et al., 2002; Miller et al., 2004).

Cognitive interventions. Cognitive models propose cognitive treatment of command hallucinations (Beck and Rector, 2003; Byrne et al., 2003; Beck-Sander, et al. 1997; Chadwick and Birchwood, 1994). Chadwick and Birchwood (1994) reorted a broad plan for the use of cognitive therapy with patients experiencing auditory hallucinations. According to these authors, compliance and affective responses are related to patients' beliefs about the amount of power possessed by the voices. They suggested that lessening the patients' fears of disobedience, refuting the voices' utility, and increasing the patients' perceived level of control could serve to minimize the occurrence of hallucinations. Specifically, treatment should involve carefully establishing a supportive, therapeutic relationship with patients, disputing the patients' beliefs via hypothetical contradictions, and verbal challenges and "empirically testing" the beliefs. These cognitive techniques could assist in the treatment of patients whose voices mandate harm to self or others.

Byrne et al. (2003) developed a two-stage cognitive treatment protocol for patients experiencing command hallucinations. In the first stage, clinicians are urged to spend a great deal of time actively listening, encouraging, and emphasizing a commitment to patients' treatment priorities. Building rapport in this manner is vital because it may be very difficult to engage individuals experiencing command hallucinations in a way that allows for sustained treatment. The initial assessment should be used to identify the parameters of the hallucinations (e.g., voice identity, benevolence/malevolence, voice omnipotence, degree of compliance), and to begin bolstering the patients' perceived control.

Secondly, the intervention involves employing cognitive strategies to help the patients manipulate the occurrence of command hallucinations. Thus, clinicians help the patients begin to challenge their beliefs, question the evidence, conduct reality testing, and refute the commands. Patients are further coached regarding the benefits of resisting commands and are encouraged to take a more detached view of their experience - all of which serve the ultimate goal of empowering patients and enhancing mastery.

Expanding cognitive therapy to include behavioral and social skills training is another potential treatment approach (Granholm et al, 2002). McQuaid et al. (2000) noted that cognitive-behavioral therapy and social skills training may improve functioning among people with schizophrenia by lessening cognitive vulnerabilities such as self-defeating beliefs, increasing coping skills, and improving treatment adherence. It is likely that patients with command auditory hallucinations might benefit in many of the same ways by learning to identify, monitor and "check" their symptoms.

We needed further empirical research regarding cognitive treatments for the positive symptoms of schizophrenia (Chadwick and Birchwood, 1994; McQuaid et al, 2000), and Byrne et al. (2003) reported that a randomized controlled trial has been undertaken. We recommend emphasizing the overall assessment of the effectiveness of psychotherapeutic treatments for command hallucinations and, specifically, their ability to improve suicidal behavior.

Conclusion

This review of the research on the association between hallucinations and suicidal behaviour indicates that the prevalence of suicidal ideation, suicide attempts and completed suicide among people with schizophrenia is high. Several researchers have argued that the presence of command hallucinations is relevant to the increased rate of suicide in people with schizophrenia. However, the exact nature of the association of command hallucinations and suicidal behaviour is unclear, and the findings of the studies were quite contradictory.

Although most empirical studies find no statistically significant relationship between command hallucinations and suicidal behaviour, we argue that the occurrence of command hallucinations is clinically significant. Every clinician should investigate the presence of command hallucinations, and the clinical management of command hallucinations may play a role in preventing suicidal behavior.

References

Allebeck, P. (1989). Schizophrenia: A life-shortening disease. *Schizophrenia Bulletin, 15,* 81-89.

Allebeck, P. & Wistedt, B. (1986). Mortality in schizophrenia: A ten-year follow-up based on the Stockholm County inpatient register. *Archives of General Psychiatry, 43,* 650-653.

American Psychiatric Association (1994). *Diagnostic and Statistical Manual of Mental Disorders, 4th ed.* Washington, DC: American Psychiatric Association.

American Psychiatric Association (1997). Practice guidelines for the treatment of patients with schizophrenia. *American Psychiatric Association, 154,* 1-63.

American Psychiatric Association (2003). Practice guideline for the assessment and treatment of patients with suicidal behavior. *American Journal of Psychiatry, 160.*

Barraclough, B., Bunch, J., Nelson, B., & Sainsbury, P. (1974) A hundred cases of suicide: clinical aspects. *British Journal of Psychiatry, 125,* 355-373.

Beautrais, A. L., Joyce, P. R., Mulder, R. T., Fergusson, D. M., Deavoll, B. J., & Nightingale, S. K. (1996). Prevalence and comorbidity of mental disorders in persons making serious attempts: a case– control study. *American Journal of Psychiatry., 153,* 1009-1014.

Beck, A. T., & Rector, N. A. (2003). Cognitive model of hallucinations. *Cognitive Therapy and Research, 27,* 19-25.

Beck-Sander, A., Birchwood, M., & Chadwick, P. (1997). Acting on command hallucinations: a cognitive approach. *British Journal of Clinical Psychology, 36,* 139-148.

Breier, A., & Astrachan, B. M. (1984). Characterization of schizophrenic patients who commit suicide. *American Journal of Psychiatry, 141,* 206-209.

Breier, A., Schreiber, J. L., Dyer, J., & Pickar, D. (1991). National Institute of Mental Health longitudinal study of chronic schizophrenia: Prognosis and predictors of outcome. *Archives of General Psychiatry, 48,* 239-246.

Buckley, P. F., Hrouda, D. R., Friedman, L., Noffsinger, S. G., Resnick, P. J., & Camlin-Shingler, K. (2004). Insight and its relationship to violent behavior in patients with schizophrenia. *American Journal of Psychiatry, 161,* 1712-1714

Byrne, S., Trower, P., Birchwood, M., Meaden, A., & Nelson, A. (2003). Command hallucinations: Cognitive theory, therapy, and research. *Journal of Cognitive Psychotherapy: An International Quarterly, 17,* 67-84.

Caldwell, C. B., & Gottesman, I. I. (1992). Schizophrenia--a high risk factor for suicide: Clues to risk reduction. *Suicide and Life-Threatening Behavior, 22,* 479-493.

Caldwell, C. B., & Gottesman, I. I. (1990). Schizophrenics kill themselves too: A review of risk factors for suicide. *Schizophrenia Bulletin, 16,* 571-589.

Chadwick, P., & Birchwood, M. (1994). The omnipotence of voices: A cognitive approach to auditory hallucinations. *British Journal of Psychiatry, 164,* 190-201.

Chakos, M., Lieberman, J., Hoffman, E., Bradford, D., & Sheitman, B. (2001). Effectiveness of second-generation antipsychotics in patients with treatment-resistant schizophrenia: a review and meta-analysis of randomized trials. *American Journal of Psychiatry, 158,* 518-526.

Cheng, K. K., Leung, C. M., Lo, W. H., & Lam, T. H. (1990). Risk factors of suicide among schizophrenics. *Acta Psychiatrica Scandinavica, 81,* 220-224.

Cheung, P., Schweitzer, I., Crowley, K., & Tuckwell, V. (1997). Violence in schizophrenia: role of hallucinations and delusions. *Schizophria Research, 26,* 181-190.

Citrone, L., Volavka, J., Czobor, P., Sheitman, B., Lindenmayer, J., McEvoy, J., Cooper, T.B., Chakos, M., & Liberman, J. (2001). Effects of clozapine, olanzapine, Risperidone, and haloperidol on hostility among patients with schizophrenia. *Psychiatric Services, 52,* 1510-1514.

Conner, K. R., Conwell, Y., Duberstein, P. R., & Eberly, S. (2004). Aggression in suicide among adults age 50 and over. *American Journal of Geriatric Psychiatry, 12,* 37-42.

Conwell, Y., Duberstein, P. R., & Caine, E. D. (2002). Risk factors for suicide in later life. *Biological Psychiatry, 52,* 193-204.

Cotton, P. G., Drake, R. E., & Gates, C. (1985). Critical treatment issues in suicide among schizophrenics. *Hospital and Community Psychiatry, 36,* 534-536.

Davis, J. M., Chen, N., & Glick, I. D. (2003). A meta-analysis of the efficacy of second-generation antipsychotics. *Archives of General Psychiatry, 60,* 553-564.

Delespaul, P., DeVries, M., & van Os, J. (2002). Determinants of occurrence and recovery from hallucinations in daily life. *Social Psychiatry and Psychiatric Epidemiology, 37,* 97-104.

Drake, R. E., Gates, C., Whitaker, A., & Cotton, P. G. (1985). Suicide among schizophrenics: A review. *Comprehensive Psychiatry, 26,* 90-100.

Erkwoh, R., Willmes, K., Eming-Erdmann, A., & Kunert, H. J. (2002). Command hallucinations: who obeys and who resists when? *Psychopathology, 35,* 272-279.

Essock, S. M., Frisman, L. K., Covell, N. H., & Hargreaves, W. A. (2000). Cost-effectiveness of clozapine compared with conventional antipsychotic medication for patients in state hospitals. *Archives of General Psychiatry, 57*, 987-994.

Frances, A., Docherty, J. P., & Kahn, D. A. (1996). Expert Consensus Guidelines Series: Treatment of schizophrenia. *Journal of Clinical Psychiatry, 12B*, 5-58.

Granholm, E., McQuaid, J. R., McClure, F. S., Pedrelli, P. & Jeste, D. V. (2002). A randomized controlled pilot study of cognitive behavioral social skills training for older patients with schizophrenia. *Schizophrenia Research, 53*, 167-169.

Harkavy-Friedman, J. M., Kimhy, D., Nelson, E. A., Venarde, D. F., Malaspina, D., & Mann, J. J. (2003). Suicide attempts in schizophrenia: the role of command auditory hallucinations for suicide. *Journal of Clinical Psychiatry, 64*, 871-874.

Harris, E. C., & Barraclough, B. (1997). Suicide as an outcome for mental disorders. A meta-analysis. *British Journal of Psychiatry, 170*, 205-228.

Hawton, K., Sutton, L., Haw, C., Sinclair, J., & Deeks, J. J. (2005). Schizophrenia and suicide: systematic review of risk factors. *British Journal of Psychiatry, 187*, 9-20.

Hellerstein, D., Frosch, W., & Koenigsberg, W. (1987). The clinical significance of command hallucinations. *American Journal of Psychiatry, 144*, 219-221.

Inskip, H. M., Harris, E. C., & Barraclough, B. (1998). Lifetime risk of suicide for affective disorder, alcoholism and schizophrenia. *British Journal of Psychiatry, 172*, 35-37.

Junginger, J. (1990). Predicting compliance with command hallucinations. *American Journal of Psychiatry, 147*, 245-247.

Junginger, J., & McGuire, L. (2001). The paradox of command hallucinations. *Psychiatric Services, 52*, 385-386.

Kane, J. M., Marder, S. R., Schooler, N. R., Wirshing, W. C., Umbricht, D., Baker, R. W., et al. (2001). Clozapine and haloperidol in moderately refractory schizophrenia: A 6-month randomized and double-blind comparison. *Archives of General Psychiatry, 58*, 965-972.

Kasper, M. E., Rogers, R., & Adams, P. A. (1996). Dangerousness and command hallucinations: an investigation of psychotic inpatients. *Bulletin of the American Academmy of Psychiatry and the Law, 24*, 219-224.

Kennedy, B. R., Williams, C. A., & Pesut, D. J. (1994). Hallucinatory experiences of psychiatric patients in seclusion. *Archives of Psychiatric Nursing, 8*, 169-176.

Lakeman, R. (2001). Making sense of the voices. *International Joal of Nursing Studies, 38*, 523-531.

Leucht, S., Barnes, T. R., Kissling, W., Engel, R. R., Correll, C., & Kane, J. M. (2003). Relapse prevention in schizophrenia with new-generation antipsychotics: a systematic review and exploratory meta-analysis of randomized, controlled trials. *Amerian Journal of Psychiatry, 160*, 1209-1222.

Mann, J. J. (2003). Neurobiology of suicidal behaviour. *Nature Reviews, 4*, 819-828.

Marder, S. R., Essock, S. M., Miller, A. L., Buchanan, R. W., Davis, J. M., Kane, J. M., Lieberman, J., & Schooler, N. R. (2002). The Mount Sinai Conference on the Pharmacotherapy of Schizophrenia. *Schizophrenia Bulletin, 28*, 5-16.

Margo, A., Hemsley, D. R., & Slade, P. D. (1981). The effects of varying auditory input on schizophrenic hallucinations. *British Journal of Psychiatry, 139*, 122-127.

McNiel, D. E., Eisner, J. P., & Binder, R. L. (2000). The relationship between command hallucinations and violence. *Psychiatric Services, 51*, 1288-1292.

McQuaid, J. R., Granholm, E., McClure, F. S., Roepke, S., Pedrelli, P., Patterson, T. L., & Jeste, D. V. (2000). Development of an integrated cognitive-behavioral, social skills training intervention for older patients with schizophrenia. *Journal of Psychotherapy Practice and Research, 9,* 1-8.

Meltzer, H. Y. (2004). What's atypical about atypical antipsychotic drugs? *Current Opinion in Pharmacology, 4,* 53-57.

Meltzer, H. Y., Alphs, L., Green, A. I., Altamura, A. C., Anand, R., Bertoldi, A., Bourgeois, M., Chouinard, G., Islam, M. Z., Kane, J., Krishnan, R., Lindenmayer, J. P., Potkin, S., & International Suicide Prevention Trial Study Group. (2003). Clozapine treatment for suicidality in schizophrenia: International Suicide Prevention Trial (InterSePT). *Archives of General Psychiatry, 60,* 82-91.

Meltzer, H. Y., & Okayli, G. (1995). Reduction of suicidality during clozapine treatment of neuroleptic-resistant schizophrenia: Impact on risk-benefit assessment. *American Journal of Psychiatry, 152,* 183-190.

Miles, C. P. (1977). Conditions predisposing to suicide: A review. *Journal of Nervous and Mental Disease, 164,* 231-246.

Miller, A. L., Chiles, J. A., & Chiles, J. K. (1999). The Texas Medication Algorithm Project (TMAP) schizophrenia algorithms. *Journal of Clinical Psychiatry, 60,* 649-657.

Miller, A. L., Hall, C. S., Buchanan, R. W., Buckley, P. F., Chiles, J. A., Conley, R. R., Crismon, M. L., Ereshefsky, L., Essock, S. M., Finnerty, M., Marker, S. R., Miller del, D., McEvoy, J. P., Rush, A. J., Saeed, S. A., Schooler, N. R., Shon, S. P., Stroup, S., & Tarin-Godoy, B. (2004). The Texas Medication Algorithm Project antipsychotic algorithm for schizophrenia: 2003 update. *Journal of Clinical Psychiatry, 65,* 500-508.

Modestin, J., Zarro, I., & Waldvogel, D. (1992). A study of suicide in schizophrenic inpatients. *British Journal of Psychiatry, 160,* 398-401.

Nasrallah, H. A., & Smeltzer, D. J. (2002). *Contemoporary Diagnosis and Management of The Patient with Schizophrenia.* Newton, PA: Handbooks in Health Care.

Nelson, B. (1997). *Cognitive Behavioural Therapy with Schizophrenia: A Practice Manual.* Cheltenham, UK: Stanley Thornes (Publishers) Ltd.

Nordentoft, M., Jeppesen, P., Abel, M., Kassow, P., Petersen, L., Thorup, A., Krarup, G., Hemmingsen, R., & Jorgensen, P. (2002). OPUS study: suicidal behaviour, suicidal ideation and hopelessness among patients with first-episode psychosis. One-year follow-up of a randomised controlled trial. *British Journal of Psychiatry, 43,* s98-s106.

O'Connor, F. W. (1991). Symptom monitoring for relapse prevention in schizophrenia. *Archives of Psychiatric Nursing, 5,* 193-201.

O'Connor, F. W. (1994). A vulnerability-stress framework for evaluating clinical interventions in schizophrenia. *Image--the Journal of Nursing Scholarship, 26,* 231-237.

Pinikahana, J., Happell, B., & Keks, N. A. (2003). Suicide and schizophrenia: a review of literature for the decade (1990-1999) and implications for mental health nursing. *Issues in Mental Health Nursing, 24,* 27-43.

Planansky, K., & Johnston, R. (1973) Clinical setting and motivation in suicidal attempts of schizophrenics. *Acta Psychiatrica Scandinavica, 49,* 680-690.

Pompili, M., Amador, X.F., Girardi, P., Harkavy-Friedman, J., Harrow, M., Kaplan, K., Krausz, M., Lester, D., Meltzer, H.Y., Modestin, J., Montross, L.P., Mortensen, P.B., Munk-Jorgensen, P., Nielsen, J., Nordentoft, M., Saarinen, P.I., Zisook, S., Wilson, S.T.,

& Tatarelli, R. (2007).Suicide risk in schizophrenia: learning from the past to change the future. *Annals of General Psychiatry*, 6,10

Pompili, M., Lester, D., Innamorati, M., Tatarelli, R.. & Girardi P. (2008). Assessment and treatment of suicide risk in schizophrenia. *Expert Review of Neurotherapeuthics*, 8, 51-74.

Preti, A., Tondo, L., Sisti, D., Rocchi, M. B., & de Girolamo, G. (2010). Correlates and antecedents of hospital admission for attempted suicide: a nationwide survey in Italy. *European Archives of Psychiatry and Clinical Neuroscience, 260*(3), 181-190.

Raymont, V. (2001). Suicide in schizophrenia - how can research influence training and clinical practice? *Psychiatric Bulletin*, 25, 46-50.

Rogers, D. R. (1988). Autoamputation of the left arm--a bizarre suicide. *The American Journal of Forensic Medicine and* Pathology, 9, 64-65.

Rogers, P., Watt, A., Gray, N. S., MacCulloch, M., & Gournay, K. (2002). Content of command hallucinations predicts self-harm but not violence in a medium secure unit. *American Journal of Forensic Psychiatry*, 13, 251-262.

Rogers, R., Gillis, R., Turner, E., & Frise-Smith, T. (1990). The clinical presentation of command hallucinations in a forensic population. *American Journal of Psychiatry*, 147, 1304-1307.

Roy, A. (1986). Depression, attempted suicide, and suicide in patients with chronic schizophrenia. *Psychiatric Clinics of North America*, 9, 193-206.

Roy, A., & Pompili, M. (2009). Management of schizophrenia with suicide risk. *Psychiatric Clinics of North America*, 32:863-83

Rudnick A. Relation between command hallucinations and dangerous behavior. *Journal of the American Academy of Psychiatry and the Law*, 1999, 27:253-257

Shaffer, D., Gould, M. S., Fisher, P., Trautman, P., Moreau, D., Kleinman, M., & Flory, M. (1996). Psychiatric diagnosis in child and adolescent suicide. *Archives of General Psychiatry, 53(4)*, 339-48.

Siris, S. G. (2001). Suicide and schizophrenia. *Journal of Psychopharmacology*, 15, 127-135.

Slade, P. D. (1976). Towards a theory of auditory hallucinations: outline of an hypothetical four-factor model. *The British Journal of Social and Clinical Psychology*, 15, 415-423.

Tarrier, N., Goodinga, P., Gregga, L., Johnsona, J., & Drakeb, R. (2007). The Socrates Trial Group. Suicide schema in schizophrenia: The effect of emotional reactivity, negative symptoms and schema elaboration *Behaviour Research and Therapy, 45*, 2090-2097.

Wasserman, D. (2001). *Suicide - an unnecessary death*. London: Martin Dunitz Publishers.

World Health Organization. (1973). *International pilot study of schizophrenia*. Geneva: World Health Organizaton.

Zisook, S., Byrd, D., Kuck, J., & Jeste, D. V. (1995). Command hallucinations in outpatients with schizophrenia. *Journal of Clinical Psychiatry*, 56, 462-465.

In: Hallucinations: Types, Stages and Treatments
Editor: Meredith S. Payne, pp. 179-193
ISBN: 978-1-61728-275-1
© 2011 Nova Science Publishers, Inc.

Chapter 10

Behavioral Symptoms of Dementia

Ladislav Volicer and Elizabeth Vongxaiburana
School of Aging Studies, University of South Florida, Tampa, FL, USA

Abstract

Behavioral symptoms of dementia are often more difficult to manage than consequences of cognitive impairment. They may lead to caregiver burn-out or need for institutionalization. It is important to distinguish two types of behavioral symptoms: those which occur when the patient is solitary and those which occur when the patient is interacting with others. When patients are solitary they may develop agitation or apathy; very often these symptoms alternate in the same patient. When the patients are interacting with their caregivers, they may resist their care efforts because they do not understand why they need the care. If the caregiver persists in providing care despite patient's resistiveness, the patients may defend themselves, become combative and their behavior may be called abusive. Behaviors labeled abusive are often the most difficult behaviors of nursing home residents to manage. Resistiveness to care, related to lack of understanding, depression, hallucinations and delusions, are strongly related to abusive behaviors. Presence of depressive symptoms and delusions is also related to abusive behaviors independent of resistiveness to care. Very few residents who understand others and are not depressed are abusive. Behavioral interventions preventing escalation of resistiveness to care into combative behavior and the treatment of depression can be expected to decrease or prevent abusive behavior of many nursing home residents with dementia. Therefore, antidepressants should be used initially when non-pharmacological interventions are not effective.

Introduction

Behavioral symptoms of dementia are often more difficult to manage than consequences of cognitive impairment. They may lead to caregiver burn-out or need for institutionalization [1]. Research and treatment of behavioral symptoms of dementia are hindered by inconsistent and confusing terminology of these symptoms. Some research uses one term encompassing all symptoms, e.g. "behavioral and psychological symptoms of dementia (BPSD)" [2], "agitation" [3] or "obstreperous behavior". Several conceptual frameworks were developed to classify and describe behavioral symptoms of dementia on the basis of nursing, psychological, or psychiatric concepts [4]. They include Need-Driven Dementia-Compromised Behavior (NDB) [5], Progressively Lowered Stress Threshold (PLST) [6], Antecedent-Behavior-Consequence model (ABC) [7], Habilitation Approach [8], and the Psychobehavioral Metaphor model [9]. Although these models provide some guidance for management of behavioral symptoms of dementia, none of them were generally accepted and all of them have some drawbacks. For instance, the NDB model does not recognize the importance of caregiver behavior in escalation of resistiveness to care to combative behavior [10]; limited daytime napping by episodes of exercise decreased agitation contrary to the PLST assumption [11]; and interventions based on the ABC model did not reduce disruptive behavior [12]. Although the Psychobehavioral Model stresses use of other psychoactive medications than antipsychotics, it did not succeed in decreasing the use of antipsychotics in demented nursing home residents.

The main problem with most of these terms and conceptual frameworks is failure to clearly differentiate between behaviors that are present when the patient is solitary, and behaviors that are present when the patient is interacting with others. This distinction is very important because non-pharmacological interventions for these two types of behaviors are quite different. Behaviors that occur when the patient is solitary require intervention of the caregiver; preferably involvement in meaningful activities but sometimes pharmacological management is also required. In contrast, behaviors that occur when the patient is interacting with others require modification of the behavior of the individual who is interacting with the patient. Common examples of these two types of behaviors are agitation defined in a narrow sense below as a solitary behavior, and resistiveness to care that occurs when the patient interacts with a care provider. These two types of behaviors have very different relationships with dementia severity (Figure 1)[13]. Agitation occurs quite frequently even in individuals with borderline cognitive impairment, while resistiveness to care occurs rarely in individuals with mild dementia but increases significantly with progression of dementia. Therefore, this chapter will describe separately behaviors occurring when the patient is solitary and behaviors occurring when the patient interacts with others.

Behaviors While the Patient Is Solitary

Several behaviors may occur when the patient is not interacting with others. They include hoarding, inappropriate dressing or disrobing, eating or drinking inedible substances, hiding things, and collecting items belonging to others. Some of these behaviors are very important because they may lead to decreased dignity of the patient (e.g., disrobing, eating inedible substances) or to undesirable interaction with other residents of a long-term facility (e.g., invading other residents' rooms or collecting items belonging to others). However, the most common behaviors that occur when the patient is solitary are agitation as defined below and apathy.

Agitation

Agitation in the narrow sense of the word may be described as "behaviors that communicate to others that the person with dementia is experiencing an unpleasant state of excitement and that are unrelated to known physical needs of the patient that can be remedied and are without known motivational intent." [14] The symptoms of agitation may include restlessness, repetitive verbalization, and repetitive physical movements. However as will be described below, there is not a complete agreement which symptoms should be included under this narrow definition of agitation. It is important to realize that these symptoms could be evoked by either physical needs of the patient (e.g., pain, hunger, thirst) or by environmental factors (e.g., noise, too high or low temperatures). Therefore, it is very important to exclude these factors before behaviors indicating agitation can be ascribed to the dementing process itself.

The confusion related to the term of "agitation" is clearly documented by inappropriate use of this term in the Neuropsychiatric Inventory (NPI) [15] and inconsistent inclusion of Minimum Data Set (MDS) items in MDS-based scales for measurement of agitation. One of the behavioral areas measured by NPI is labeled "Agitation/Aggression" but the probing question is "Does subject have periods when he/she refuses to cooperate or won't let people help him/her? Is he/she hard to handle?". Thus, this behavioral area is actually measuring problems occurring during interaction with a caregiver, not behavior exhibited when the patient is solitary. An MDS-based scale for measuring agitation was recently developed using factor analysis of MDS items [16]. This analysis identified four behavioral domains: Conflict, Withdrawal, Agitation and Attention Seeking. The Attention Seeking domain contains some items that could be considered symptoms of agitation (repetitive questions and complaints). Its separation from symptoms included in the Agitation domain could be due to the degree of verbal impairment caused by dementia. Alternative selection of items was used for the study represented in Figure 1. (Table 1).

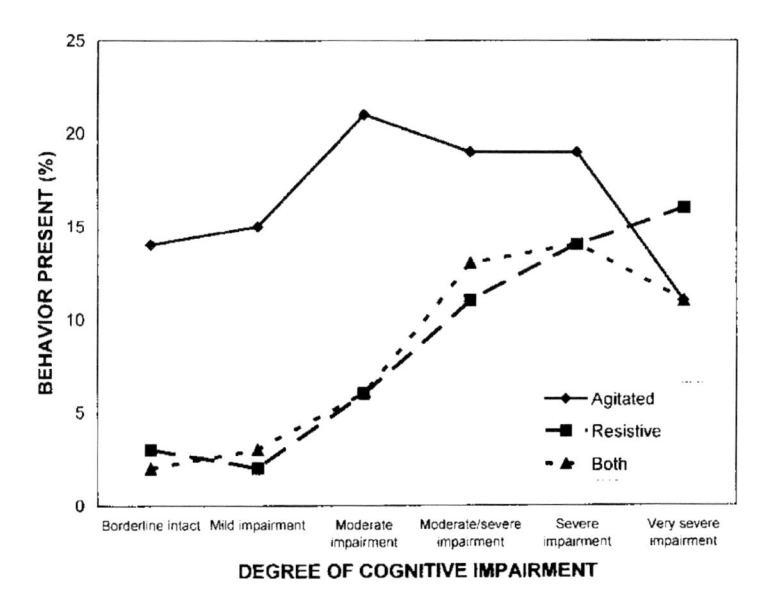

Figure 1. Prevalence or agitation and resistiveness in nursing home residents with different degree of cognitive impairment (reprinted with permission from [13])

Table 1. Items from the Minimum Data Set (MDS) proposed for measurement of agitation

Gerritsen et al. [16]	Volicer et al. [13]
Periods of restlessness (B5d) Repetitive physical movements (E1n) Wandering (E4aa) Socially inappropriate/disruptive behavior (E4da)	Repetitive questions (E1b) Repetitive verbalization (E1c) Expression of what appear to be unrealistic fears (E1f) Repetitive health complaints (E1b) Repetitive anxious complaints or concerns (E1j) Repetitive physical movements (E1n)
Alpha = 0.70	Alpha = 0.71

Reports from the literature indicate that agitation is one of the most common behavioral symptoms of dementia; however, most of these studies used the broad definition of agitation including practically all behavioral symptoms of dementia. Rowe et al. found verbal agitation in 86% and physical agitation in 55% of community dwelling persons with dementia [17]; Cohen-Mansfield reported that two agitated behaviors at least once a week were present in 87% of nursing home residents with dementia [18]. Agitation has similar prevalence in different etiologies of progressive dementias and is associated with more neurofibrillary tangles in the orbitofrontal cortex [19].

Apathy

Apathy is a symptom different from depression [20]. It may be diagnosed by responses to the Apathy/Indifference domain of NPI where the probing questions are: "Has subject lost interest in the world around him/her? Has she/he lost interest in doing things or lack motivation for starting new activities? Is he/she more difficult to engage in conversation or doing chores? Is subject apathetic or indifferent?" The MDS has two items that are related to the presence of apathy located in Section E, "Mood and Behavior Patterns"; "Indicators of Depression, Anxiety, Sad Mood"; "Loss of Interest"):*Withdrawal from activities of interest* and *Reduced social interaction*.

Apathy is also a very common behavioral symptom of dementia, present in 27% of individuals with dementia living in the community [21] and up to 92% of patients with advanced dementia [22]. It is less common in individuals with dementia who lived with their spouses than in individuals who lived with others [23]. Apathy characteristics differ in individuals with less severe and more severe dementia. In less severe individuals, apathy was associated with worse quality of life and decreased functional abilities but there was no correlation between apathy and depression. In more severe individuals, apathy was associated with depression, and decreased functional abilities but not with worse quality of life [24]. Unfortunately, apathy is very often not diagnosed and treated because apathetic patients do not cause a disturbance that would attract caregivers' attention. Incidence of apathy is related to the presence of neurofibrillary tangles in anterior cingulate cortex [25] and to reduced perfusion in the left anterior cingulated, right inferior and medial gyrus frontalis, left orbitofrontal gyrus and right gyrus lingualis [26].

Apathy very often coexists with agitation. Analysis of MDS data from Dutch nursing homes using the scales described above [16] showed that 45% of residents have symptoms of agitation, 37% symptoms of apathy and 25% have symptoms of both apathy and agitation (unpublished results). These residents switch from agitation to apathy sometimes several times a day; furthermore, they are difficult to treat with medication because sedating medications increase apathy and stimulating medications increase agitation. The best treatment for these residents and for all other residents with either apathy or agitation is involvement in meaningful activities [27].

A randomized study found that involvement in music therapy significantly decreased agitation and apathy in patients with moderate-severe dementia [28]. Multi-sensory behavior therapy using Snoezelen added to standard pharmacological and occupational therapy decreased both agitation and apathy and improved activities of daily living [29]. An open-labeled study recently reported that administration of methylphenidate improved apathy, and also depression Mini-Mental Examination score and functional status [30].

Behaviors While Patient Is Interacting with Others

Behavioral symptoms that occur when the patient is interacting with others may be more difficult to manage than symptoms occurring when the patient is solitary. Patients may interact with caregivers or, if the patients reside in a long-term care facility, with other residents. This interaction may involve grabbing somebody's hand to get a companion for wandering, sexual advances, or entering somebody else's room. However, the most common behavior that causes problems for the caregivers is resistiveness to care, which may escalate into combativeness and abusive behavior.

Resistiveness to care

Resistiveness to care may be defined as "Behaviors that are used by a person with dementia to withstand or oppose care" [31]. Resistiveness to care occurs most frequently during hands on care when activities of daily living are provided by a caregiver, during administration of medications, and when redirecting the patient. A survey of 110 physicians providing services to nursing home residents identified resisting care as to most common symptom present in 71% or residents, more common than restlessness reported to be present in 50% of residents [32].

Resistiveness to care mainly happens because the patient does not understand the intent of the caregiver and the need for care. Therefore, the patient resists unwanted attention of the caregiver and may even strike out if the caregiver insists on providing the care. This explanation is supported by the increased prevalence of resistiveness to care in patients who lack understanding because of cognitive impairment (Figure 2). However, resistiveness to care is also increased by presence of hallucinations and delusions and by depression. The escalation of resistiveness to care into combative behavior is sometimes labeled "aggression" and persons with dementia are considered "aggressive". In fact, the person with dementia may consider the caregiver to be the aggressor; labeling somebody who exhibits resistiveness to care "aggressive" is actually blaming the patient, someone who has been victimized by inappropriate caregiver approaches.

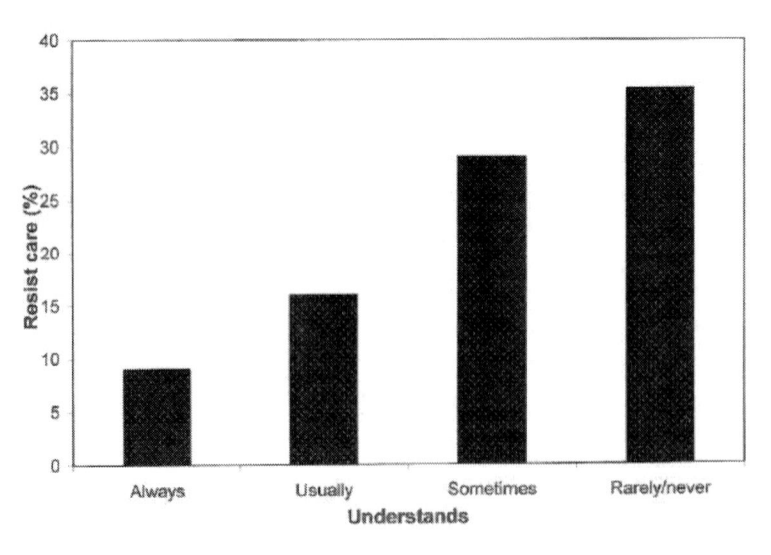

Figure 2. Prevalence of resistiveness to care in nursing home residents with different ability to understand others (reprinted with permission from [13])

It is important to prevent escalation of resistiveness to care into combative behavior that may result in injury to the patient or caregiver. Sometimes it is possible to gain the patient's cooperation by using white lies or "fiblets"; e.g., saying that the patient has to take a bath because his/her relative is coming for a visit. In other cases, it may help if the caregiver leaves and comes back after a short time because the patient may forget that he/she did not want to accept care and will become cooperative. Distraction during care may be also useful, such as reminiscing with the patient. Resistiveness during bathing is difficult to manage, but the most effective intervention is to change the care strategy: development of person-centered showering, or replacement of shower bath by bed bath [33].

Abusive behavior

Abusive behavior of an individual with dementia may be directed towards a caregiver or another resident and could be either verbal or physical. Not all abusive behaviors are due to escalation of resistiveness to care. Analysis of MDS data from residents of Dutch nursing homes showed that depression may cause both verbal and physical abuse independent of resistiveness to care, and delusions may cause verbal abuse independent of resistiveness to care (Figure 3). The importance of depression for development of abusive behavior, which is often labeled "aggression", is supported by correlation of aggression with abnormalities of the serotoninergic system.

Aggression before death was found to be related to decreased density of serotonin (5-HT) 1A receptors found on autopsy [34] and aggressive subjects exhibited supersensitivity of 5-HT receptors indicating less serotoninergic activity [35]. Polymorphism of 5-HT_{2A} receptors was correlated with aggressive behavior in two studies [36;37] while in another study the same polymorphism was related just to hallucinations and delusions [38]. Similarly, two studies found relationship between polymorphism of the 5-HT transporter that may result in increased reuptake of 5-HT and aggressive behavior [39;40] while one study found relationship only with psychosis [41]. The relationship between serotoninergic function and aggressive behavior may not be unique for Alzheimer's disease because decreased serotoninergic activity is present also in frontotemporal dementia [42].

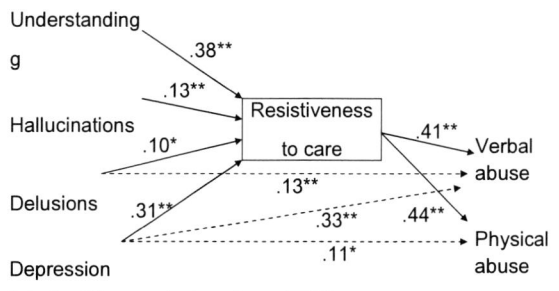

** p<.000, *p<.005 (reprinted with permission from [43]).

Figure 3. Model of risk factors for abusive behavior based on statistically significant relationships of antecedent factors to resistiveness to care and verbal and physical abuse. The dotted lines show partial correlation coefficients when resistiveness to care is controlled for

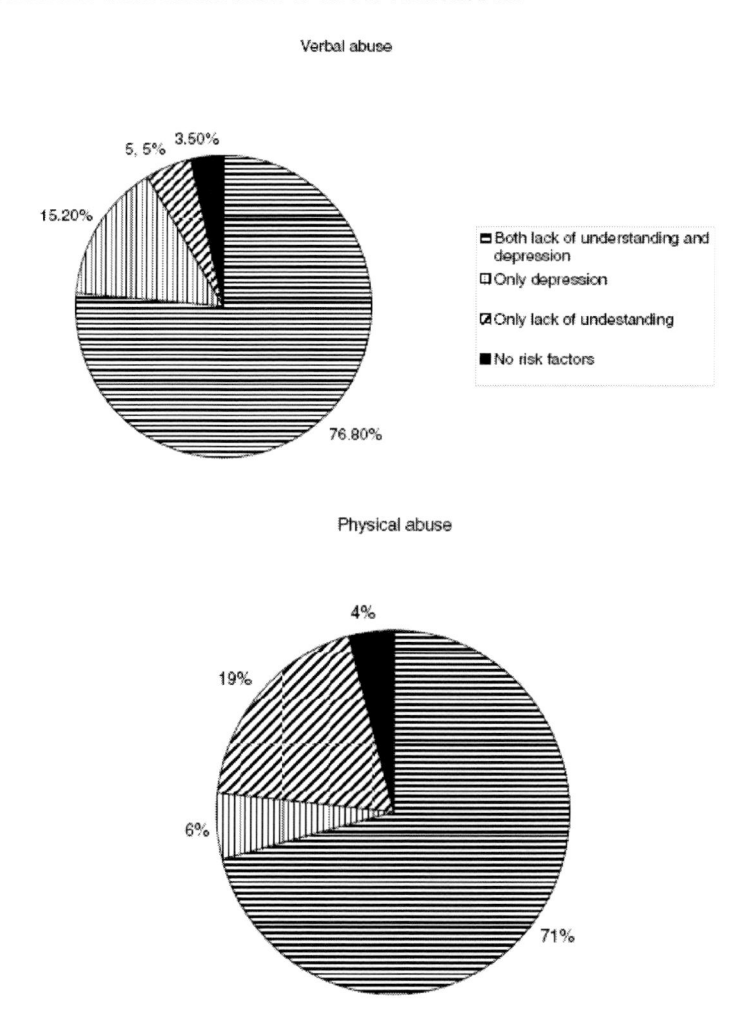

Figure 4. Presence of two main risk factors for abusive behavior in nursing home residents with dementia

Analysis of MDS data from Dutch nursing homes indicated that abusive behavior is strongly correlated with resistive behavior and presence of depression [43], Delusions and hallucinations were also related to abusive behavior but the correlation was lower (Figure 3). This finding agrees with some previous data showing that physically aggressive behavior is associated with depression, male gender, and impairment in ADLs after adjustment for delusions, hallucinations, sleep disturbance and severity of dementia. In addition, after adjustment for depression, gender and impairment of ADLs, there was no association of abusive behavior with either delusions or hallucinations [44]. Similarly, analysis of MDS data from a national sample of nursing home residents found that both physical and verbal aggressions were correlated more strongly with presence of depression than with presence of delusions or hallucinations [45].

Lack of understanding and depression are the two most important risk factors for development of abusive behaviors, because resistive behavior is strongly correlated with, and in most cases caused by the lack of understanding, [43]. Analysis of MDS data indicated that less than 4% of residents who are labeled as abusive do not have either of these two risk factors (Figure 4). Therefore, improvement of communications between caregivers and residents and effective treatment of depression may eliminate most episodes of abusive behavior.

Depression in Dementia

Depression in AD is often unrecognized and overlooked [46]. Prevalence rates range from 15 percent to as high as 50 percent [47]. One reason for highly variable prevalence rates of depression in AD is due to difficulties in diagnosis. Major overlap between symptoms of depression and symptoms of dementia complicate accurate diagnosis [48]. Additional reasons for the wide range of prevalence include differences in researchers' focus on symptoms versus specifically defined depressive disorders, diverse study samples varying in causes of dementia, stage of illness, country of residence, and placement of patient, as well as variation in the instruments used to assess depressive symptoms and disorders. Furthermore, disagreement over diagnostic criteria for depression in AD is another reason why prevalence rates are so variable; no general consensus on the most valid method to assess and diagnose depression in AD exists [48].

Recently, a consensus was reached regarding diagnostic criteria. Criteria for diagnosis of depression in individuals with Alzheimer's disease (Depression in AD) should be different from criteria for diagnosis of depression in cognitively intact individuals [49]. Although the provisional diagnostic criteria were derived from those for Major Depressive Episode, there are several significant differences. First, Depression of AD requires the presence of three or more symptoms (vs. five or more for Major Depressive Episode). Second, this diagnosis does not require the presence of symptoms nearly every day, as is the case for Major Depressive Episode. Third, criteria for the presence of irritability and for the presence of social isolation or withdrawal were added. Fourth, the criteria for loss of interest or pleasure were revised to reflect decreased positive affect or decreased pleasure in response to social contact and usual activities

(Table 2). Depression in individuals with Alzheimer's disease may be also measured on the basis of several MDS items [50].

High prevalence of depression in individuals with Alzheimer's disease can be expected because Alzheimer's disease causes serotoninergic deficit [51]. Therefore, treatment with antidepressants that potentiate the effect of serotonin may be similar to treatment with cholinesterase inhibitors that potentiate the effect of acetylcholine. Of course, non-pharmacological treatment of depression in Alzheimer's disease may be also effective especially in patients with mild or moderate dementia. Nonpharmacologic therapies specifically targeting depression or its symptoms can be roughly categorized as emotion-oriented therapies, brief psychotherapies, and sensory stimulation therapies [52].

Table 2. Provisional diagnostic criteria for depression of alzheimer Alzheimer's disease

A.	Three (or more) of the following symptoms have been present during the same 2-week period and represent a change from previous functioning: at least one of the symptoms is either 1) depressed mood or 2) decreased positive affect or pleasure.
\multicolumn{2}{l	}{Note: Do not include symptoms that, in your judgment, are clearly due to a medical condition other than Alzheimer disease, or are a direct result of non-mood-related dementia symptoms (e.g., loss of weight due to difficulties with food intake).}
1)	Clinically significant depressed mood (e.g., depressed, sad, hopeless, discouraged, tearful)
2)	Decreased positive affect or pleasure in response to social contacts and usual activities
3)	Social isolation or withdrawal
4)	Disruption in appetite
5)	Disruption in sleep
6)	Psychomotor changes (e.g., agitation or retardation)
7)	Irritability
8)	Fatigue or loss of energy
9)	Feelings of worthlessness, hopelessness, or excessive inappropriate guilt
10)	Recurrent thoughts of death, suicidal ideation, plan or attempt
B.	All criteria are met for Dementia of the Alzheimer Type (DSM-IV-TR).
C.	The symptoms cause clinically significant distress or disruption in functioning.
D.	The symptoms do not occur exclusively during the course of a delirium.
E.	The symptoms are not due to the direct physiological effects of a substance (e.g., a drug of abuse or a medication).
F.	The symptoms are not better accounted for by other conditions such as major depressive disorder, bipolar disorder, bereavement, schizophrenia, schizoaffective disorder, psychosis of Alzheimer disease, anxiety disorders, or substance-related disorder.
\multicolumn{2}{l	}{*Specify if:*}
\multicolumn{2}{l	}{**Co-occuring Onset:** if onset antedates or co-occurs with the AD symptom}
\multicolumn{2}{l	}{**Post-AD Onset**: if onset occurs after the AD symptoms}
\multicolumn{2}{l	}{*Specify:*}
\multicolumn{2}{l	}{**With Psychosis of Alzheimer Disease**}
\multicolumn{2}{l	}{**With Other Significant Behavioral Signs or Symptoms**}
\multicolumn{2}{l	}{**With Past History of Mood Disorder**}
\multicolumn{2}{l	}{Modified from [49]}

Antipsychotic Therapy

Antipsychotics are currently the most commonly used medications to treat behavioral symptoms of dementia. A survey of physicians practicing in nursing homes indicated that they consider resistiveness to care the most common problem occurring in 71% of nursing home residents with behavioral problems and that they use antipsychotics in 70% of residents with behavioral problems [32]. Antidepressants were not even listed separately and were included in a large group of other medications that were used in 12% of these residents. This prevalent use of antipsychotics mostly continues despite recent warning about serious side effects of antipsychotic medications. Antipsychotics increase the risk of stroke and sudden cardiac death [53], triple the incidence of serious events in community dwelling individuals and double the incidence in nursing home residents [54], increase incidence of hip fractures [55] and overall mortality rate [56].

Despite FDA "black box" warnings of these adverse consequences of antipsychotic use, there was relatively small decrease in the use of these medications. The use of atypical antipsychotics fell in the year following the advisory by 2% overall, although by 19% among those with dementia [57]. Unfortunately, since this warning was originally issued just for atypical antipsychotics, some of this decrease may represent a switch from atypical to typical antipsychotics, though it is now recognized that typical antipsychotics represent the same dangers [58]. Antipsychotics are used frequently despite several meta-analysis studies indicating a moderate effect of only some antipsychotics, namely olanzepine and risperidone in one study [59], and aripiprazole and risperidone in another [60]. A nationwide study found that 32% of antipsychotic drug users had no identified clinical indication for this therapy and that prevalence of antipsychotic use differ significantly in different facilities [61].

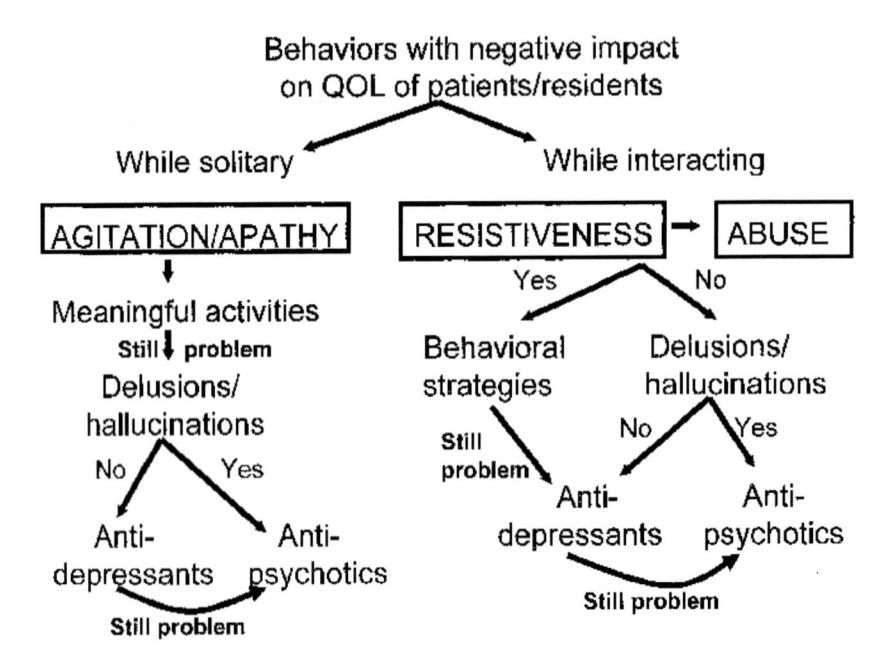

Figure 5. Algorithm for management of behavioral symptoms of dementia

What are the alternatives of antipsychotic use? A double-blind randomized study indicated that citalopram is as effective as risperidone in treatment of agitation and psychotic symptoms in patients with dementia [62]. In another study, citalopram decreased irritability and apathy scores by 60% without sedation in a group of behaviorally disturbed patients with Alzheimer's disease [63]. However, these effects require effective antidepressant doses and duration of therapy as indicated by the DIADS study where NPI score was improved only in those patients who obtained antidepressant effect after treatment with sertraline [64]. There is also some evidence that inhibitors of cholinesterase have small beneficial effects on behavioral symptoms of dementia [59] and one double-blind randomized study found that behavioral symptoms of dementia were improved by administration of prazosin [65].

Conclusion

An algorithm for management of behavioral symptoms of dementia based on information in this chapter is presented in Figure 6. Non-pharmacological management is the first step for both agitation/apathy and resistiveness/abusive behavior. However, the non-pharmacological approaches are different in these two types of symptoms. Agitation/apathy is best treated by providing meaningful activities in a continuous activity programming. Resistiveness should be diminished by improved communication with the patient; this may prevent escalation into combative behavior. Changes in care providing strategy are also very effective. If behavioral symptoms cannot be controlled by non-pharmacological interventions alone, antidepressants should be used as the first line medication choice. Antipsychotics should only be used as the first medication choice if the patient has hallucinations or delusions that are bothering the him/her and causing behavioral symptoms. Antipsychotics may be added if treatment with sufficient doses of an antidepressant is not effective. They may potentiate the antidepressant effect of antidepressants; aripiprazole was specifically approved by FDA for this purpose. The need for medications should be re-evaluated periodically and the non-pharmacological strategies should be continued even though the patient may be medicated.

References

[1] Phillips, V. L. & Diwan, S. (2003). The incremental effect of dementia-related problem behaviors on the time to nursing home placement in poor, frail, demented older people. *J Am Geriatr Soc*; *51*, 188-193.

[2] Thompson, C., Brodaty, H., Trollor, J. & Sachdev, P. (2009). Behavioral and psychological symptoms associated with dementia subtype and severity. *Int Psychogeriatrics*.

[3] Cohen-Mansfield, J., Werner, P. & Marx, M. S. (1989). An observational study of agitation in agitated nursing home residents. *Int Psychogeriatrics, 1*, 153-165.

[4] Volicer, L. & Hurley, A. C. (2003). Management of behavioral symptoms in progressive degenerative dementias. *Journal of Gerontology: Medical Sciences*; 58A, 837-845.

[5] Algase, D. L., Beck, C., Kolanowski, A., Whall, A., Berent, S. & Richards, K. et al. (1996). Need-driven dementia-compromised behavior: an alternative view of disruptive behavior. *Am J Alzheim Dis*; *11*, 10-19.

[6] Hall, G. R. & Buckwalter, K. C. (1987). Progressively lowered stress threshold: a conceptual model for care of adults with Alzheimer's disease. *Arch Psych Nurs, 1*, 399-406.

[7] Smith, M. & Buckwalter, K. (2005). Back to the A-B-C's: Understanding & Responding to Behavioral Symptoms in Dementia. University of Iowa, School of Nursing. 2005. http://www.nursing.uiowa.edu/hartford/nurse/back_abc.htm retrieved on 2-12-2010.

[8] Raia, P. (1999). Habilitation therapy: a new starscape. In: Volicer L, Bloom-Charette L, editors. *Enhancing the Quality of Life in Advanced Dementia*. Philadelphia: Taylor & Francis, 21-37.

[9] Tariot, P. N. (1999). Treatment of agitation in dementia. *J Clin Psychiatry, 60*, (suppl 8), 11-20.

[10] The measurement (1999). of Need-Driven Dementia-Compromised Behavior: achieving higher level of interrater reliability. *J Gerontol Nursing, 25*, 33-37.

[11] Alessi, C. A., Yoon, E. J., Schnelle, J. F., Al-Samarrai, N. R. & Cruise, P. A. (1999). A randomized trial of a combined physical activity and environmental intervention in nursing home residents: do sleep and agitation improve? *JAGS, 47*, 784-791.

[12] Beck, C. K., Vogelpohl, T. S., Rasin, J. H., Uriri, J. T., O'Sullivan, P. & Walls, R. et al.(2002). Effects of behavioral interventions on disruptive behavior and affect in demented nursing home residents. *Nurs Res, 51*, 219-228.

[13] Volicer, L., Bass, E. A. & Luther, S. L. (2007). Agitation and resistiveness to care are two separate behavioral syndromes of dementia. *Journal of the American Medical Directors Association, 8*, 527-532.

[14] Hurley, A. C., Volicer, L., Camberg, L., Ashley, J., Woods, P. & Odenheimer, G. et al. (1999). Measurement of observed agitation in patients with Alzheimer's disease. *J Mental Health Aging, 5*, 117-133.

[15] Cummings, J. L., Mega, M., Gray, K., Rosenberg-Thompson, S., Carusi, D. A. & Gornbein, J. (1994). The neuropsychiatric inventory: Comprehensive assessment of psychopathology in dementia. *Neurology, 44*, 2308-2314.

[16] Gerritsen, D. L., Achterberg, W. P., Steverink, N., Pot, A. M., Frijters, D. H. M. & Ribbe, M. W. (2008). The MDS Challenging Behavior Profile for long-term care. *Aging Mental Health, 12*, 116-123.

[17] Rowe, M. A., Straneva, J. A., Colling, K. B. & Grabo, R. (2000). Behavioral problems in community dwelling people with dementia. *Journal of Nursing Scholarship, 32*, 55-56.

[18] Cohen-Mansfield, J. (1988). Agitated behavior and cognitive functioning in nursing home residents: preliminary results. *Clin Gerontol, 7*(3/4), 11-22.

[19] Tekin, S., Mega, M. S., Masterman, D. M., Chow, T., Garakian, J. & Vinters, H. V. et al.(2001). Orbitofrontal and anterior cingulate cortex neurofibrillary tangle burden is associated with agitation in Alzheimer disease. *Ann Neurol, 49*, 355-361.

[20] Levy, M. L., Cummings, J. L., Fairbanks, L. A., Masterman, D., Miller, B. L., Craig, A. H. et al.(1998). Apathy is not depression. *Journal of Neuropsychiatry, 10*, 314-319.

[21] Lyketsos, C. G., Steinberg, M., Tschanz, J. T., Norton, M. C., Steffens, D. C. & Breitner, J. C. S. (2000). Mental and behavioral disturbances in dementia: Findings from the Cache County Study on Memory in Aging. *Am J Psychiatry, 157*, 708-714.

[22] Mega, M. S., Cummings, J. L., Fiorello, T. & Gornbein, J. (1996). The spectrum of behavioral changes in Alzheimer's disease. *Neurology, 46*, 130-135.

[23] Clarke, D. E., van Reekum, R., Simard, M., Streiner, D. L., Conn, D. & Cohen, T. et al. (2008). Apathy in dementia: clinical and sociodelmographic correlates. *Journal of Neuropsychiatry and Clinical Neuroscience, 20*, 337-347.

[24] Yeager, C. A. & Hyer, L. (2008). Apathy in dementia: relations with depression, functional competence, and quality of life. *Psychol Rep, 102*, 718-722.

[25] Marshall, G. A., Fairbanks, L. A., Tekin, S., Vinters, H. V. & Cummings, J. L. (2006). Neuropathologic correlates of apathy in Alzheimer's disease. *Dement Geriatr Cogn Disord, 21*, 144-147.

[26] Benoit, M., Koulibaly, P. M., Migneco, O., Darcourt, J., Pringuey, D. J. & Robert, P. H. (2002). Brain perfusion in Alzheimer's disease with and without apathy: a SPECT study with statistical parametric mapping analysis. *Psychiatry Res Neuroimaging, 114*, 103-111.

[27] Volicer, L., Simard, J., Pupa, J. H., Medrek, R. & Riordan, M. E. (2006). Effects of continuous activity programming on behavioral symptoms of dementia. *Journal of the American Medical Directors Association, 7*, 426-431.

[28] Raglio, A., Bellelli, G., Traficante, D., Gianotti, M., Ubezio, M. C. & Villani, D. et al. (2008). Efficacy of music therapy in the treatment of behavioral and psychitric symptoms of dementia. *Alzheimer Dis Assoc Disord, 22(2)*, 158-162.

[29] Staal, J. A., Sacks, A., Matheis, R., Collier, L., Calia, T. & Hanif, H. et al.(2007). The effects of Snoezelen (multi-sensory behavior therapy) and psychiatric care on agitation, apathy, and activities of daily living in dementia patients on a short term geriatric psychiatric inpatient unit. *Int J Psychiatry Med, 37*, 357-370.

[30] Padala, P. R., Burke, W. J., Shostrom, V. K., Bhatia, S. C., Wengel, S. P. & Potter, J. F. et al.(2010). Methylphenidate for apathy and functional status in dementia of the Alzheimer type. *American Journal of Geriatric Psychiatry*.

[31] Mahoney, E. K., Hurley, A. C., Volicer, L., Bell, M., Gianotis, P. & Hartshorn, M. et al.(1999). Development and testing of the resistiveness to care scale. *Res Nurs Health, 22*, 27-38.

[32] Cohen-Mansfield, J. & Jensen, B. (2008). Assessment and treatment approaches for behavioral disturbances associated with dementia in the nursing home: self-reports of physician practices. *Journal of the American Medical Directors Association, 9*, 406-413.

[33] Hoeffer, B., Talerico, K. A., Rasin, J., Mitchell, C. M., Stewart, B. J. & McKenzie, D. et al. (2006). Assisting cognitively impaired nursing home residents with bathing: effects of two bathing interventions on caregiving. *The Gerontologist, 46*, 524.

[34] Lai, M. K. P., Tsang, S. W. Y., Francis, P. T., Esiri, M. M., Keene, J. & Hope, T. et al. (2003). Reduced serotonin 5-HT$_{1A}$ receptor binding in the temporal cortex correlates with aggressive behavior in Alzheimer disease. *Brain Res, 974*, 82-87.

[35] Lanctôt, K. L., Herrmann, N., Eryavec, G., van Reekum, R., Reed, K. & Naranjo, C. A. (2002). Central serotonergic activity is related to the aggressive behaviors of Alzheimer's disease. *Neuropsychopharmacology, 27*, 646-654.

[36] Assal, F., Alarcon, M., Solomon, E. C., Masterman, D., Geschwind, D. H., Cummings, J. L. (2004). Association of the serotonin transporter and receptor gene polymorphism in neuropsychiatric symptoms in Alzheimer disease. *Arch Neurol, 61*, 1249-1253.

[37] Lam, L. C., Tang, N. L., Ma, S. L., Zhang, W. & Chiu, H. F. (2004). 5-HT2A T102C receptor polymorphism and neuropsychiatric symptoms in Alzheimer's disease. *Int J Ger Psychiat, 19*, 523-526.

[38] Pritchard, A. L., Harris, J., Pritchard, C. W., Coates, J., Hague, S. & Holder, R. et al. (2008). Role of 5HT 2A and 5HT 2C polymorphisms in behavioral and psychological symptoms of Alzheimer's diesease. *Neurobiol Aging, 29*, 341-347.

[39] Ueki, A., Ueno, H., Sato, N., Shinjo, H. & Morita, Y. (2007). Serotonin transporter gene polymorphism and BPSD in mild Alzheimer's disease. *Journal of Alzheimers Disease, 12*, 245-253.

[40] Sukonick, D. L., Pollock, B. G., Sweet, R. A., Mulsant, B. H., Rosen, J. & Klunk, W. E. et al.(2001). The *5-HTTPR*S/*L* polymorphism and aggressive behavior in Alzheimer disease. *Arch Neurol, 58*, 1425-1428.

[41] Pritchard, A. L., Pritchard, C. W., Bentham, P. & Lendon, C. L. (2007). Role of serotonin transporter polymorphisms in th behavioral and psychological symptoms in probable Alzheimer disease patients. *Dement Geriatr Cogn Disord, 24*, 201-206.

[42] Huey, E. D., Putnam, K. T. & Grafman, J. (2006). A systematic review of neurotransmitter deficits and treatments in frontotemporal dementia. *Neurology, 66*, 17-22.

[43] Volicer, L., Van der Steen, J. T. & Frijters, D. (2009). Modifiable factors related to abusive behaviors in nursing home residents with dementia. *Journal of the American Medical Directors Association, 10*, 622.

[44] Lyketsos, C. G., Steele, C., Galik, E., Rosenblatt, A., Steinberg, M. & Warren, A. et al.(1999). Physical aggression in dementia patients and its relationship to depression. *Am J Psychiatry, 156*, 66-71.

[45] Leonard, R., Tinetti, M. E., Allore, H. G. & Drickamer, M. A. (2006). Potentially modifiable resident characteristics that are associated with physical or verbal aggression among nursing home residents with dementia. *Arch Intern med, 166*, 1295-1300.

[46] Thakur, M. & Blazer, D. G. (2008). Depression in long-term care. *Journal of the American Medical Directors Association, 9*, 82-87.

[47] Olin, J. T., Katz, I. R., Meyers, B. S., Schneider, L. S. & Lebowitz, B. D. (2002). Provisional diagnostic criteria for depression of Alzheimer disease: rationale and background. *Am J Geriatr Psychiatry, 10*, 129-141.

[48] Starkstein, S. E., Mizrahi, R. & Power, B. D. (2008). Depression in Alzheimer's disease: Phenomenology, clinical correlates and treatment. *International Review of Psychiatry, 20*, 382-388.

[49] Olin, J. T., Schneider, L. S., Katz, I. R., Myers, B. S., Alexopoulos, G. S. & Breitner, J. C et al. (2002). Provisional diagnostic criteria for depression of Alzheimer disease. *American Journal of Geriatric Psychiatry, 10*, 125-128.

[50] Gerritsen, D., Ooms, M., Steverink, N., Frijters, D., Bezemer, D. & Ribbe, M. (2004). Three new observational scales for use in Dutch nursing homes: scales from the Resident Assessment Instrument for Activities of Daily Living, cognition and depression (in Dutch). *Tijdschr Gerontol Geriatr, 35*, 55-64.

[51] Yamamoto, T. & Hirano, A. (1985). Nucleus raphe dorsalis in Alzheimer's disease: neurofibrillary tangles and loss of large neurons. *Ann Neurol, 17*, 573-577.

[52] Gellis, Z. D., McClive-Reed, K. P. & Brown, E. L. (2009). Treatments for depression in older persons with dementia. *Annals of Long-Term Care, 17*, 29-36.

[53] Ray, W. A., Chung, C. P., Murray, K. T., Hall, K. & Stein, C. M. (2009). Atypical antipsychotic drugs and the risk of sudden cardiac death. *N Engl J Med, 360*, 225-235.

[54] Rochon, P. A., Normand, S. L. & Gomes, T. et al (2008). Antipsychotic therapy and short-term serious events in older adults with dementia. *Arch Intern med, 168*, 1090-1096.

[55] Jalbert, J. J., Eaton, C. B., Miller, S. C. & Lapane, K. L. (2010). Antipsychotics use and the risk of hip fracture among older adults afflicted with dementia. *Journal of the American Medical Directors Association, 11*, 120-127.

[56] Schneider, L. S., Dagerman, K. S. & Insel, P. (2005). Risk of death with atypical antipsychotic drug treatment for dementia: meta-analysis of randomized placebo-controlled trials. *JAMA, 294*, 1934-1943.

[57] Dorsey, E. R., Rabbanni, A., Gallagher, S. A., Conti, R. M. & Alexander, G. C. (2010). Impact of FDA Black Box advisory on antipsychotic medications. *Archives Internal Medicine, 170*, 96-103.

[58] Rochon, P. A. & Anderson, G. M. (2010). Prescribing optimal drug therapy fo older people. *Arch Intern med, 170*, 103-106.

[59] Sink, K. M., Holden, K. F. & Yaffe, K. (2005). Pharmacological treatment of neuropsychiatric symptoms of dementia: a review of the evidence. *JAMA, 293*, 596-608.

[60] Schneider, L. S., Dagerman, K. & Insel, P. S. (2010). Efficacy and adverse effects of atypical antipsychotics for dementia: meta-analysis of randomized, placebo-controlled trials. *American Journal of Geriatric Psychiatry, 14*, 191-210.

[61] Chen, Y., Briesacher, B. A., Field, T. S., Tjia, J., Lau, D. T. & Gurwitz, J. H. (2010). Unexplained variation across US nursing homes in antipsychotic prescribing rates. *Arch Intern med, 170*, 89-95.

[62] Pollock, B. G., Mulsant, B. H., Rosen, J., Mazumdar, S., Blakesley, R. E. & Houck, P. R. et al. (2007). A double-blind comparison of citalopram and risperidone for the treatment of behavioral and psychotic symptoms associated with dementia. *American Journal of Geriatric Psychiatry, 15*, 942-952.

[63] Siddique, H., Hynan, L. S. & Weiner, M. F. (2009). Effect of serotonin reuptake inhibitor on irritability, apathy, and psychotic symptoms in patients with Alzheimer's disease. *Journal of Clinical Psychiatry, 70*, 915-918.

[64] Lyketsos, C. G., DelCampo, L., Steinberg, M., Miles, Q., Steele, C. D. & Munro, C. et al. (2003). Treating depression in Alzheimer disease - Efficacy and safety of sertraline therapy, and the benefits of depression reduction: The DIADS. *Arch Gen Psychiatry, 60*, 737-746.

[65] Wang, L. Y., Shofer, J. B., Rohde, K., Hart, K. L., Hoff, D. J. & McFall, Y. H. et al. (2009). Prazosin for the treatment of behavioral symptoms in patients with Alzheimer disease with agitation and aggression. *American Journal of Geriatric Psychiatry, 17*, 744-751.

Chapter 11

Analysis and Relevance of Psychotic-Like Experiences: Repercussions on the Continuity Model of Hallucinations

*J. Adolfo Cangas
and I. Álvaro Langer*
University of Almería, Spain

There are currently many works that focus on the possible continuity of psychotic symptoms, that is, on the consideration of behaviors traditionally associated with schizophrenia (such as hallucinations and delusions) as not being exclusive to this condition, and being related to other alterations, and even manifesting in an attenuated form in the general population.

Many studies confirm the presence of psychotic symptoms in various psychopathological disorders (depression, dissociative disorders, posttraumatic stress disorder, etc.) (Altman, Collins, & Mundy, 1997; Dhossche, Ferdinand, van der Ende, Hostra, & Verhulst, 2002; Romme & Escher, 1996; Ohayon, 2000; Tien, 1991) and also in the general population (Baker & Morrison, 1998; Barret & Etheridge, 1992; Bentall & Slade, 1985; Johns & van Os, 2001; Kot & Serper, 2002; Morrison, 2001; Morrison & Wells, 2003; Ohayon, 2000; Pearson et al., 2008; Serper, Dill, Chang, Kot, & Elliot, 2005; Slade & Bentall, 1988; Tien, 1991; Verdoux & van Os, 2002). Likewise, diverse laboratory investigations have shown that hallucinatory or pseudohallucinatory experiences can be generated by means of mechanisms that include suggestion, sensory deprivation, or classic conditioning (Barber & Calverley, 1964; Bryant & Mallard, 2003; Zukerman & Cohen, 1964).

In some people from the general population, this type of experience may lead to mental disorders or, contrariwise, hallucinatory experiences may become pseudohallucinatory experiences (they are not assigned the same meaning, the people disagree with their "authenticity", etc.) as time goes by.

However, in the literature, there are diverse models of continuity and the changeover in these types of experiences is not clear. Likewise, there is some debate about the mechanisms that are common to these behaviors in diverse populations (clinical and nonclinical) and their essential differences. The analysis of these aspects is the goal of this chapter.

Hallucination-like Experiences in Clinical and General Population

There is a long tradition in Ppsychiatry of the study of hallucinations in the general population (Mckellar, 1968; Sidgewick, 1894; Straus, 1969; West, 1948). In recent years, one of the most notable lines of research is that originated by Launay and Slade (1981) with the elaboration of the Launay Slade Hallucinatory Scale (LSHS) to measure the predisposition to hallucinations. Concepts like predisposition, tendency, proclivity, or high risk mental state are used to group a series of investigations that assess hallucination-like experiences (hereafter HLEs), both in clinical (Kot & Serper, 2002; Levitan, Ward, Catts, & Hemsley, 1996; Singh, Sharan, & Kulhara, 2003; Young, Bentall, Slade, & Dewey, 1987) and in nonclinical samples (Aleman, Nieuwenstein, Bocker, & de Haan, 2001; Feelgood & Rantzen, 1994, Laroi, Marczewski, & van der Linden, 2004; Paulik, Badcock, & Maybery, 2006; Waters, Badcock, & Maybery, 2003).

With regard to the factor structure of the LSHS, various studies propose it to be a multifactor scale (with between 2 and 4 factors), with clinical and subclinical items (Aleman et al., 2001; Laroi et al., 2004; Levitan et al., 1996; Paulik et al., 2006; Waters et al., 2003). Likewise, it has been proposed that clinical samples tend to respond more to clinical items than to subclinical ones, in contrast to the distribution of the responses in nonclinical samples (Levitan et al., 1996; Serper et al., 2005). In other words, HLEs are measured as a multidimensional construct, with clinical and subclinical components, related to vivid daydreams, intrusive thoughts, perceptual disturbance, and hallucinatory experiences typical of psychosis (Cangas, Langer, & Moriana, in press). However, although most investigators propose their multidimensional nature, few studies have assessed the diverse dimensions separately. Not all the dimensions may present the same degree of vulnerability to develop a clinical hallucination and they may not be related in the same way to other relevant factors such as anxiety, depression, or stress.

In this sense, Paulik et al. (2006), using a sample of university students, analyzed the relation of three components (vivid mental events, perceptual hallucinatory experiences, and religious hallucinatory experiences) with depression, anxiety, and stress, finding that anxiety was the most relevant variable of the three components. However, the study of Paulik et al. (2006) only used nonclinical samples, and they did not analyze these subcomponents in samples with mental disorders. The study of Langer, Cangas and Serper (in press) analyze the differences and similarities in the distribution of responses to hallucinatory predisposition in clinical and nonclinical populations and to determine the relation of HLEs with various clinical symptoms. These groups included hallucinating schizophrenic patients, nonpsychotic clinically disordered patients, and a group of individuals with no psychiatric diagnoses. The results revealed that HLEs are related to various clinical symptoms across diverse groups of individuals, although, vivid daydreams obtained a weaker relation than the other three factors.

Regression analysis found that the Psychoticism dimension of Symptom Check List-90-R (Derogatis, 1994) was the most important predictor of HLEs. Additionally, increased auditory and visual clinical hallucination predisposition was the only subcomponent that differentiated schizophrenic patients from other groups. These distributions of responses in the dimensions of HLEs suggested that not all the dimensions are characteristic of people who hear voices. Vivid daydreams, intrusive thoughts, and visual distortions and auditory perceptual distortion may represent a state of general vulnerability unlikely to be a specific risk experience for predisposition to clinical hallucinations. Likewise, Yung et al. (2006) assessed HLEs in nonpsychotic help-seekers, identifying three subtypes: bizarre experiences, persecutory ideas and magical thinking. The first two were associated with distress, depression, and poor functioning, but not magical thinking. The investigators reassessed HLEs in a community sample (secondary students), finding four subtypes (in addition to those identified in the previous study, they added Perceptual Abnormalities). However, the subtypes were related in the same way as in the previous study, again finding that magical thinking did not have an important relation with hallucinations in a clinical population (Yung et al., 2009).

These studies show that the HLEs are a multidimensional concept, and there are differences in the vulnerability of each one of them. It is advisable to study them individually because there may be components that are unrelated or very weakly related to distress or disability, and which may be a part of normality, and there may be other components that are more specific to people with clinical disorders.

Methodological Aspects

Another important aspect to consider is how hallucinatory experiences are assessed. One of the problems of the continuity paradigm may be overdetermination of the phenomenon (Nelson & Yung, 2008). There may be false positives due to the misinterpretation of HLEs. Most of the studies were based on self-applied scales and were cross-sectional. The impact or repercussion of these experiences on people has often not been assessed, so we do not know whether or not they have any clinical relevance. In order to decrease misinterpretation and, thereby, false positives and negatives and the risk of stigmatization, investigators have analyzed other variables or have used diverse assessment methods.

One of the ways to reduce misinterpretation is to understand the meaning of these experiences. In other words, it is important to know precisely how people understand the different situations posed in the questionnaires. Thus, for the same item or situation, such as, "I have been worried by voices I hear in my head," two people might both report that they have had that experience, but each referring to a very different experience. For example, a person with a psychopathological disorder will probably attribute it to forces outside of him- or herself, which will cause an intense emotional reaction that the person tries to avoid, whereas a person with no psychopathological disorder might consider the experience "curious," and attribute it to "normal" causes (tiredness, noisy environment, etc.), and it would not cause any intense emotional reaction. Therefore, the repercussion and personal experience in this type of behavior may vary enormously, not only in the clinical population, but also with regard to the normal one (Chadwick & Birchwood, 1994; Romme & Escher, 2000). It is therefore important to know, not only whether there are experiences related to hallucinations, but also the emotional reaction they cause and to what the person attributes them. In other words, it is important to consider the psychological mechanisms involved in the response to the experience, which would be influenced by beliefs and appraisals (Bentall, Haddock, & Slade, 1994; Chadwick, Birchwood, & Trower, 1996; Morrison, 2001).

In order to determine the beliefs associated with hallucination-like experiences, Cangas et al. (in press) applied the *Revised Hallucination Scale* (RHS, Morrison, Wells, & Nothard, 2000) to 265 university students and found the presence of four factors, which are basically attributed to six types of beliefs: personal difficulties, psychological explanations, dreamlike experiences, vivid thoughts, perceptive distortions, and personal desires. The results about beliefs have, in turn, allowed us to find other factors related to hallucinations. That is, sleep-related experiences, suggestion-related states (such as personal desires), experiences that are explained by specific situations (such as poor light, physical exhaustion, boredom, etc.), and stressful situations (such as personal difficulties and problems). This last point has been studied in other psychotic experiences such as delusions, in which the degree of discomfort and worry is what differentiates healthy and unhealthy individuals (Peters, Days, McKenna, & Orbach, 1999). Concluding, the beliefs associated with HLEs also followed a multidimensional pattern. Some beliefs are related to a degree of distress and others are derived from experiences without much emotional involvement or clinical relevance. Nevertheless, these data contrast with hallucinatory experiences in the population with psychosis, which are frequently associated with a high degree of distress, impact on life, delusional ideation, bizarre ideas, etc., and a loss of "common sense" and hyper-reflectivity in these people is also characteristic (Stanghellini & Ballerini, 2007).

Another aspect to take into account to distinguish between a clinically relevant experience or true hallucination is the clinicians' (clinical psychologists and psychiatrists) perception of the psychotic experiences; and clinicians should ask patients exactly what they are referring to. The clinical criteria will determine, among other factors, whether or not a population is considered clinical, with the consequent classification and diagnosis. In this sense, the study of Langer, Berrio, Ibañez-Rojo, & Cangas (2010) assessed whether or not, by analyzing two clinicians' responses to HLEs, they could distinguish the clinical relevance of the experiences of three groups of participants; people without a psychopathological diagnosis, nonpsychotic clinical population, and patients with a diagnosis of schizophrenia. As the results show, although the general population reports having hallucinatory experiences, when analyzed by clinicians, such responses are mostly assessed as being typical of people without a clinical diagnosis, without any clinical relevance, and the rest of the responses were classified as having clinical but not psychotic relevance. In the nonpsychotic clinical group, a major variability was identified in the classification, fluctuating between typical characteristics of the clinical group (e.g., anxiety, low mood) and without clinical relevance, nevertheless, a very small percentage (5%) was classified as having psychotic relevance. In contrast, the experiences described by people who hear voices, indicating a strong relation with psychotic clinical relevance. Although in a low percentage, nonpsychotic clinically relevant responses were found, and even some without clinical relevance (see Figure 1).

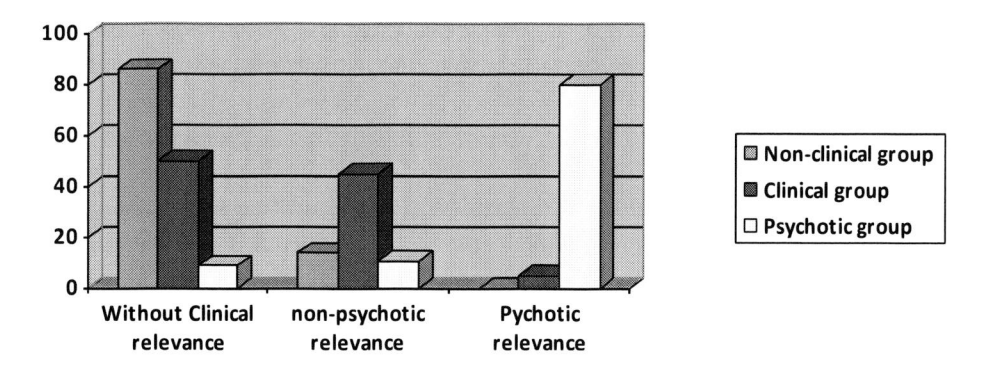

Figure 1. Percentage of responses assigned in each dimension of clinical relevance by groups

Concerning the reasons for assigning a dimension without clinical relevance, the responses revolve around: occasional situations, specific occurrences (including anecdotes), daydreams, and magical thinking. But this had no impact on their personal life. Typical characteristics in the clinical relevance dimension were: low self-esteem, low mood, emotional instability. Nevertheless, these are occasional experiences with a subjective internal explanation. Finally, with regard to the psychotic dimension, the following responses were assigned: the direct allusion to voices, different types of delusional ideation, loss of control over the experience, and distortion of reality.

Thus, at least from a clinical viewpoint, the experiences described by the general population do not share characteristics or aspects that may be considered typical of psychotic patients. However, psychotic experiences may be catalogued as "clinical nonpsychotic," that is, they tend to be "normalized." In any event, in this study, it should also be taken into account that the only information provided to the clinicians was the participants' written self-reports, that is, the professionals did not get to see them or interview them. Otherwise, variability might decrease, because the clinicians would have more information about them.

In fact, there is also some discrepancy about the validity of self-applied questionnaires. For some authors, they have adequate concurrent validity, because they contrast the information obtained in the questionnaires with interviews that confirm the experiences (Konings, Bak, Hanssen, van Os, & Krabbendam, 2006; Liraud, Droulout, Parrot, & Verdoux, 2004); however, other studies show that when interviewing the participants who reported having psychotic experiences, the percentage of those who really had a psychotic disorder decreased considerably. For example, in the study of Kendler, Gallagher, Abelson, and Kessler. (1996), of the sample analyzed, 28% stated they had some psychotic experiences ; however, when interviewed, the percentage of psychotic disorders was less than 1%. Probably, approximations that use both self-applied questionnaires and interviews are more efficient to detect psychotic experiences that really have a risk of leading to a psychotic disorder, thus reducing false positives.

Factors Related to HLEs

The studies that have assessed the course of these experiences longitudinally are scarce (e.g., Chapman, Chapman, Kwapil, Eckblad, & Zinser, 1994; Escher, Romme, Buiks,

Delespaul, & van Os, 2003; Poulton et al., 2000; Rösller et al., 2007). These works indicate that psychotic experiences tend to decrease over time, that is, only a small percentage leads to the complete manifestation of the disorder. However, the people who inform they have such experiences are more vulnerable to having some psychopathological problem than those who do not report such experiences. These results are reflected in a recent meta-analysis (van Os, Linscott, Myin-Germeys, Delespaul, & Krabbendam, 2009), in which it was reported that in approximately 75-90% of the people who had a psychotic experience, these experiences were transitory and disappeared over time. This coincides with the results of Yung et al. (2009) in that the HLEs are infrequent and intermittent experiences, and an unspecific risk for the development of a psychotic disorder in community samples.

Although most psychotic experiences are transitory, there is a percentage that leads to a clinical syndrome. The diverse models proposed indicate that the changeover depends on the existence of other concomitant environmental factors: among these variables are isolation and the lack of social support, consumption of psychoactive drugs (cannabis), traumas, migration, and age (adolescence and early adulthood) (Kilcommons & Morrison 2005; van Os et al., 2009).

Likewise, hearing an inner voice should not be a problem unless the person considers it "dangerous," something that necessarily must be eliminated, or a sign that something bad will happen (for example, if a person hears a voice saying "die" and thinks that it necessarily means that what will happen is than "I will die"). These elements have currently been studied, under the denomination of "meta-cognitions," where, in fact, people with hallucinations have more beliefs related to superstition and punishment and about the dangerousness of their own thoughts (Morrison, 2001; Morrison & Wells, 2003). For this fusion between thinking and action to occur, on the one hand, this type of beliefs must be socially present—for example, superstitious beliefs are fairly common nowadays (García-Montes, Pérez-Álvarez, Sass, & Cangas, 2008)—and, also, it is more likely for people to present some kind of emotional alterations or social difficulty (Cangas, García, López, & Olivencia, 2003). It is different, for instance, to think that "I am going to die" when one is depressed or stressed than when one does not feel that way (probably in the first case, this kind of experiences would have more credibility, thinking would be more ruminative, it could generate different consequences, etc.). Therefore, people with emotional alterations may be more likely to have this type of meta-cognitive beliefs associated with hallucinations.

Conclusions

Hallucinations are a relatively habitual behavior in a clinical population, and can also manifest in the general population. Nevertheless, there are noteworthy differences thatn indicate their greater or lesser clinical relevance. Thus, having the experience of hearing voices may not be a problem in itself, unless the person is in an altered emotional situation or is socially isolated. Contrariwise, if a person with hallucinations begins to normalize their life (without directly intervening in the hallucinations), they may cease to have any effect or may even disappear (Husting & Hafner, 1990).

Therefore, to study this phenomenon, it is not so relevant to analyze whether or not it is possible for them to occur, but instead under what circumstances they do occur. Likewise, as mentioned above, there are also diverse dimensions that make it impossible to consider this phenomenon uniform.

These aspects are essential in the research of the continuity of hallucinatory experiences. In this sense, it is not appropriate to separate the factors that are concomitant to the experiences because, as mentioned, these factors can cause an experience to be considered a problem that requires attention, or, in contrast, an aspect or normal variant in a person's life. Likewise, the works on HLEs indicate that it is preferable to analyze their dimensions separately because some factors may have no relation to psychopathological aspects.

On the one hand, although most of these experiences are occasional and ephemeral, some percentage lead to the complete manifestation of the symptom or clinical disorder, which may account for underlying problems of the self, which involves all the vital areas (Nelson, Yung, Bechdolf, & McGorry, 2008; Sass & Parnas, 2003). Ultimately, the model of continuity of hallucinations has generated a fair amount of research; however, to study the symptom isolatedly, both of the person who undergoes it and the social and cultural context in which it is undergone has not favored the development of a model that explains this type of phenomena without committing the methodological and theoretical errors currently observed. Future approximations should incorporate the above-mentioned aspects in their analysis and so, be able to better determine when this type of experiences will lead to a clinical problem. Thus they will avoid cataloguing daily and innocuous experiences as being hallucinatory or psychotic, with the risk of stigmatization involved.

References

Aleman, A., Nieuwenstein, M. R., Böcker, K. B. & de Haan, E. H. (2001). Multi-dimensionality of hallucinatory predisposition: Factor structure of the Launay-Slade Hallucination Scale in a normal sample. *Personality and Individual Differences, 30*, 287-292.

Altman, H., Collins, M. & Mundy, P. (1997). Subclinical hallucinations and delusions in nonpsychotic adolescents. *Journal of Child Psychology and Psychiatry, 38,* 413-420.

Baker, C. & Morrison, A. P. (1998). Metacognition, intrusive thoughts and auditory hallucinations. *Psychological Medicine, 28,* 1199-1208.

Barber, T. X. & Calverley, D. S. (1964). An experimental study of "hypnotic" (auditory and visual) hallucinations. *Journal of Abnormal and Social Psychology, 68*, 13-20.

Barret, T. R. & Etheridge, J. B. (1992). Verbal hallucinations in normals I: People who hear "voices". *Applied Cognitive Psychology, 6,* 379-387.

Bentall, R. P. & Slade, P. D. (1985). Realibility of a scale measuring disposition towards hallucinations: A brief report. *Personality and Individual Differences, 6,* 527-529.

Bentall, R. P., Haddock, G. & Slade, P. D. (1994). Pychological treatment for auditory hallucinations: From theory to therapy. *Behavior Therapy, 25,* 51-66.

Bryant, R. A. & Mallard, D. (2003). Seeing is believing: The reality of hypnotic hallucinations. *Consciousness and Cognition, 12*, 219-230.

Cangas, A. J., Langer, A. I. & Moriana, J. A. (in press). Hallucinations and related perceptual disturbance in a non-clinical Spanish population. *International Journal of Social Psychiatry.*

Cangas, A. J., García-Montes, J. M., López, M. & Olivencia, J. (2003). Social and personality variables related to the origin of auditory hallucinations. *International Journal of Psychology and Psychological Therapy, 3,* 181-194.

Chadwick, P. & Birchwood, M. (1994). The omnipotence of voices. A cognitive approach to auditory hallucinations. *British Journal of Psychiatry, 164,* 190-201.

Chadwick, P., Birchwood, M. & Trower, P. (1996). *Cognitive therapy for delusions, voices and paranoia.* New York: Wiley.

Chapman, L. J., Chapman, J. P., Kwapil, T. R., Eckblad, M. & Zinser, M. C. (1994). Putatively psicosis-prone subjects 10 years later. *Journal of Abnormal Psychology, 103,* 171-183.

Derogatis, L. R. (1994). *Symptom checklist-90-R (SCL-90-R): Administration, scoring and procedures manual.* Minneapolis, MN: National Computer Systems.

Dhossche, D., Ferninand, R., van der Ende, J., Hofstra, M. B. & Verhulst, F. (2002). Diagnostic outcome of self-reported hallucinations in a community sample of adolescents. *Psychological Medicine, 32,* 619-627.

Escher, S., Romme, M., Buiks, A., Delespaul, P. & Van Os, J. (2002). Independent course of childhood auditory hallucinations: A sequential 3-year follow-up study. *British Journal of Psychiatry, 181,* 10-18.

Feelgood, S. R. & Rantzen, A. J. (1994). Auditory and visual hallucinations in university students. *Personality and Individual Differences, 17,* 293-296.

García-Montes, J. M., Pérez-Álvarez, M. Sass, L. & Cangas, A. J. (2008). The role of superstition in psychopathology. *Philosophy, Psychiatry, & Psychology, 15,* 227-237.

Husting, H. H. & Hafner, R. J. (1990). Persistent auditory hallucinations and their relationship to delusions and mood. *Journal of Nervous and Mental Disease, 178,* 264-267.

Johns, L. C. & van Os, J. (2001). The continuity of psychotic experiences in the general population. *Clinical Psychology Review, 21,* 1125-1141.

Kendler, K. S., Gallagher, T. J., Abelson, J. M. & Kessler, R. C. (1996). Lifetime prevalence demographic risk factors, and diagnostic validity of nonaffective psychosis assessed in a US community sample: The National Comorbidity Survey. *Archives of General Psychiatry, 53,* 1022-1031.

Kilcommons, A. & Morrison, A. P. (2005). Relationships between trauma and psychosis: An exploration of cognitive and dissociative factors. *Acta Psychiatrica Scandinavica, 112,* 351-359.

Konings, M., Bak, M., Hanssen, M., van Os, J. & Krabbendam, L. (2006). Validity and reliability of the CAPE: A self-report instrument for the measurement of psychotic experiences in the general population. *Acta Psychiatrica Scandinavica, 114,* 55-61.

Kot, T. & Serper, M. (2002). Increased susceptibility to auditory conditioning in hallucinating schizophrenic patients: A preliminary investigation. *Journal of Nervous and Mental Disease, 190,* 282-288.

Langer, A. I., Cangas., A. J. & Serper, M. (in press). Analysis of the multidimensionality of hallucination-like experiences in clinical and nonclinical Spanish samples and their relation to clinical symptoms: Implications for the model of continuity. *International Journal of Psychology.*

Langer, A. I., Berrio,V., Ibañes-Rojo., V. & Cangas, A. J. (2010). *Is it possible to distinguish hallucination-like experiences between clinical and general population?* Poster presented at the 18th European Congress of Psychiatry, Munich, Germany.

Larøi, F., Marczewski, P. & van der Linden, M. (2004). Further evidence of the multi-dimensionality of hallucinatory predisposition: Factor structure of a modified version of the Launay-Slade Hallucination Scale in a normal sample. *European Psychiatry, 19,* 15-20.

Launay, G. & Slade, P. D. (1981). The measurement of hallucinatory predisposition in male and female prisoners. *Personality and Individual Differences, 2,* 221-234.

Levitan, C., Ward, P. B, Catts, S. V. & Hemsley, D. R. (1996). Predisposition toward auditory hallucinations: The utility of the Launay-Slade Hallucination scale in psychiatric patients. *Personality and Individual Differences, 21,* 287- 290.

Liraud, F., Droulout, T., Parrot, M. & Verdoux, H. (2004). Agreement between self-rated and clinically assessed symptoms in subjects with psychosis. *Journal of Nervous and Mental Disease, 192,* 352-356.

Mckellar, P. (1968). *Experience and behaviour.* Harmondsworth: Penguin Press.

Morrison, A. P. (2001). The interpretation of intrusions in psychosis: An integrative cognitive approach to hallucinations and delusions. *Behavioural and Cognitive Psychotherapy, 29,* 257-276.

Morrison, A. P. & Wells, A. (2003). A comparison of metacognitions in patients with hallucinations, delusions, panic disorder and non-patient controls. *Behaviour Research and Therapy, 41,* 251-256.

Morrison, A. P., Wells, A. & Nothard, S. (2000). Cognitive factors in predisposition to auditory and visual hallucinations. *British Journal of Clinical Psychology, 39,* 67-78.

Nelson, B. & Yung, A. R. (2008). Psychotic-like experiences as overdetermined phenomena: When do they increase risk for psychotic disorder? *Schizophrenia Research, 108,* 303-304.

Nelson, B., Yung, A. R., Bechdolf, A. & McGorry, P. D. (2008). The phenomenological critique and self-disturbance: Implications for ultra-high risk ("prodrome") research. *Schizophrenia Bulletin, 34,* 381-392.

Ohayon, M. M. (2000). Prevalence of hallucinations and their pathological associations in the general population. *Psychiatry Research, 97,* 153-164.

Paulik, G., Badcock, J. C. & Maybery, M. T. (2006). The multifactorial structure of the predisposition to hallucinate and associations with anxiety depression and stress. *Personality and Individual Differences, 41,* 1067-1076.

Pearson, D., Samlley, M., Ainsworth, C., Cook, M., Boyle, J. & Flury, S. (2008). Auditory hallucinations in adolescent and adult student: Implications for continuums and adult pathology following child abuse. *The Journal of Nervous and Mental Disease, 196,* 634-638.

Peters, E., Days, S., McKenna, J. & Orbach, G. (1999). Delusional ideation in religious and psychotic populations. *British Journal of Clinical Psychology, 38*, 83-96.

Poulton, R., Caspi, A., Moffitt, T. E., Cannon, M., Murray, R. & Harrington, H. (2000). Children's self-reported psychotic symptoms and adult schizophreniform disorder: A 15 year longitudinal study. *Archives of General Psychiatry, 57,* 1053-1058.

Romme, M. A. & Escher, S. (1996). Empowering people who hear voices. In G. Haddock and P.D. Slade (Eds.), *Cognitive-Behavioural interventions with psychotic disorders*. Londres: Routledge.

Romme, M. & Escher, S. (Eds.). (2000) *Making sense of voices*. London: Mind.

Rössler, W., Riecher-Rössler, A., Angst, J., Murray R., Gamma, A. & Eich D, et al. (2007). Psychotic experiences in the general population: A twenty-year prospective community study. *Schizophrenia Research, 92,* 1-14

Sass, L. A. & Parnas, J. (2003). Schizophrenia, consciousness, and the self. *Schizophrenia Bulletin, 29,* 427-444.

Serper, M., Dill, C. A., Chang, N., Kot, T. & Elliot, J. (2005). Factorial structure and classification of hallucinations: Continuity of experience in psychotic and normal individuals. *Journal of Nervous and Mental Disease, 193,* 265-272.

Sidgewick, H. A. (1894). Report on the consensus of hallucinations. *Proc Soc Psychical Res. 26,* 259-394.

Singh, G., Sharan, P. & Kulhara, P. (2003). Phenomenology of hallucinations: a factor analitic approach. *Psychiatry and Clinical Neurosciences, 57,* 333-336.

Slade, P. D. & Bentall, R. P. (1988). *Sensory deception: A scientific analysis of hallucination*. Baltimore: The Johns Hopkins University.

Stanghellini, G. & Ballerini, M. (2007). Values in persons with schizophrenia. *Schizophrenia Bulletin, 33,* 131-141.

Strauss, J. S. (1969). Hallucinations and delusions as points on continua functions. *Archives of General Psychiatry, 21,* 581-586.

Tien, A. (1991). Distributions of hallucinations in the population. *Psychiatric Epidemiology, 26,* 287-292.

Van Os, J., Linscott, R. J., Myin-Germeys, I., Delespaul, P. & Krabbendam, L. (2009). A sistematic reviuw and meta-analysis of the psychosis continumm: Evidence for a psychosis proneness-persistence-impairment model of psychotic disorder. *Psychological Medicine, 39,* 179-195.

Verdoux, H. & van Os, J. (2002). Psychotic symptoms in non-clinical populations and the continuum of psychosis. *Schizophrenia Research, 54,* 59-65.

Waters, F. A. V., Badcock, J. C. & Maybery, M. T. (2003). Revision of the factor structure of the Lauany-Slade Hallucination Scale (LSHS-R). *Personality and Individual Differences, 35,* 1351-1357.

West, D. J. (1948). A mass observation questionnaire on hallucinations. *J Sos Psychical Res, 34,* 187-196.

Young, H. F., Bentall, R. P., Slade, P. D. & Dewey, M. E. (1987). The role of brief instructions and suggestibility in the elicitation of auditory and visual hallucinations in normal and psychiatric subjects. *The Journal of Nervous and Mental Disease, 175,* 41-48.

Yung, A. R., Nelson, B., Baker, K., Buckby, J. A., Baksheev, G. & Cosgrave, E. M. (2009). Psychotic-like experiences in a community sample of adolescents: Implications for the continuum model of psychosis and prediction of schizophrenia. *Australian and New Zealand Journal of Psychiatry, 43,* 118-128.

Yung, A. R., Buckby, J. A., Cotton, S. M., Cosgrave, E. M., Killackey, E. J., Stanford C., et al,. (2006). Pyschotic-like experiences in nonpsychotic help-seekers: Associations with distress, depression, and disability. *Schizophrenia Bulletin, 32,* 352-359.

Zuckerman, M. & Cohen, N. (1964). Sources of reports of visual and auditory sensations in perceptual-isolation experiments. *Psychological Bulletin, 62,* 1-20.

Chapter 12

Hallucinatory Disorder: A Clinical Entity?

Massimo Carlo Mauri[*,1], *Filippo Dragogna*[1], *Isabel Valli*[2], *Giancarlo Cerveri*[3], *Lucia S. Volonteri*[3] *and Giorgio Marotta*[4]

[1]Clinical Neuropsycopharmacology Unit, Fondazione IRCCS Ca'Granda, Ospedale Maggiore Policlinico, Milan, Italy
[2]Psychological Medicine and Psychiatry, Institute of Psychiatry, King's College, London, United Kingdom
[3]Ospedale Fatebenefratelli e Oftalmico, Milan, Italy
[4]Nuclear Medicine Department, Fondazione IRCCS Ca' Granda, Ospedale Maggiore Policlinico, Milan, Italy

Abstract

Chronic Hallucinatory Psychosis (CHP) is a disease that has long been considered in the French literature, but is neglected by the current Anglo-Saxon classification systems, which generally classifies it among the atypical forms of Schizophrenia.

Various authors have described the disorder, attributing it different characteristics. In 1911, Gilbert Ballet (1985) first described CHP, which has been subsequently considered by De Clérambault (1923), Ey (1934) and Pull (1987). These Authors underlined the central nature of the hallucinatory symptoms and suggested the nosographic autonomy of the syndrome, but each hypothesized different underlying pathogenetic mechanisms and disagreed about the prognosis.

The French concept of "Psychose Hallucinatoire Chronique" is characterized by late-onset psychosis, predominantly in females, with rich and frequent hallucinations, but almost no dissociative features or negative symptoms.

---

[*] Corresponding author: Clinical Psychiatry, Clinical Neuropsychopharmacology Unit, University of Milan Medical School, IRCCS Ospedale Maggiore Policlinico, Via F. Sforza 35, 20122 Milano, Italy, Tel. +39.0255035997, Fax +39.0250320310, E-mail: maurimc@policlinico.mi.it

We propose the definition of "Hallucinatory Disorder" (HD) in order to underline the differences between the clinical picture we observed and the psychopathological profile of Chronic Hallucinatory Psychosis proposed by the French Authors.

Auditory verbal hallucinations are the prevalent psychopathological phenomena in HD, appearing in the absence of other types of hallucinations and of thought or behavioral disorganization.

History

Gilbert Ballet, in 1911, described Chronic Hallucinatory Psychosis (CHP), a disorder characterized by auditory verbal hallucinations (AVHs) as the core feature and a long-standing, often chronic, time course (Ballet, 1911). Gilbert Ballet also identified as characteristic features of the disorder a strong family history and a distressful state of restlessness followed by a rich hallucinatory symptomatology and persecutory ideation, usually accompanied by grandiose delusions. Prognosis was reported as severe, with a frequent evolution towards a milder, but chronic, clinical picture including cognitive impairment.

Years later, De Clerembault (1923) underlined the specificity of this clinical picture, classifying it within the Delusional psychoses group; the author suggested that CHP was conceivable as a Chronic Delusional psychosis sustained by a "syndrome of mental automatism" and followed by a delusional structure, that was considered secondary to the hallucinatory phenomena. In other words, delusions were conceived as a cognitive phenomenon, a way to explain hallucinations. Therefore, hallucinatory phenomena were considered the primum movens of the delusional symptomatology. De Clerembault hypothesized an organic cause, such as an endocrine disorder, or a previous infective illness.

A different causal relationship was supported by Ey (1934) who suggested that hallucinations belonged to the delusional structure: hallucinatory phenomena were the effect as opposed to the cause of the delusions. According to Ey, hallucinations were the "voice" of the delusion. Therefore, CHP would not be conceivable as an autonomous nosographical entity but should be either included among chronic delusional psychoses or among well-structured delusions or considered as a peculiar kind of schizophrenia.

According to Ey, the clinical picture was generally characterized by sudden onset, patients themselves appearing surprised by the hallucinatory phenomena. Patients also developed depressive-like or dissociative symptoms as a prodromal aspect of the delusions and the AVHs. Given the stable clinical picture and well-preserved functioning, Ey considered prognosis to be more favorable than Ballet: during the evolution of the most typical form of the illness, patients were spared cognitive impairment and other typical symptoms of schizophrenia, such as negative symptoms or conceptual disorganization.

We observed in clinical practice a clinical picture that meets some of the criteria described by French authors and have used the term "Hallucinatory Disorder" (HD) (Mauri et al., 2006, 2008) to underline some differences between this clinical picture and the definitions of CHP proposed in the past. HD seems to be characterized by hallucinations as a primary and relatively isolated phenomenon (as in the definition of Ballet), whereas the favorable prognosis seems to correspond to that described by Ey (Figure 1).

Hallucinatory Disorder

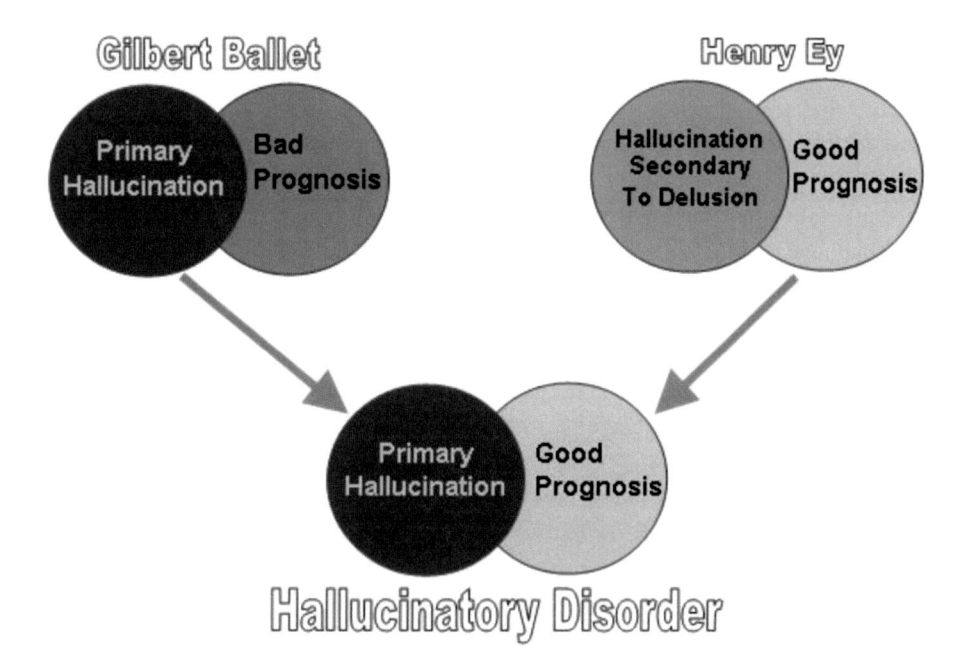

Figure 1. Clinical Characteristics of Hallucinatory Disorder

We chose the term "disorder" rather than "psychosis" to highlight a parallel with Delusional Disorder, a condition in which delusions appear as an isolated symptom, although they can also be a symptom of Schizophrenia, like hallucinations.

Hallucinatory Disorder: Clinical Picture

Hallucinatory Disorder is characterized by a clinical picture briefly defined by the following criteria:

a) Chronic AVHs that during acute phases interfere with everyday living activities
b) Absence of thought or behavioral disturbances
c) Depressive and negative symptoms, if present, appear to be secondary and consequential to the hallucinatory picture
d) Persecutory or reference delusions, if present, appear to be secondary to the hallucinatory picture, often as an interpretation of their occurrence or as an attempt to rationalize them.
e) Sudden onset
f) Poor response to treatment with first and second generation antipsychotics

g) Favorable prognosis and good social functioning, due to the absence of deterioration and integration, at a later stage of the disorder, of hallucinatory phenomena in everyday living activities
h) Partial to full insight
i) Tendency to chronicity of hallucinatory symptomatology

The onset of HD seems to appear suddenly, and patients frequently show an attitude of perplexity that may mimic a depressive psychomotor block. However, once they have overcome this first phase, they can relate again to the environment, to the point that patients describe their hallucinations, which become a disturbing but often tolerable part of their familial, social and working lives. Hallucinations in HD patients are generally experienced as entirely real, even if impossible to understand. Patients are nevertheless often directly aware of their illness and complain about the disturbance caused by the voices, which are a source of suffering and hinder them from pursuing a normal life (Mauri et al., 2006).

In a study comparing a group of patients meeting HD criteria and a group of patients with schizophrenia, Mauri and colleagues (Mauri et al., 2008) reported some significant differences in terms of symptoms, that were discussed, considering the three dimensions of Schizophrenia proposed by Liddle (Liddle,1987). The authors used various clinical rating scales (PANNS, SANS, SAPS, BPRS), to assess psychopathology and interpreted the data by considering the three different syndromes of schizophrenia proposed by Liddle (Liddle, 1984, 1987). They reported a significant ($p=0.004$) difference in the *negative symptoms* cluster, that includes poverty of speech, blunted affect and reduced spontaneous movements, with higher scores for the schizophrenia patients. The same was true for *the disorganization syndrome* that is defined by positive formal thought disorder ($p=0.006$) and inappropriate affect ($p=0.027$). The analysis also revealed a significant between-group difference in the reality distortion dimension characterized by delusions ($p=0.050$) and hallucinations ($p<0.001$), due to HD patients scoring high on the hallucinations item but significantly lower for delusions. The clinical picture of HD patients seemed to be dominated by hallucinatory symptoms. Conversely, in the group of schizophrenic patients, greater global impairment led to a higher PANSS total and general psychopathology scores.

It seems therefore, that all three dimensions contribute to the psychopathological picture of Schizophrenia, while the clinical profile of HD patients reveals a prevalent polarization on a single dimension.

The poor response to treatment with antipsychotics seems to be another factor that differentiates HD from Schizophrenia, in which positive symptoms are among the most sensitive to pharmacological treatment (Mauri et al., 2006).

The two groups were well-matched in terms of some sociodemographic variables such as age, gender, age at onset, and duration of illness, but there were some significant differences in other sociodemographic characteristics: the HD patients had a higher average educational level ($p=0.028$) and were more frequently employed ($p=0.003$) (Mauri et al., 2006, 2008).

These findings, together with their significantly higher Global Assessment of Functioning (GAF) score, can be considered a consequence of the different severity of the two clinical pictures, and indicate that HD patients have a better quality of life and prognosis (Mauri et al.,2006, 2008).

Consistent with the literature, persistent auditory hallucinations could be considered a specific dimension of treatment resistance (Gonzalez et al., 2006; Persaud and Marks, 1995).

Several authors (Tien, 1991; Choong et al., 2007; Verdoux et al., 2002) reported the occurrence of auditory hallucinations in the general population to such an extent that they cannot be considered to be pathognomonic of psychiatric illness. However, there are fundamental differences in the characteristics of these experiences. In the psychiatric population, these tend to be frequent, intrusive, and distressing. In contrast, in the nonclinical population, these are predominantly positive and nonthreatening (Choong et al., 2007).

Romme and Escher (1989) described a 3 step process occurring in people who chronically hear voices, in a way similar to the HD concept:

1) Startling phase: usually sudden onset, mainly as a frightening experience.
2) Organization phase: the process of selection, coping and *communication* with voices.
3) Stabilization phase: the period in which people who learned to cope with the voice consolidated their coping strategy.

In other words, this process is conceivable as a process of learning to cope with the voices. The authors described this "clinical" pattern from a cohort of people who learned to handle their voices, similarly to HD patients.

Finally, a diagnosis of Hallucinatory Disorder can be less stigma-inducing than one of Schizophrenia and can be considered as a further step toward a dimensional view of Schizophrenia and Psychotic Disorder (Van Os, 2009).

Neurocognitive Aspects

A deficit in either auditory imagery, self-monitoring, or episodic memory is reported to be insufficient, in itself, to account for the generation of auditory verbal hallucinations. Nevertheless, there is evidence that auditory verbal hallucinations are associated with impaired verbal self-monitoring and impaired memory for one's own speech, an abnormal influence of top-down processing on perception, and an externalizing response bias in the form of a tendency to claim that unfamiliar or unrecognized material originated from an external source (Seal et al., 2004).

However, despite many psychological investigations, the cognitive mechanisms that transform self-generated mental events into the experience of perceived speech remain unclear (Johns & Van Os, 2001). Recent reviews have emphasized the benefits of employing a multidimensional approach to understanding the cognitive processes involved in psychosis. This approach highlights the social and psychological aspects of the experience and emphasizes the importance of cognitive biases in the generation and maintenance of auditory verbal hallucinations (Rector, 2003; Garety et al., 2001).

Neuroimaging Data

Neuroimaging investigations of auditory verbal hallucinations have implicated an extensive network of cortical and subcortical regions that normally mediate auditory perception and imagery, as well as other regions involved in monitoring behavior and memory retrieval (Copolov et aI., 2003; Shergill et al., 2000; Weiss & Heckers, 2001).

However, no studies have yet defined a model that exhaustively explains AVHs and it remains to be established to what extent impairments in these regions produce AVHs or whether they are merely epiphenomena.

A related but distinct question is whether the impairments are specific to AVHs, positive psychotic symptoms, or to Schizophrenia in general. AVHs in Schizophrenia are typically experienced together with delusions, and have been consistently identified as part of the *reality distortion syndrome* (Liddle et al.,1992). Data from studies of patients with prominent AVHs may also be related to the presence of delusions. Cahill *et al.* (Cahill et al.,1996) found that self-monitoring deficits were more associated with the severity of delusions than with AVHs. A parsimonious explanation for their co-occurrence is that delusions and hallucinations reflect a common impairment in appraising external stimuli: the former being due to the misinterpretation of innocuous behaviors or events, and the latter to the misinterpretation of auditory perceptions (Fleminger,1992). The relevance of impaired appraisal may explain why it is unusual to find individuals with Schizophrenia who experience AVHs but not delusions.

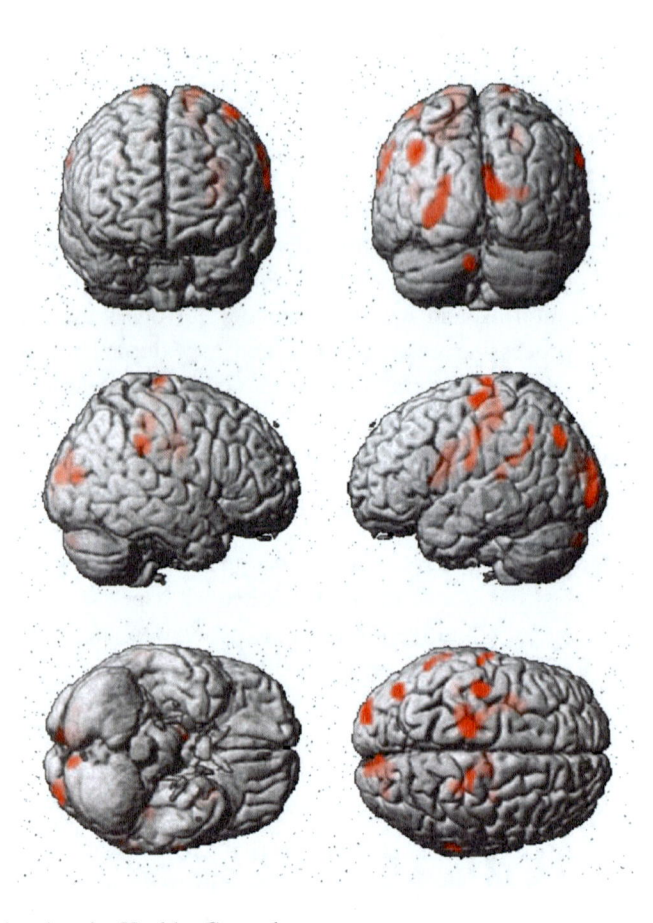

Figure 2. rCBF Schizophrenia<Healthy Controls

Mauri et al. (2008), used SPECT and EEG to compare schizophrenic subjects, patients experiencing AVHs without a diagnosis of schizophrenia and healthy controls. In terms of diagnosis, (defined using DSM-III-R SCID) 100% of the SCH patients met DSM-III-R criteria for Schizophrenia, whereas the diagnosis in the HD group was Psychotic Disorder Not Elsewhere Classified.

The basal EEG data, performed with the aim of excluding the possibility that the symptoms presented by the HD patients could be secondary to a temporal lobe epileptic focus, revealed no significant differences between the two patients groups.

SPECT data showed the following results: in comparison with the healthy subjects, the SCH patients showed a reduction in regional cerebral blood flow (rCBF) in some areas of the right frontal lobe (medial frontal gyrus and superior frontal gyrus) (Figure 2), whereas the HD patients did not show any area of reduced perfusion in comparison with either the SCH patients or the healthy subjects.

The perfusion pattern in the SCH patients seems to be in line with the finding of resting hypofrontality previously reported in some studies of Schizophrenia (Vita et al.,1995 – Lawrie et al.,2002), but not replicated in a similar number of others (Kling et al.,1986). Studies of the clinical correlates of resting hypofrontality have revealed a strong association with negative symptoms (Liddle et al.,1992), therefore the pattern of frontal hypoperfusion we found exclusively in SCH patients could be related to the clinical results showing that negative symptoms are a significantly more relevant feature of Schizophrenia than that of HD ($p=0.004$).

The SPECT data showed that, in comparison with the healthy subjects, the HD patients had a rather complex activation pattern, characterized by increased rCBF in cortical and subcortical areas, listed below (Figure 3).

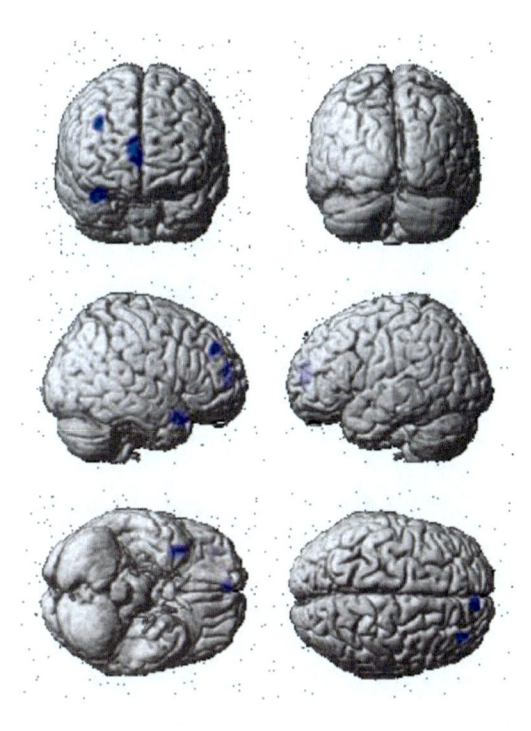

Figure 3. rCBF Hallucinatory Disorder>Healthy Controls

The pattern of activation we observed is similar to the one reported by Shergill *et al.* (2000) in a study of hallucinations in Schizophrenia, in which a diffuse activation network characterized by the involvement of areas of the temporal, inferior parietal, premotor and inferior frontal cortex was observed. However, in the fMRI study by Shergill *et al.* (2000) signal was greater in patients than controls in areas that were mainly in the right hemisphere, whereas we found greater activation in similar regions but in the left hemisphere.

The lateralization of our findings to the left hemisphere seems to reflect the characteristic linguistic content of the hallucinations, and has also been found in McGuire's studies on inner speech and auditory verbal imagery (McGuire et al.,1996). The analogy between the areas of greater rCBF in HD patients compared to controls and those found by McGuire *et al.* is particularly clear considering McGuire's data concerning auditory verbal imagery in healthy volounteers and in schizophrenic patients with and without a strong history of auditory verbal hallucinations. In both studies, greater rCBF in HD and SCH patients compared to controls was found in the left inferior frontal gyrus (BA 44/45), middle temporal gyrus (BA 21), superior temporal gyrus and the parietal operculum (BA 43), and bilaterally in the insula and supplementary motor area (BA 6).

The most significant difference between these patterns of activation observed in HD and SCH patients was that HD patients showed no significant increase in perfusion in the inferior frontal gyrus (Broca's area, BA 44). However, compared to controls HD patients showed increased rCBF in the superior temporal gyrus, which includes Wernicke's area, that is active during both passive listening (Wise et al., 1991) and the processing of the phonological and semantic aspects of words (Demonet et al.,1992). Furthermore, the significant greater perfusion of the inferior parietal lobule observed in our HD patients showed a trend towards higher values in normal subjects engaged in tasks relating to inner speech (McGuire et al., 1996).

The observed analogies between the regions involved in inner speech and auditory verbal imagery, and those activated by hallucinations (Liddle et al.,1992 – Shergill et al.,2000 – McGuire et al.,2000), seem to be in line with the pathogenetic hypothesis by Frith and Done (Frith, Done,1988). The authors propose that inner speech is not altered in hallucinating subjects, but a defect in the mechanisms of self-monitoring which prevents the recognition of the endogenous nature of verbal thoughts, which are then erroneously considered as having an external origin (Copolov et al., 2000).

The activation of the primary motor area, as well as the higher flow in the supplementary motor area observed in HD patients in comparison with healthy controls, could perhaps be interpreted on the basis of what some authors have previously suggested: the production of mental images may involve the reconstruction of remembered perceptions (Kosslyn et al., 1993), and the motor area activity may correspond to the creation of a phonological representation (McGuire et al., 1996).

We also observed significant differences between HD patients and SCH patients (Figure 4). Some of these differences were due to a reduced rCBF in the schizophrenic patients rather than an increase in those with HD.

It is believed that BA 46 is the site of working memory (GoldmanRakic, 1991), and various authors have suggested that a dysfunction in this area may be involved in the pathogenesis of the hallucinations associated with Schizophrenia. An increase in rCBF at this level in subjects with HD compared to SCH patients may therefore be interpreted by hypothesizing that analogous areas may subtend the hallucinations associated with both diseases.

Thalamic increases in rCBF (compared to healthy subjects and SCH patients) may also be related to the pathogenesis of the hallucinations because it has been hypothesized that the pulvinar may be involved in language processing (Ojemann et al.,1968) and the processing of impulses related to multiple sensory modalities (Ingram, 1976).

The increasing in rCBF in HD patients compared to SCH patients at the level of amygdala and right parahippocampal gyrus, seems to be particularly interesting because the perihippocampal region is normally activated when an unexpected stimulus is encountered (Stern et al, 1996), and psychological models of self-monitoring suggest that it may be involved whenever there is a discrepancy between the expected and perceived results of cognitive activity (Gray et al, 1991).

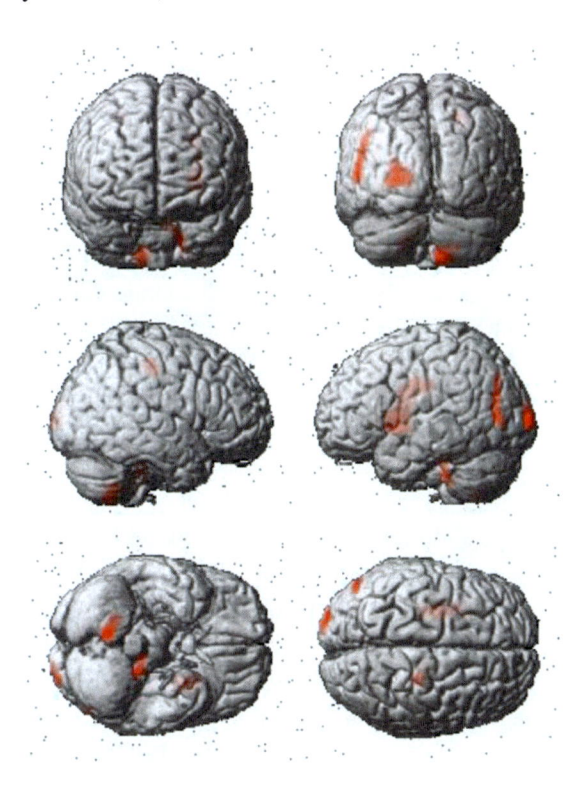

Figure 4. rCBF Hallucinatory Disorder>Schizophrenia

Compared to controls, SCH patients showed a significant increase in rCBF in the left middle temporal gyrus (BA 39) and left middle occipital gyrus (BA 18). This result may be attributable to the fact that the SCH patients were not selected on the basis of any additional criterion such as the presence of a psychopathological dimension. The group was heterogeneous precisely because of the different presentations of Schizophrenia, which vary widely depending on the weight contributed by each of the psychopathological dimensions to the clinical picture. Therefore, this clinical variability can possibly be considered the basis of a corresponding variability in the perfusion pictures, which was probably responsible for the finding of an exiguous number of significantly activated regions in the group of schizophrenic patients as a whole.

Conclusion

On the bases of clinical and imaging data, it seems possible to propose that HD and schizophrenic patients present significant differences capable of supporting the proposed hypothesis of HD as an independent clinical entity.

The proposed differentiation could be important because of the better quality of life and prognosis for HD patients.

Furthermore, a diagnosis of Hallucinatory Disorder can be less stigma-inducing than one of Schizophrenia and can be considered as a further step toward a dimensional view of Schizophrenia and Psychotic Disorder.

Finally, the definition of a specific clinical entity might be essential to allow the investigation of pharmacological responses in more homogeneous groups of patients.

References

Ballet, G. La psychose hallucinatoire chronique. *Encephale*, 1985, 11, 401-11.

Cahill, C; Silbersweig, D; Frith, C. Psychotic experiences induced in deluded patients using distorted auditory feedback. *Cogn Neuropsy.*, 1996, 1, 201-211.

Choong, C; Hunter, MD; Woodruf, PW. Auditory hallucinations in those populations that do not suffer from schizophrenia. *Curr Psychiatry Rep.*, 2007, 9, 206-12.

Copolov, DL; Seal, ML; Maruff, P; Waite, M; Wong, MTH; Ulusoy, R; Egan, GF. A PET study of brain activation in response to auditory hallucinations and external speech in schizophrenic patients. *Biol Psychiatry*, 2000, 47, 122.

Copolov, DL; Seal, ML; Maruff, P; Ulusoy, R; Wong, MT; Tochon-Danguy, HJ; Egan, GF. Cortical activation associated with the experience of auditory hallucinations and perception of human speech in schizophrenia: a PET correlation study. *Psychiatry Res.*, 2003, 122, 139-52.

De Clérambault, G. Les psychoses hallucinatoires chroniques. Paris : *Soc. Méd. Mentale*, 1923.

Demonet, JF; Chollet, F; Ramsay, S; Cardebat, D; Nespoulous, JL; Wise, R; et al. The anatomy of phonological and semantic processing in normal subjects. *Brain*, 1992, 115, 1753-68.

Ey, H. *Traité des hallucinations*. Paris: Masson, 1934.

Fleminger, S. Pre-conscious perceptual processing. *Br J Psychiatry*, 1992, 161, 572-573.

Frith, CD; Done, DJ. Towards a neuropsychology of schizophrenia. *Br J Psychiatry*, 1988, 153, 437-443.

Garety, PA; Kuipers, E; Fowler, D; Freeman, D; Bebbington, PE. A cognitive model of the positive symptoms of psychosis. *Psychol Med.*, 2001, 31, 189-95

Goldman-Rakic, PS. Prefrontal cortical dysfunction in schizophrenia: the relevance of working memory. In: *Psychopathology and the Brain*. Carroll BJ, Barrett JE (eds), 1991. New York: Raven Press, 1-23.

Gonzalez, JC; Aguilar, EJ; Berenguer, V; Leal, C; Sanjuan, J. Persistent auditory hallucinations. *Psychopathology*, 2006, 39, 120-125.

Gray, JA; Feldon, J; Rawlins, JNP; Hemsley, DR; Smith, AD. The neuropsychology of schizophrenia. *Behav Brain Sci.*, 1991, 14, 1-84.

Johns, LC; van Os, J. The continuity of psychotic experiences in the general population. *Clin Psychol Rev.*, 2001, 21, 1125-41.

Ingram, WR. A review of Anatomical Neurology. University Park Press: *Baltimore Md*, 1976.

Kling, AS; Metter, EJ; Riege, WH; Kuhl, DE. Comparison of PET measurement of local brain glucose metabolism and CAT measurement of brain atophy in chronic schizophrenia and depression. *Am J Psychiatry*, 1986, 143, 175-180.

Kosslyn, SM; Alpert, NM; Thompson, WL; et al. Visual mental imagery activates topographically organized visual cortex: PET investigations. *J Cognitive Neurosci.*, 1993, 5, 263-287.

Lawrie, SM; Buechel, C; Whalley, HC; Frith, CD; Friston, KJ; Johnstone, EC. Reduced frontotemporal functional connectivity in schizophrenia associated with auditory hallucinations. *Biol Psychiatry*, 2002, 51, 1008-1011.

Liddle, PF. The symptoms of chronic schizophrenia: a re-examination of the positive-negative dichotomy. *Br J Psychiatry*, 1987, 151, 145-151.

Liddle, PF; Friston, KJ; Frith, CD; Hirsch, SR; Jones, T; Frackowiak, RS. Patterns of cerebral blood flow in schizophrenia. *Br J Psychiatry*, 1992, 160, 179-186.

Mauri, MC; Valli, I; Ferrari, VMS; Regispani, F; Cerveri, G; Invernizzi, G. Hallucinatory disorder: Preliminary data for a clinical diagnostic proposal. *Cogn Neuropsy.*, 2006, 11, 480-492.

Mauri, MC; Gaietta, M; Dragogna, F; Valli, I; Cerveri, G; Marotta, G. Hallucinatory disorder, an original clinical picture? Clinical and imaging data. *Prog Neuropsychopharmacol Biol Psychiatry*, 2008, 32, 523-30.

McGuire, PK; Shergill, S; Brammer, M; Williams, S; Murray, RM. Functional MRI studies of auditory hallucinations. *Biol Psychiatry*, 2000, 47, 122.

McGuire, PK; Silbersweig, DA; Murray, RM; David, AS; Frackowiak, RSJ; Frith, CD. Functional anatomy of inner speech and auditory verbal imagery. *Psychol Med.*, 1996, 26, 29-38.

Ojemann, GA; Fedio, P; Van Buren, JM. Anomia from pulvinar and subcortical parietal stimulation. *Brain*, 1968, 91, 99-116.

Persaud, R; Marks, I. A pilot study of exposure control of chronic auditory hallucinations in schizophrenia. *Br J Psychiatry*, 1995, 167, 45-50.

Pull, MC; Pull, CB; Pichot, P. Des criteres empiriques francais pour les psychoses. III. Algorithmes et arbre de decision. *L'Encephale,* 1987, 13, 59-66.

Rector, NA; Seeman, MV; Segal, ZV. Cognitive therapy for schizophrenia: a preliminary randomized controlled trial. *Schizophr Res.*, 2003, 63, 1-11.

Romme, MA; Escher, AD. Hearing voices. *Schizophr Bull.*, 1989, 15, 209-16.

Seal, ML; Aleman, A; McGuire, PK. Compelling imagery, unanticipated speech and deceptive memory: neurocognitive models of auditory verbal hallucinations in schizophrenia. *Cogn neuropsychiatry*, 2004, 9, 43-72.

Shergill, SS; Bullmore, E; Simmons, A; Murray, RM; McGuire, PK. Functional Anatomy of Auditory Verbal Imagery in Schizophrenic Patients with Auditory Hallucinations. *Am J Psychiatry*, 2000, 157, 1691-1693.

Shergill, SS; Brammer, MJ; Williams, SR; Murray, RM; McGuire, PK. Mapping auditory hallucinations in schizophrenia using functional magnetic resonance imaging. *Arch Gen Psychiatry*, 2000, 57, 1033-8.

Stern, CE; Corkin, S; Gonzalez, RG; Guimaraes, AR; Baker, JR; Jennings, PJ; et al. The hippocampal formation participates in novel picture encoding : evidence from functional magnetic resonance imaging. *Proc Natl Acad Sci,* USA1996, 93, 8660-8665.

Tien, AY. Distributions of hallucinations in the population. *Soc Psychiatry Psychiatr Epidemiol.*, 1991, 26, 287-92.

Van Os, J. "Salience sindrome" replaces Schizophrenia» in DSM-V and ICD-11 : psychiatry's evidence-based entry into the 21st century? *Acta Psychiatr Scand.*, 2009, 120, 363-372.

Verdoux, H; van Os, J. Psychotic symptoms in non-clinical populations and the continuum of psychosis. *Schizophr Res.*, 2002, 54, 59-65.

Vita, A; Bressi, S; Perani, D; Invernizzi, G; Giobbio, GM; Dieci, M; et al. High-resolution SPECT study of regional cerebral blood flow in drug-free and drug-naive schizophrenic patients. Am J Psychiatry 1995, 152, 876-882.Weiss AP, Heckers S. Neuroimaging of declarative memory in schizophrenia. *Scand J Psychol.*, 2001, 42, 239-50.

Wise, R; Chollet, F; Hadar, U; Friston, K; Hoffner, E; Frackowiak, RSJ. Distribution of cortical neural networks in word comprehension and word retrival. *Brain*, 1991, 114, 1803-1817.

Chapter 13

The Neurobiological Basis of Hallucinations

Jitka Bušková[*]
Department of Neurology, 1st Faculty of Medicine and General
Teaching Hospitál, Charles University, Pratur, Czech Republic

Abstract

Hallucinations are perceptions in the absence of an external stimulus and are accompanied by a compelling sense of their reality. They can occur in healthy individuals but they are a diagnostic feature of several illness. The differential diagnosis includes psychiatric diseases (e.g., schizophrenia, bipolar disorder), neurologic diseases (e.g., Alzheimer disease, Parkinson´s disease, Lewy Body disease), Charles Bonnet syndrome. Hallucinations may also be prominent in delirium, drug-intoxication states and drug-withdrawal states (particularly alcohol withdrawal) and may also occur as an adverse effect of medication. Hallucinations may also occur in the hypnagogic (before sleep) and hypnopompic periods (after sleep). We present an overview of current understanding of neurobiologic / pathophysiologic mechanisms for these symptoms in healthy people and in mentioned diseases.

Hallucinations are defined as false sensory perceptions that arise in the absence of an external stimulus of the relevant sensory organ and are accompanied by a compelling sense of their reality [1].

Hallucinations can occur in healthy individuals [2, 3, 4, 5] or can be associated with neurologic diseases (e.g. Alzheimer´ disease, Parkinson´s disease, Lewy Body disease, metabolic and neurodegenerative disorders) and psychiatric diseases (e.g. schizophrenia, bipolar disorder). Hallucinations may also be prominent in delirium, drug-intoxication states and drug-withdrawal states (particularly alcohol withdrawal) and may occur as an adverse effect of medication. Hallucinations may also occur in the hypnagogic (before sleep) and

---

[*] Corresponding author: Department of Neurology, 1st Faculty of Medicine and General Teaching Hospital, Charles University, Kateřinská 30, Pratur 2, 120 00., Tel. +420-732 325 637, e-mail: vankjit@seznam.cz

hypnopompic (after sleep) periods. At present it is still unknown whether they are generated by similar mechanisms in patiens and in healthy people or not.

As a first approach to studing the mechanism of hallucinations, psychologically normal individuals with hallucinations due to lesions have been studied, and the lesion was generally found to be in the brain pathway of the sensory modality (e.g. visual, auditory, somatic/tactile, gustatory, olfactory, minor hallucinatory phenomena and their combinations) of the hallucinations [6]. For example, the complex visual hallucinations seen in Charles Bonnet syndrome are most often cause by damage to the visual system such as macular degeneration or lesions to the central nervous system pathway between the eye and the visual cortex [7]. After a lesion, hallucinations seems to be caused also by compensatory overactivation of tissue in the nearby brain sensory pathway. This type of hallucinations may be termed a „release" form.

The neurobiological basis of hallucinations has most frequently been investigated in patiens with schizophrenia. It might be expected that the basis for auditory hallucinations would be found in the brain regions known to subserve normal audition, language percention and language production (primary and secondary auditory cortex, middle temporal gyrus, Wernicke and Broca areas, anterior cingulate cortex and dorsolateral prefrontal cortex). The most consistent finding of structural neuroimaging studies of patients with auditory hallucinations is reduced gray matter volume in the superior temporal gyrus, including the primary auditory cortex [8]. One fairly large study also reported volume reduction in the dorsolateral prefrontal cortex, suggesting that faulty frontotemporal interactions may contribute to the experience of hallucinations being involuntary [9].

It has been also assumed altered connectivity among temporal, prefrontal and anterior cingulate regions involved in the genesis of hallucinations. One major concept on the origin of hallucinations is the idea that hallucinating individuals may misattribute internally generated speech (or sensory stimuli) as coming from an external source [10]. In support of this concept, several studies have found evidence for reduced functional frontotemporal connectivity in patients with schizophrenia who were asked to speak or complete sentences, and this was particularly pronounced in those with auditory hallucinations [11]. Blakemore and colleagues [12] have provided experimental evidence that another required element enabling one to discriminate between self-produced and external stimuli is the correct placement of sensory stimuli in space and time.

However, the major question of how this altered activity arises is still unanswered. Behrendt has provided a thought-provoking hypothesis based on the idea that perceptual experience arises from synchronization of gamma oscillations thalamocortical network [13]. This oscillatory activity is normally constrained by sensory imput and also by prefrontal and limbic attentional mechanisms. There is evidence that in patients with schizophrenia there is impaired modulation of thalamocortical gamma activity by external sensory imput, allowing attentional mechanisms to play a preponderant role in the absence of sensory imput. This may lead to hallucinations. Moreover, conditions of stress/hyperarousal and neurochemical alterations characteristic of schizophrenia (e.g. dopaminergic hyperactivity, nicotinic receptor abnormalities) may be factors that predispose toward this uncoupling of sensory imput from thalamocortical activity and pathological activation of thalamocortical circuits by attentional mechanisms.

Another interesting approach that has been used to study hallucinations is rapid eye movement (REM) sleep, since hallucinations are regular features of REM [14]. Gottesmann has described a hypothesis related to the neurochemical background of sleep-waking mental activity. Acetylcholine, which mainly activates cortical neurons, is released at the maximal rate during waking and REM sleep. Its importance in mental functioning is well –known. However, brainstem-generated monoamines, which mainly inhibit cortical neurons, are only released during waking. Both kinds of influences contribute to the organized mentation of waking. During REM sleep, the monoaminergic neurons became silent except for the dopaminergic ones. This results in a large disinhibition and the maintained dopamine influence may be involved in the familiar psychotic-like mental activity of dreaming. Indeed, in this original activation-disinhibition state, the increase of dopamine influence at the prefrontal cortex level could explain the most total absence of negative symptoms of schizophrenia during dreaming, while an increase in the nucleus accumbens is possibly responsible for hallucinations, which is regular feature of mentation during this sleep stage.

Described quasi-total cortical disinhibition during REM sleep is complicated by yet another neurochemical phenomenon which no doubt contributes to the weird nature of dreams. The typical features of dreams (sensorimotor hallucinations, bizzare imagery, diminished self-reflective awareness, orientational instability, intensification of emotion, instinctual behaviors) [15] are highly reminiscent of schizophrenic symptoms. It happens that the only monoaminergic neurotransmiter which continues to function during REM sleep is dopamine, which is known to be dysfunctional in psychosis, and especially among schizophrenic patients. In a normal subject, when the dopamine level increases in the extracellular enviroment of the brain, under the influence, for example of amphetamines, nightmares occur [16, 17]. Conversaly, in schizophrenic patients, when the action of dopamine is diminished by the administration of neuroleptics, the delirium and hallucinations vanish [18]. Gottesmann also suggest that the silence of the noradrenergic neurons during REM sleep might enhance the impact of dopamine on the cortex.

Braun et al. reviewed single case reports of post-lesion psychosis involving hallucinations [6] and found that the temporal lobe was the most common lesion site followed by the frontal lobe and, then, tissue around the third ventricle. We hesitate to believe that this is indicative of a predilection for lesion loci to be located within dopaminergic pathways. Interestingly, Cochen et al. found hallucinations associated with autonomic dysfunction in patients with Guillain-Barré syndrome [19] and they assume that the putative central target of the antibodies may be in the lateral hypothalamus, which is (i) close to the third ventricle, where the blood-brain barier is weaker and thereby more exposed to autoimmune attack; (ii) where hypocretin neurons controlling wake/non-REM/REM sleep transition are located and where the paraventricular nucleus and the median preoptic nucleus controlling the autonomous system are located. They suggest that hallucinations in Guillain-Barré syndrome are manifestations of a sleep and dream-related disorder.

Hallucinations in Parkinson's disease has been study during the past decade, but a numer of questions still remain. Hallucinations in this desease are now seen as resulting from complex interactions between pharmacologic and disease-related factors. Complex visual hallucinations are associated with abnormal activity in the ventral extrastriate visual cortex, which may result from various and probably concomitant machanisms, including dopaminergic overactivity and/or imbalance in monoaminergic (relatively preserved) and cholinergic (altered) neurotransmission; alteration of brainstem sleep/wake and dream regulation; dysfunction of the visual pathways, nonspecific (coincidental ocular disease) and /or specific, such as Parkinson's disease-associated retina dysfunction and functional alterations in the ventral stream of visual cortical pathways; dysfunction of top-down mechanisms of vision, such as impaired attentional focus; and finally, antiparkinsonian drugs and other farmacologic agents may interfere with the preceding mechanisms at many levels [20].

Some patients suffering from hallucinations has been successfully treated with antipsychotics, tricyclic antidepressants, monamine oxidace (MAO) type-A inhibitors, selective serotonin reuptake inhibitors (SSRIs), noradrenergic uptake inhibitors and venlafaxine. Nevertheless, it has been also described drug-induced hallucinations [21]. Especially antidepressants have been noted to cause hallucinations, often with drug overdose, but also in rare instance as a side effect at therapeutic dose. Among the risk factors, the more common is old age, neurodegenerative diseases, head injurie and depression.

In conclusion, although useful insight has been gained, we still have a long way to go to fully understand what causes hallucinations. It is hoped that this brief review will provoke increased interest on this subject.

References

[1] American Psychiatric Association. *DSM-IV-TR*; Washington D.C., 2000.
[2] Grimby, A. Bereavement among elderly people: grief reactions, post-bereavement hallucinations and quality of life. *Acta Psychiatr Scand*, 1993, 87, 72-80.
[3] Johns, LC; van, Os, J. The continuity of psychotic experiences in the general population. *Clinical Psychology Review*, 2001, 21, 1125-1141.
[4] Stip, E; Letourneau, G. Psychotic symptoms as a kontinuum between normality and patology. *Can J Psychiatry*, 2009, 140-151.
[5] Scott, J; Martin, G; Bor, W; et al. The prevalence and correlates of hallucinations in Australian adolescents: results from a national survey. *Schizophr Res*, 2009, 107, 179-185.
[6] Braun, CM; Dumont, M; Duval, J; et al. Brain modules of hallucination: an analysis of multiple patients with brain lesions. *J Psychiatry Neurosci*, 2003, 28, 432-449.
[7] Rovner, BW. The Charles Bonnet syndrome: a review of recent research. *Curr Opin Ophtalmol*, 2006, 17, 275-7.
[8] Allen, P; Laroi, F; McGiure, PK; et al. The hallucinating brain: a review of structural and functional neuroimaging studies of hallucinations. *Neurosci Biobehav Rev*, 2008, 32, 175-91.
[9] Boksa, P. On the neurobiology of hallucinations. *J Psychiatry Neurosci*, 2009, 34, 260-262.
[10] Frith, CD; Done, DJ. Towards a neuropsychology of schizophrenia. *Br J Psychiatry*, 1988, 153, 437-43.
[11] Ford, JM; Mathalon, DH. Corollary discharge dysfunction in schizophrenia: can it explain auditory hallucinations? *Int J PSychophysiol*, 2005, 58, 179-89.
[12] Blakemore, SJ; Frith, CD; Wolpert, DM. Spatio-temporal prediction modulates the perception of self-produced stimuli. *J Cogn Neurosci*, 1999, 11, 551-559.
[13] Behrendt, RP. Dysregulation of thalamic sensory "transmission" in schizophrenia: neurochemical vulnerability to hallucinations. *J Psychopharmacol*, 2006, 20, 356-72.

[14] Gottesmann, C. The neurochemistry of waking and sleeping mental activity: the disinhibition-dopamine hypothesis. *Psychiatry Clin Neurosci*, 2002, 56, 345-54.

[15] Hobson, JA; Stickgold, R. Pace-Schott, EF. The neuropsychology of REM sleep dreaming. *Neuroreport*, 1998, 9, R1-R14.

[16] Pehek, EA. Comparison of effects of haloperidol administration on amphetamine-stimulated dopamine release in the rat media prefrontal cortex and dorsal striatum. *J Pharmacol Exp Ther*, 1999, 289, 14-23.

[17] Thompson, DF; Pierce, DR. Drug-induced night mares. *Ann Pharmacother*, 1999, 33, 93-98.

[18] Kinon, BJ; Lieberman, JA. Mechanisms of action of atypical antipsychotic drugs: a critical analysis. *Psychopharmacology*, 1996, 124, 2-34.

[19] Cochen, V; Arnulf, I; Demeret, S; et al. Vivid dreams, hallucinations, psychosis and REM slep in Guillain Barré syndrome. *Brain*, 2005, 128, 2535-2545.

[20] Fénelon, G. Psychosis in Parkinson's disease: phenomenology, frequency, risk factors, and current understanding of pathophysiologic mechanism. *CNS Spectr*, 2008, 3, 18-25.

[21] Cancelli, I; Marcon, G; Balestrieri, M. Factors associated with complex visual hallucinations during antidepressant treatment. *Hum Neuropharmacol Clin Exp*, 2004, 19, 577-584.

Chapter 14

Social Variables Related to the Origin of Hallucinations

Adolfo J. Cangas, Álvaro I. Langer, José M. García-Montes, José A. Carmona, and Luz Nieto
University of Almería (Spain)

Hallucinations are very dramatic behavior that today is considered to be a distinguishing characteristic of a group of serious mental disorders, as is the case of schizophrenia. Despite the seemingly bizarre nature of this type of behavior, it should not be misconstrued that hallucinations hold no functionality for the person experiencing them or that they cannot be understood through different psychological or social mechanisms (Layng & Andronis, 1984).

To study this behavior, is it not only worthwhile to analyze people that suffer from schizophrenia, it is also useful to involve people with other disorders who experience voices (such as mood, dissociative and personality disorders, and posttraumatic stress) (Altman, Collins & Mundy, 1997; Dhossche, Ferdinand, van der Ende, Hostra & Verhulst, 2002; Romme & Escher, 1989; Ohayon, 2000; Tien, 1991), or even individuals within the normal population that may have similar experiences (Baker & Morrison, 1998; Cangas, Langer & Moriana, in press; Morrison & Wells, 2003; Serper, Dill, Chang, Kot & Elliot, 2005).

The study of hallucinations has also garnered significant interest from the classic works of Bentall, Jackson and Pilgrim (1988) and of Person (1986), who showed the utility of focusing on specific symptoms (rather than general syndromic characteristics such as schizophrenia), given that they are better related to etiological variables, can aid in the study of the continuity of psychotic symptoms, can improve reliability, etc.

The reality today is that the symptom of hallucinations is sufficient for a diagnosis of schizophrenia. However, its significance in diagnosis has not always been as it is in present times. In fact, for Bleuler (1911) (who introduced the term "schizophrenia"), hallucinations were a secondary symptom of other more basic disorders (the famous four As: changes in Association, Affection, Autism and Ambivalence). It would be later in history, particularly under the influence of Kurt Schneider and the propositions of formal diagnostic systems that sought to offer a more reliable system of classification, which would lead to the dominant role that hallucinations have today.

Since the 1960s a fundamental problem of psychopathological diagnosis was its low grade of reliability. To site an example, the famous *United States-United Kingdom study* (Cooper, Kendell, Gurland *et al.,* 1972) found that there were numerous discrepancies between the diagnoses made in the U.S.A. and those made in England after an analysis of psychiatric interviews that were recorded by professionals in both continents. These differences were attributed to the diagnostic systems used that were seen as too generalized or vague. It was also in this same period that the famous Rosenhan (1973) study took place when group of students who pretended to hear voices were admitted to a psychiatric institution. What is notable about this case is that, once inside, the group of people stopped pretending the original behavior but continued to be held in the center for six months, and when they were discharged the diagnosis that had been given to them was "residual schizophrenia."

In 1959, Kurt Schneider was interested in finding what was specific about schizophrenia, that is, what symptoms might be pathognomonic of this disorder or what behaviors would indicate a case of schizophrenia and not another type of disorder. His interest was not in looking for the etiology of psychosis, but in finding its distinctive characteristics. That was how he came to differentiate between first-rank symptoms and symptoms of second rank. The first rank would be characteristics of schizophrenia and would include diverse types of hallucinations and delusions such as voices arguing, experiences of somatic passivity or delusional perceptions. In contrast, the second-rank symptoms, such as confusion, depressive or euphoric states, and feelings of emotional impoverishment, could be present in many disorders. This proposal is what finally prevailed in the diagnostic systems of our current times (ICD and DSM).

It should also be taken into consideration that, since the 60s, antipsychotic medication has acted specifically against hallucinations and delusions, eliminating or alleviating their effects in a significant percentage of cases (about one half of patients). The existence of a drug that acts against these behaviors is therefore more likely to become *essential*.

We must also take into account the spectacular and dramatic nature of hallucinatory behavior, which is why it is a cause of great concern. Hallucinations are configured as a fundamental behavior in current Psychopathology; but what is their origin? In the next section we will focus on the social aspects involved in their origin and maintenance.

Social Factors Associated with the Origin of Hallucinations

Drawing from the introduction, it appears that hallucinations may be consequences of very basic situations (as previously noted by Bleuler). In this sense, social components will take a leading role. Clearly then, to analyze this behavior, cultural variables must first be taken into account. Schizophrenia is a disorder specifically of modern times. Even though in other epochs there have been cases of hallucinations, their significance, origin and consequences are markedly different from the cases of schizophrenia in the present times and therefore should not be likened. For example, the visions of mystics in the Middle Ages are very different from the voices of schizophrenics today (Cangas, Sass & Perez, 2008; Sarbin & Juhasz, 1967), not only because in the Middle Ages it was more common that people experienced visions and today it is the auditory hallucination that predominates, but because of the very different consequences present in each historic period (in the Middle Ages one could increase their social status by associating the hallucinations with a religious origin, while in present times hallucinations represent a significant social stigma associated with mental illness). In times past, a person's life was not paralyzed, whereas today, the experience of hallucinations represents an obstacle to basic life projects (studies, family, etc.).

Today, a central aspect of our society is the "medicalization" of any behavior that is considered "abnormal." It is from the nineteenth century forward that hallucinations acquired this particular character (Berrios, 1996). In other times and in other cultures hallucinations were closely related to religious or mystical activities and were not regarded as they are now.

Coexisting with the medical concept of psychopathological behavior is the social role of the mentally ill. The existence of hallucinations in a person often produces stigma, fear or rejection in others, which in turn affects the very way that person feels about him or herself. When someone begins to manifest this kind of behavior they are likely to think: am I going crazy? – which then contributes to an ever-accelerating emotional reaction (Cangas, Garcia, López & Olivencia, 2003).

It is also important to take into account that in the western world we are less familiar with the internal events that are related to feeling different, behaving in different ways, or having intense emotional experiences; unlike some Eastern traditions which are more embracing of these types of experiences (Al-Issa, 1977, 1995; Wahass & Kent, 1997a, 1997b). Thus, to the extent that our society is increasingly "rational" it rejects experiences that are not strictly within this construct, fostering the need to explain everything in a rational way (the logic possibly being that for people the "thought" is first and then the "emotion"). This means that hallucinatory experiences in our society, different than in other cultures, provoke an intense emotional reaction, a desire to control those experiences, and a different way of confronting them.

Another aspect that is characteristic of modern times is "hyperreflexivity" or exaggerated self-consciousness of processes that usually go unnoticed (Pérez, 2008; Sass, 1992). Both positive and negative symptoms in psychosis can be understood as an excess of hyperreflexivity, of being trapped in thought processes that generally the person cannot distance him or herself from. This aspect is related to studies that have focused on the analysis of metacognitive beliefs, that is, the ideas that people have about their own thoughts and thought processes. Findings from these studies have showed that patients who hear voices score higher than the normal population in: low cognitive confidence (e.g., "I don't have much memory"); negative beliefs about the controllability of thoughts and the risk involved in not controlling them (e.g., "when I start to worry I can't stop"); positive thoughts about the act of worrying ("I need to be worried in order to stay organized"); and cognitive self-awareness ("I am aware of how my mind works") (Baker & Morrison, 1998; Morrison & Wells, 2003). Though, above all, it is the superstitious beliefs about mental events that are of fundamental importance (García, Pérez, Soto, Perona & Cangas, 2006; García, Pérez, Sass & Cangas, 2008). It is common for patients with psychosis who hear voices to inbue them with great power, a power established by chance or biased associations: "because they were able to foretell the death of my father," "because they know everything about me..." There is an important fusion between thought and action, that is, a person believes that having a certain type of thought will provoke that thought in the form of action (García, Pérez & Cangas, 2006).

Hyperreflexivity in psychosis is also associated with another essential factor, the "loss of common sense" (Sass, 2003; Stanghellini, 2004), which means, to the extent that a person questions every-day, commonplace processes, it is likely that they will distance themselves from common ways of behaving. For instance, if a person is continually asking: "is this world real?", "am I the only one who sees the supernatural beings that are invading us?", "why do we have to have relationships with other people?", etc. (questions that could indeed make sense, but that we generally do not pose to ourselves), it may be a form of social "paralysis," the experience of seeing difficulties in a unique way and feeling "different" than other people.

Where does this hyperreflexivity or loss of common sense in schizophrenia come from? Its emergence is related to the social factors that begin during key evolutionary moments in our society, such as adolescence. At this stage, the person not only changes their ways of behaving (leaving behind the infant world), but also begins to frame their future as a person (in the workplace as well as within emotional and social spheres). During the stage of adolescence (which is relatively long in our society) new roles appear that the person has to assimilate, such as the need to have greater autonomy outside of the home (although, paradoxically, they may be required to remain dependent or compliant within the sphere of the family). It is a stage of new activities: the first romantic relationships, sexual discovery, and the first heartbreaks. This also corresponds with a greater critical capacity, with the realization of the many inconsistencies in the "adult world," and with awareness that the rules that had previously governed behavior are now changed and more complex. These are the multiple processes that can contribute to an adolescent's "unhappiness-in-the-world." Difficulties of adaptation can spawn feelings of not fitting in with the ways of everyone else, with other people's values, with the desires of others, etc. This, in turn, produces a constant questioning of common behavior and ways of seeing things. Using the words of Laing (1960), in psychosis the person would feel as if they have been "swallowed" by the world. Hence, subjectivity now plays an important role, or, from the writings of Sass (1992), "the external world, supposedly objective, becomes subjective and de-realized, while the inner self, which is supposedly subjective, becomes objective and deified" (Sass, 1992, p. 338).

In this new stage it is crucial to look at how the personality has developed, which has, in part, been modulated by processes of family dynamics. In schizophrenia, the influence of high expressed emotion as a predictor of relapse has been emphasized, though it is also important to recognize that this type of emotion may be an influencing factor in the very origin of this disorder together with other communication disorders within the family network (Read, Seymor & Mosher, 2004). From childhood, through interactions with others (family relationships of course playing an important role), the personality is taking shape, which will then determine ways of being, ways of meeting demands, and ways facing social difficulties. In this regard, it is well documented that people who have develop schizophrenia have previously shown signs of having a vulnerable personality with schizotypal or schizoid personality components. It is common for these people to describe their childhood as more solitary than the rest of their companions and characterized by strange behavior or by different types of behavior than that of the other boys and girls of their age (Parnas & Handest, 2003; Stanghellini, 2004b). There are more difficulties in dealing with people as well as difficulties in social adjustment. Also, studies that have investigated the personality of people most prone to hallucinations found that they scored higher in emotional instability and avoidance components (Barrett & Ehteridge, 1994).

It is important to add to this picture the specific circumstances of an individual's development that may contain components of social isolation or stress. One might recall the famous studies on sensory deprivation where students without psychopathological problems were put into chambers void of any type of stimulation, and after a time, began to experience hallucinations. In patients with psychosis, as mentioned before, it is very common that there are difficulties in interacting with others. It might be argued that hallucinations in some way "supplant" natural speech; to the extent that there is little interaction with others, there is a greater presence of thoughts in the form of dialogues. Hallucinations can be seen as "breaking the silence of the inner dialogue" (Stanghellini & Cutting, 2003).

It is also common that the onset of hearing voices is linked to experiences of stress. Romme and Escher (1989) identified six triggers, most of them having to do with the themes discussed in this section, such as intolerable or adverse situations (divorce, job loss, etc.), recent trauma especially when not expected (e.g., the death of a loved one), conflicting aspirations (goals that are not met), threats, childhood trauma, and the denial of emotions.

We must nevertheless take into consideration that hallucinations are not merely a "passive" reaction to adverse situations; they are also a compensatory mechanism or attempt to overcome the adversity. Clearly, hallucinatory behavior is probably not the best solution; furthermore, it can be reinforced behavior – which, in fact, helps to keep it going. Hallucinations may very well alleviate the feeling of discomfort, ease the responsibility for having certain thoughts, help to recognize a specific sensation, contribute to feeling special, etc. This is why many patients (especially in the early stages of the disorder) have commented that hallucinations provide them with company or help them to make a decision, and so on (Knudson & Coyle, 1999). Recently it has been postulated that a fundamental aspect in the explanation of this behavior is experiential avoidance, where the person does not engage or enter into contact with aversive subjective elements (thoughts, images, feelings) because of the suffering they generate. This obviously offers the person the advantage of alleviating the initial stress, but it also paralyzes that person from participating in and realizing activities that could be valuable to them (Veiga-Martínez, Pérez-Álvarez & García-Montes, 2008).

Hallucinations may also contain components of positive reinforcement, though these may be more difficult to detect. In this case, as proposed by Layng and Andronis (1984), to understand hallucinatory behavior we must bear in mind the array of possible behaviors available to a person, and recognize the instances when hallucinations are probably the "least bad" of the possibilities and when the reinforcers cannot be easily identified (because of being delayed in time, for having to do with forms of personal avoidance, for being controlled by different audiences, etc.).

In the explanation of hallucinations is important to differentiate between the variables involved in the onset, or origin, of the experiences and those that have a function in their maintenance; at the first stage, one set of variables may be involved, and in a subsequent stage, there may be other variables. For example, high stress situations can be key in the onset of hallucinations, but once the hallucinations are established, lesser degrees of stress or more common adversities can serve as triggers.

In sum, in the emergence of hallucinations, multiple social factors are involved. Together with contributing components of today's society – an emphasis on the medical, little familiarity with internal events, the presence of social stigma – the person who hears voices is likely to be in a situation of significant social isolation and likely to be affected by personality characteristics such as avoidance and schizotypal components, and emotional disorder. In this context, when subjected to different key stressors, it is likely that one's behavior (thoughts, feelings) is interpreted incorrectly and is considered not to be one's own or not self-generated (this would be, then, the hallucinations). This behavior would have a number of important repercussions in the form of either positive or negative reinforcement. Later in time, the presence of intense stressors or difficulties is no longer necessary for this behavior to be maintained given that a habitual way of acting will have been established in relations (or the lack thereof) with others.

Psychological Treatment of Hallucinations

From the previous section we can see the importance that different social aspects can have, not only in the etiology of hallucinations, but also relating to the types of interventions used for this behavior. Although the principally known treatment for hallucinations (and of widespread use in the western world) is pharmacological treatment, psychological intervention, which has shown clearly favorable results, is also essential. Moreover, it is important not to refer to the relationship of the psychological to the pharmacological as merely complementary, because where pharmacological treatment has failed to reach, psychological intervention has had an affect (Cuevas-Yust, 2006).

Various therapeutic strategies have been designed that are specific for the treatment of the positive symptoms of schizophrenia. Among them, the most consolidated proposals are the cognitive behavioral techniques for hallucinations and delusions. The early procedures employed the basic principles of behavior analysis, such as positive reinforcement of incompatible behaviors, extinction, or punishment procedures such as time-out (e.g., Lindsley, 1959; Haynes & Geddy, 1973). Subsequently, standard procedures in the treatment of anxiety and depression have been used and adapted to this population, procedures such as systematic desensitization, detection of thought, self-monitoring, or counterstimulation (Chadwick, Birchwood & Trower, 1996; Farhall, Greenwood & Jackson, 2007). According to Slade and Bentall (1988), the variability of these proposals can be reduced to three essential elements: focusing on or centering on a person's own voice, with the help of the therapist, in order for it to reclaim its effect in that person's own experience (not that of external agents); anxiety reduction techniques, such as systematic desensitization; and, distraction (such as counterstimulation techniques, or as Slade and Bentall propose, the reinforcement of incompatible behaviors).

In general, the results of these procedures have been positive. However, there are also a number of limitations, such as the fact that many of these works are case studies, or that several of the studies (especially the earliest research) were realized within an institutionalized population (where, for example, it is easier to control the contingencies), or the lack of analysis of the significance of the different components introduced. But perhaps even more important is that when the results of these interventions were compared with other psychosocial treatments such as social skills training, family intervention or assertive community treatment, no significant differences were found. It may be the non-specific factors contained in all psychological interventions that explain such results (Cuevas-Yust, 2006; Gaudiano, 2005).

More recently, what are known as third-generation interventions are being used. The therapeutic goal here is not to eliminate the symptom, but that it affects the person in a different way and therefore does not paralyze his or her life. The basis of the idea is that trying to deliberately suppress private events such as feelings, thoughts, and images, can paradoxically produce an increase in this type of activity. Within this philosophy different techniques of acceptance have been used. Procedures for achieving mindfulness techniques, for example, make the person aware of cognitive and emotional processes, but without trying to change them, merely letting them "flow." The results show that when using these techniques patients improve in the post-treatment evaluation, although differences are not significant when compared with the control group (Chadwick, Hughes, Russell & Dagmar, 2009).

Acceptance and Commitment Therapy also seeks the acceptance of private events (which are being avoided) by using metaphors and a series of experiential exercises. The intent is that the person does not fight the symptoms, but that they change the socio-verbal framework within which are they are generated. Furthermore, the idea is no longer to merely accept the symptoms, but to act according to what can be valuable to the person. This is indeed an essential aspect of the therapy and particularly important in the area of psychosis. Schizophrenia is usually characterized precisely by a marked apathy and anhedonia. Unraveling valuable aspects that are important for the person and then directing behavior toward these aspects is key. This activity is not only effective for the positive symptoms but also for the negative symptoms of schizophrenia (García-Montes & Pérez-Álvarez, in press; Pérez-Álvarez, García-Montes, Perona & Vallina, 2008).

The two randomized studies that exist to this date on the effectiveness of Acceptance and Commitment Therapy (Bach & Hayes, 2002; Gaudiano & Herbert, 2006) found that there were fewer re-hospitalizations in the people that received this type of treatment, although they did not show a reduced frequency of hallucinations (which, as has been discussed, is not the objective). After this procedure people became more active and engaged, the voices were not paralyzing the people's lives in the same way that had been previously experienced. This can be seen as an important change in people's relationship with these symptoms. The assumptions made about this intervention are also consistent with the idea that sometimes it is not necessary to focus directly on hallucinations in order to modify them and that other related behaviors can be treated (behaviors related to mood states, social isolation, etc.) to diminish their effect.

The favorable data drawn from the results of third-generation psychotherapies are beginning to glean importance. Although more randomized studies are still needed, there seems to be an opening of new perspectives, not only related to the usefulness of these therapeutic techniques, but also related to the explanation of various processes involved in hallucinatory behavior.

References

Al-Issa, I. (1977). Social and cultural aspects of hallucinations. *Psychological Bulletin, 84*, 167-176.

Al-Issa, I. (1995). The illusion of reality or the reality of illusion: Hallucinations and culture. *British Journal of Psychiatry, 166*, 368-373.

Altman, H., Collins, M., & Mundy, P. (1997). Subclinical hallucinations and delusions in nonpsychotic adolescents. *Journal of Child Psychology and Psychiatry, 38*, 413-420.

Bach, P.A., & Hayes, S.C. (2002). The use of Acceptance and Commitment Therapy to prevent the rehospitalization of psychotic patients: A randomized controlled trial. *Journal of Consulting and Clinical Psychology, 70*, 5, 1129-1139.

Baker, C., & Morrison, A.P. (1998). Metacognition, intrusive thoughts and auditory hallucinations. *Psychological Medicine, 28*, 1199-1208.

Barret, T.R. & Etheridge, J.B. (1994). Verbal hallucinations in normals. III: dysfunctional personality correlates. *Personality and Individual Difference, 16*, 57-62.

Bentall, R. P., Jackson, H.F., & Pilgrim, D. (1988). Abandoning the concept of schizophrenia some implications opf validity arguments of psychological research into psychotic phenomena. *British Journal of Clinical Psychology, 27*, 303-314.

Berrios, G. (1996). *The history of mental symptoms. Descriptive psychopathology since the nineteenth century.* Cambridge: Cambridge University Press.

Bleuler, E. (1911). Dementia praecox or the group of schizophrenias. New Yor: International University Press.

Cangas, A.J., Langer, A., & Moriana, J.A. (in press). Hallucinations and related perceptual disturbances in a non-clinical Spanish population. *International Journal of Social Psychiatry*.

Cangas, A.J., García-Montes, J.M., López, M., & Olivencia, J.J. (2003). Social and personality variables related to the origin of auditory hallucinations. *International Journal of Psychology and Psychological Therapy, 3*, 195-208.

Cangas, A.J., Sass, L., & Pérez, M. (2008). From the hallucinations of the Saint Teresa of Jesus to the voices of schizophrenics. *Philosophy, Psychiatry, Psychology, 15*, 239-250.

Chadwick, P., Birchwood, M., & Trower, P. (1996). *Cognitive therapy for delusions, voices and paranoia.* Chichester: Wiley.

Chadwick, P., Hughes, S., Russell, D., Russell, I., & Dagnan, D.(2009). Mindfulness for distressing voices and paranoia: a replication and randomized feasibility trial. *Behavior and Cognitive Psychotherapy. 37,* 403-412.

Cooper, J. E., Kendell, R. E., Gurland, B. J., et. Al. (1972). *Psychiatric Diagnosis in New York and London.* Maudsley Monograph 20. Oxford: Oxford University Press.

Cuevas-Yust, C. (2006). Terapia cognitiva conductual para los delirios y alucinaciones resistentes a la medicación en pacientes psicóticos ambulatorios. *Apuntes de Psicología 24*, 267-292.

Dhossche, D., Ferninand, R., van der Ende, J., Hofstra, M.B., & Verhulst, F. (2002). Diagnostic outcome of self-reported hallucinations in a community sample of adolescents. *Psychological Medicine, 32*, 619-627.

Farhall, J., Greenwood, K. M., & Jackson, H. J. (2007). Coping with hallucinated voices in schizophrenia: a review of sel-initiated strategies and therapeutic interventions. *Clinical Psychology Review, 27*, 476-493.

García-Montes, Pérez-Álvarez, M., & Cangas, A.J. (2006). Aproximación al abordaje de los síntomas psicóticos desde la aceptación. *Apuntes de Psicología, 24*, 293-307

García Montes, J.M., & Pérez Álvarez, M. (en prensa). Exposition in existential terms of a case of 'negative schizophrenia' approached by means of Acceptance and Commitment Therapy. *International Journal of Existential Psychology and Psychotherapy*.

García-Montes, J.M., Pérez-Álvarez, M. Sass, L., & Cangas, A.J. (2008). The role of superstition in psychopathology. *Philosophy, Psychiatry, Psychology, 15*, 227-237.

García Montes, J.M., Pérez-Alvarez, M., Soto-Balbuena, C., Perona-Garcelán, S., & Cangas-Díaz, A. (2006). Metacognitions in patients with hallucinations and obsessive-compulsive disorder: the superstition factor. *Behaviour Research and Therapy, 44*, 1091-1104.

Gaudiano, B.A. (2005). Cognitive behavior therapies for psychotic disorders: Current empirical status and future directions. *Clinical Psychology: Science and Practice, 12*, 33-50.

Gaudiano, B.A., & Herbert, J.D. (2006). Acute treatment of inpatients with psychotic symptoms using Acceptance and Commitment Therapy: Pilot results. *Behaviour Research and Therapy, 44*, 415-437.

Haynes, S.N., & Geddy, P. (1973). Suppression of psychotic hallucinations through timeout. *Behaviour Therapy, 4*, 123-127.

Knudson, B., & Coyle, A. (1999). Coping strategies for auditory hallucinations: a review. *Counselling Psychology Quarterly, 12*, 25-38.

Laing, R.D. (1960). *The divided self: An existential study in sanity and madness*. Hamondsworth: Penguin.

Layng, T.V.J., & Andronis, P.T. (1984). Toward a functional analysis of delusional speech and hallucinatory behavior. *The Behavior Analyst, 7*, 139-156.

Lindsley, O.R. (1959). Reduction in rate of vocal psychotic symptoms by differential positive reinforcement. *Journal of the Experimental Analysis of Behavior, 2*, 269.

Morrison, A. P., & Wells, A. (2003). A comparison of metacognitions in patients with hallucinations, delusions, panic disorder and non-patient controls. *Behaviour Research and Therapy, 41*, 251-256.

Ohayon, M.M. (2000) Prevalence of hallucinations and their pathological associations in the general population. *Psychiatry Research, 97*, 153-164.

Parnas, J., & Handest, P. (2003). Phenomenology of anomalous self-experience in early schizophrenia. *Contemporary Psychiatry, 44*, 121-134.

Pérez, M. (2008). Hyperreflexivity as a condition of mental disorder: A clinical and historical perspectiva. *Psicothema, 20*, 181-187.

Pérez Álvarez, M., García Montes, J. M., Perona-Garcelán, S., & Vallina-Fernández, O. (2008). Changing relationship with voices: new therapeutic perspectives for treating hallucinations. *Clinical Psychology and Psychotherapy, 15*, 75-85.

Persons, J. (1986). The advantages of studing psychological phenomena rather than psychiatric diagnosis. *American Psychologist, 41*, 1252-1260.

Read, J., Seymour, F., & Mosher, L.R. (2004). Unhappy families. En *J. Read, F. Seymour & L. R. Mosher . Models of madness* (pp. 253-268). New York: Routledge.

Romme, M., & Escher, S. (1989). Hearing voices. *Schizophrenia Bulletin, 15*, 109-216.

Romme, M., & Escher, S. (2000). *Making sense of voices. A mental health professional's guide to working with voices-hearer*. London: Mind.

Rosenham, D.L. (1973). On being sane in insane places. *Sciences, 179*, 250-258.

Sarbin, T.R. & Juhasz, J.B. (1967). The historical background of the concept of hallucination. *Journal of the History of the Behavioral Sciences, 3*, 339-358.

Sass, L. A. (1992). *Madness and modernism. Insanity in the light of modern art, literature, and thought*. Cambridge: Harvard University Press.

Sass, L. (2003). Negative symptoms, schizophrenia, and the self. International *Journal of Psychology and Psychological Therapy, 3*, 153-180.

Serper, M., Dill, C.A., Chang, N., Kot, T., & Elliot, J. (2005). Factorial structure and classification of hallucinations: Continuity of experience in psychotic and normal Individuals. *Journal of Nervous and Mental Disease, 193*, 265-272.

Slade, P.D., & Bentall, R.P. (1988). *Sensory deception: A scientific analysis of hallucination*. Londres: Croom Helm.

Stanghellini, G. (2004a). *Disembodied spirits and deanimated bodies. The psychopathology of common sense*. Oxford: Oxford University Press.

Stanghellini, G. (2004b). Psychopathological roots of early schizophrenia: adolescent vulnerability, hebephrenia and heboidophrenia. *Current Opinion in Psychiatry, 17*, 471-477.

Stanghellini, G., & Cutting, J. (2003). Auditory Verbal Hallucinations - Breaking the Silence of Inner Dialogue. *Psychopathology; 36*:120-128

Tien, A. (1991). Distributions of hallucinations in the population. *Social Psychiatry and Psychiatric Epidemiology, 26*, 287-292.

Veiga-Martínez, C., Pérez Álvarez, M., & García Montes, J.M. (2008). Acceptance and Commitment Therapy Applied to Treatment of Auditory Hallucinations. *Clinical Case Studies, 7*, 118-135.

Wahass, S., & Kent, G. (1997a). Coping with auditory hallucinations: A cross-cultural comparison between western (British) and non-western (Saudi Arabian) patients. *Journal of Nervous and Mental Disease, 185*, 664-668.

Wahass, S., & Kent, G. (1997b). A comparison of public attitudes in Britain and Saudi Arabian towards auditory hallucinations. *International Journal of Social Psychiatry, 43*, 175-183.

Index

A

abuse, xi, 68, 83, 132, 139, 168, 169, 170, 184, 185, 187, 203
accessibility, 86
accounting, 52, 62, 107
accuracy, 25, 101
acetylcholine, 187
acid, 106, 112, 149, 151, 153, 158, 159
adaptation, x, 114, 228
additives, 154
ADHD, 152, 158
adjustment, 186, 228
adolescent development, 116
adolescent female, 136
adolescents, xi, 27, 63, 71, 72, 73, 92, 114, 115, 118, 123, 124, 126, 127, 128, 129, 130, 132, 134, 135, 136, 137, 138, 139, 140, 142, 144, 145, 146, 201, 202, 204, 222, 232
adrenaline, 150, 160
adulthood, x, xi, 27, 113, 115, 117, 126, 132, 137, 200
advantages, 91, 233
aetiology, 103, 105
affective dimension, 40
affective disorder, 73, 80, 89, 176
aggression, 165, 173, 183, 184, 192, 193
aggressive behavior, 184, 186, 191, 192
agonist, 150, 151, 156, 159
agranulocytosis, 150
akathisia, 149
alcohol withdrawal, xiv, 219
alcoholism, 176
algorithm, 177, 189
alters, 158
alucinaciones, 232
amblyopia, 17, 19, 25

American Psychiatric Association, xii, xiii, 2, 18, 24, 34, 54, 71, 156, 163, 164, 172, 174, 222
American Psychological Association, 55, 127
amino acids, 158, 160
amphetamines, 164, 221
amygdala, 64, 71, 215
anatomy, 18, 26, 28, 29, 75, 110, 111, 216, 217
anemia, 111
anger, viii, 46, 61, 64, 65, 172
anisotropy, 5, 15, 21
antagonism, 153, 157
anterior cingulate cortex, 182, 190, 220
antibody, 159
antidepressant, 66, 70, 189, 223
antidepressant medication, 66, 70
antipsychotic, 70, 149, 150, 151, 153, 154, 155, 156, 157, 159, 164, 170, 172, 176, 177, 188, 189, 193, 223, 226
antipsychotic drugs, 149, 150, 153, 155, 156, 157, 159, 177, 193, 223
antipsychotic effect, 154
anxiety disorder, ix, 61, 62, 66, 67, 70, 78, 80, 87, 90, 115, 187
anxious mood, 66
apathy, xiii, 179, 180, 182, 183, 189, 191, 193, 231
apoptosis, 161
appetite, 187
appraisals, 66, 67, 69, 140, 198
aripiprazole, 150, 172, 188, 189
arousal, 12, 23, 64
arrest, 101
arteritis, 105, 111
artery, 105, 109
aspartate, 106, 150, 153
assertiveness, 47, 48, 51, 52, 70
assessment, x, 30, 57, 58, 59, 72, 114, 126, 129, 134, 136, 137, 158, 171, 173, 174, 177, 190, 197

assessment tools, 114
atrophy, 103
attachment, 57
attribution, ix, 12, 22, 23, 28, 51, 67, 79, 88, 89, 129, 133
attribution bias, 22, 23, 67
audition, 220
auditory cortex, 14, 15, 18, 21, 23, 54, 81, 220
auditory modality, 4, 5, 10, 22
auditory stimuli, 14
authenticity, xiv, 195
autonomic nervous system, 160
autonomy, xiv, 207, 228
avoidance, 67, 92, 108, 229, 230

B

basal ganglia, 149
baths, 155
beef, 160
behavior therapy, 92, 141, 183, 191
behavioral change, 191
behavioral problems, 188
behavioral sciences, 55
behaviors, xiii, xiv, 90, 93, 179, 180, 181, 182, 184, 186, 189, 191, 192, 195, 196, 212, 221, 226, 229, 230, 231
belief systems, 23
beneficial effect, 189
benign, 6, 139, 170, 171
bias, 5, 9, 12, 13, 22, 23, 67, 73, 87, 88, 94, 103, 211
bipolar disorder, xiv, 40, 62, 91, 94, 169, 171, 187, 219
blood flow, 30, 58, 94, 95, 106, 160, 213, 217, 218
blood plasma, 155, 158
blood pressure, 160
blood transfusion, 105
blood-brain barrier, 160
body weight, 157
borderline personality disorder, 40
brain abnormalities, 14
brain activity, 19, 20, 22, 23, 24
brain damage, 92
brain structure, 148
brainstem, 106, 108, 221

C

calcium, 106, 111, 159
cannabis, xi, 132, 138, 140, 143, 145, 200
carbohydrate, 152, 154, 158, 160
caregivers, xiii, 179, 182, 183, 186
caregiving, 191
cataplexy, 108
cataract, 98, 101, 108

catecholamines, 150, 160
categorization, 101, 102
causal relationship, 52, 208
CBS, ix, 97, 98, 99, 101, 102, 103, 104, 105, 106, 107, 108
central nervous system, 105, 133, 220
central retinal artery occlusion, 105, 109
cerebellum, 53, 81
cerebral blood flow, 30, 106, 160, 213, 217, 218
cerebral cortex, 130
cerebrospinal fluid, 153
child abuse, 203
Child Behavior Checklist, 134
Child Depression Inventory, 118
childhood, 73, 115, 116, 128, 138, 143, 144, 202, 228, 229
cholinesterase, 187, 189
cholinesterase inhibitors, 187
citalopram, 189, 193
City, 59
clarity, 99, 101
class, 77, 139, 141, 153
classroom, 136
clinical diagnosis, 8, 15, 198
clinical disorders, 197
clinical presentation, 140, 178
clinical symptoms, 140, 196, 202
clinical syndrome, 200
closure, 102
clozapine, 149, 150, 153, 157, 158, 159, 160, 172, 173, 175, 176, 177
clustering, 103, 124
cocaine, 149, 150, 154, 160
cognition, 44, 78, 84, 103, 158, 192
cognitive activity, 215
cognitive biases, vii, 1, 12, 22, 67, 87, 88, 133, 211
cognitive deficit, 12, 13, 14, 23, 62, 87, 88, 90, 92, 103, 124, 135, 139
cognitive deficits, 12, 13, 14, 23, 62, 87, 90, 92, 103, 124, 135, 139
cognitive dissonance, 66, 87
cognitive dysfunction, ix, 12, 13, 14, 23, 80, 87, 90
cognitive effort, 57
cognitive function, ix, 7, 13, 35, 92, 97, 190
cognitive impairment, xiii, 9, 22, 179, 180, 181, 183, 208
cognitive models, vii, 1, 6, 15, 115
cognitive performance, 160
cognitive process, 6, 7, 24, 90, 211
cognitive processing, 90
cognitive science, 56
cognitive system, 9
cognitive therapy, 126, 173

coherence, 15, 47
college students, 8
common sense, 198, 228, 234
common symptoms, 62
community, x, 57, 63, 66, 68, 74, 75, 103, 118, 128, 131, 142, 144, 146, 170, 182, 188, 190, 197, 200, 202, 204, 230, 232
comorbidity, 130, 174
competition, 94
complaints, 181, 182
complex interactions, 221
complexity, x, 97, 109
compliance, 69, 171, 172, 173, 176
complications, 35, 39, 43
composition, 124
comprehension, xi, 62, 95, 132, 218
computed tomography, 111
conceptual model, 190
conceptualization, ix, 79, 80, 116
conditioning, xiv, 195, 202
congruence, 73, 78, 135
connectivity, 5, 11, 12, 14, 15, 17, 21, 22, 23, 24, 124, 217, 220
connectivity patterns, 23
conscious perception, 14, 20, 31
consciousness, ix, 44, 51, 52, 56, 58, 63, 79, 83, 84, 88, 108, 144, 204, 227
consensus, 103, 186, 204
construct validity, 36, 140
consumption, 200
context memory, 62, 78
contrast sensitivity, 103, 105, 111
control group, 139, 167, 231
controlled studies, 166, 169
controlled trials, 158, 176, 193
coping strategies, 92, 138, 139
correlation, 2, 14, 35, 36, 39, 42, 48, 49, 50, 51, 85, 86, 105, 182, 184, 185, 186, 216
correlation analysis, 48, 50
correlation coefficient, 39, 185
correlations, 36, 37, 39, 42, 48, 50, 51, 68, 119, 121, 123, 141
cortex, vii, x, 2, 5, 14, 15, 16, 17, 18, 19, 20, 21, 23, 24, 25, 27, 29, 31, 53, 54, 56, 81, 97, 99, 102, 104, 105, 106, 107, 108, 111, 150, 152, 157, 158, 159, 182, 190, 191, 214, 217, 220, 221, 223
cortical neurons, 221
cortical pathway, 104, 106, 108, 222
cortisol, 160
covering, 117
creativity, 140
critical analysis, 223
criticism, 83

cross-cultural comparison, 234
cross-sectional study, 77
CSS, 161
cultural differences, 30
cytotoxicity, 161
Czech Republic, 219

D

daily living, 183, 191
dangerousness, 200
data collection, 22
data set, 14
deaths, xii, 163
declarative memory, 218
deficit, 5, 12, 14, 22, 64, 87, 88, 90, 91, 108, 133, 152, 187, 211
degenerative dementia, 189
degradation, 150
delirium, xiv, 149, 187, 219, 221
delusion, 65, 125, 133, 143, 208
delusional thinking, 127
dementia, xiii, 4, 17, 103, 179, 180, 181, 182, 183, 184, 185, 186, 187, 188, 189, 190, 191, 192, 193
demonstrations, 80
dendrites, 150
denial, 229
dependent variable, 170
depolarization, 151
depressive symptomatology, 64, 139
depressive symptoms, xiii, 66, 139, 168, 179, 186
deprivation, vii, xiv, 1, 4, 7, 16, 17, 19, 20, 21, 25, 30, 109, 133, 195, 229
desensitization, 230
detachment, 105
detection, xi, 11, 25, 55, 62, 94, 132, 140, 230
developing brain, 124
developmental process, 137
diabetes, 150, 154
diagnosis, xiv, 8, 15, 43, 62, 63, 65, 71, 98, 108, 138, 148, 178, 186, 198, 211, 213, 216, 219, 225, 226, 233
Diagnostic and Statistical Manual of Mental Disorders, 24, 71, 148, 156, 174
diagnostic criteria, 37, 80, 83, 89, 186, 187, 192
dialogues, 23, 229
diet, xii, 148, 152, 153, 154, 155, 156, 158, 160
dietary fat, 153
differential diagnosis, 108
diffusion, 14, 15, 24, 25, 28, 107
dimensionality, 201, 203
disability, 99, 139, 141, 197, 205
discomfort, 198, 229
discrimination, 10, 25, 58, 94, 125, 133

disposition, 8, 9, 11, 13, 58, 201
dissociation, 77, 112, 138
dissociative disorders, xiii, 195
dissonance, 66, 82, 87, 89
distortion, 102, 123, 133, 197, 199, 210, 212
distortions, 17, 20, 81, 121, 122, 123, 124, 125, 197, 198
distractions, 100
distress, x, 4, 34, 67, 68, 69, 70, 73, 76, 78, 82, 83, 84, 87, 89, 92, 93, 102, 114, 115, 117, 118, 119, 120, 121, 122, 123, 124, 125, 126, 138, 139, 140, 141, 143, 187, 197, 198, 205
disturbances, 11, 16, 64, 70, 83, 90, 117, 191, 209, 232
dopamine, xi, 12, 76, 108, 116, 128, 147, 148, 149, 150, 151, 152, 153, 154, 155, 156, 157, 158, 159, 160, 161, 164, 221, 223
dopamine agonist, 108
dopamine antagonists, 154
dopaminergic, xi, xii, 17, 21, 147, 148, 149, 150, 151, 153, 154, 155, 156, 157, 161, 220, 221
dorsolateral prefrontal cortex, 81, 220
dream, 39, 221
dreaming, vii, 221, 223
drug addiction, 160
drug therapy, 193
drug treatment, 193
drugs, xi, xii, 4, 6, 12, 17, 147, 148, 149, 150, 152, 153, 154, 155, 156, 157, 159, 164, 177, 193, 200, 222, 223
D-serine, 151
durability, 78
dysphoria, 74, 76, 141

E

economic evaluation, 75
editors, 111, 190
egg, 99, 160
eigenvalues, 46, 121
elaboration, 107, 155, 178, 196
embryogenesis, 99
emission, 18, 28, 105, 111
emotion, 64, 65, 66, 68, 71, 72, 73, 74, 94, 128, 187, 221, 227, 228
emotion regulation, 74
emotional disorder, 90, 115, 230
emotional distress, x, 73, 83, 113, 114, 115, 117, 123, 125
emotional experience, 64, 227
emotional processes, 23, 81, 231
emotional reactions, 51
emotional state, 133
emotional stimuli, 64

empirical studies, 64, 69, 165, 174
encephalopathy, 26
encoding, 14, 150, 218
endocrine, 208
England, 226
entrapment, 72, 127
environmental factors, xi, xii, 132, 148, 163, 181, 200
environmental stimuli, 133
epidemiology, 97, 103
epidermis, 155
epilepsy, vii, 1, 4, 12, 32, 108, 133, 152, 158
episodic memory, 85, 90, 211
etiology, 90, 135, 226, 230
euphoria, 64
event-related potential, 96
evil, 69, 109
examinations, 115
excitability, 16, 19, 20, 21, 25, 30, 106, 107
excitatory postsynaptic potentials, 150
execution, 52, 53, 55
executive function, 124
exploration, 139, 202
exposure, 20, 108, 133, 154, 160, 217
external locus of control, 14, 22

F

factor analysis, 37, 39, 46, 119, 121, 122, 181
false positive, 55, 197, 199
family history, 208
family members, 102
family relationships, 228
fantasy, 9, 29, 32
fat, 152, 153, 154, 160
faults, 139
FDA, 188, 189, 193
fears, 173, 182
feedback, 20, 44, 52, 53, 55, 81, 88, 151, 216
feelings, 38, 44, 65, 69, 71, 118, 226, 228, 229, 230, 231
female prisoners, 28, 57, 203
fever, 4
first degree relative, 65, 138
fitness, 42
five-factor model, 51, 54, 58
flashbacks, 63, 83
flavour, 98
fluctuations, 20, 76, 133, 158
fluid, 153, 159
food additives, 154
food intake, 187
Ford, 54, 56, 222
forensic patients, 167, 169

frequencies, 116
frontal cortex, 16, 21, 214
frontal lobe, 213, 221
fruits, 154
functional analysis, 233
functional imaging, 14, 21, 55
functional MRI, 26, 27, 30
fusion, 200, 227

G

galactorrhea, 160
genes, 148, 150, 151
genetic linkage, 151
genetics, 143, 156
Germany, 1, 24, 203
glaucoma, 105
glucose, 217
glutamate, 150, 151, 152, 153, 157
glycine, 151, 152, 153, 157
God, 39, 63
grading, 110
grandiose delusions, 208
gray matter, 15, 220
grotesque, 100, 101, 102

H

handedness, 23, 54
HE, 161
headache, 31
health problems, xii, 163
heart rate, 160
heat exhaustion, 161
helplessness, 28
hemisphere, 18, 26, 55, 214
heterogeneity, 90, 170
high fat, 160
high school, 136
hip fractures, 188
hippocampus, 18, 64, 150
histamine, 150
homeostasis, 158
homovanillic acid, 153
hopelessness, 177, 187
hospitalization, 169
host, 114
hostility, 173, 175
HSCT, 85
human agency, 25
human brain, 20, 29
human cerebral cortex, 130
human nature, 71
human performance, 30
human subjects, 153, 160

Hunter, 34, 55, 63, 72, 216
hyperactivity, 5, 17, 21, 152, 220
hyperarousal, 220
hyperprolactinemia, 152
hypersensitivity, 124
hyperthermia, xi, xii, 147, 148, 149, 153, 154, 155, 156, 161
hypnagogic hallucinations, 108
hypothalamus, 221
hypothesis, xiv, 5, 8, 9, 10, 11, 13, 22, 26, 36, 83, 90, 99, 107, 108, 109, 124, 125, 148, 150, 151, 152, 153, 155, 157, 207, 214, 215, 216, 220, 221, 223

I

idiosyncratic, xiii, 17, 127, 164
illusion, 25, 71, 93, 232
illusions, iv, 16, 26, 73
illusory contours, 19
image, 2, 7, 55, 58, 70, 84
imagery, vii, 1, 5, 6, 7, 8, 9, 10, 11, 14, 16, 19, 20, 21, 22, 23, 24, 25, 26, 27, 28, 29, 30, 31, 32, 59, 77, 98, 102, 108, 126, 211, 212, 214, 217, 218, 221
images, ix, 3, 5, 6, 7, 8, 9, 16, 17, 20, 24, 27, 28, 29, 30, 79, 80, 82, 83, 84, 85, 88, 91, 95, 98, 100, 101, 102, 105, 107, 110, 214, 229, 231
imagination, 38
imaging modalities, 107
immersion, xi, 147, 155
immune system, 155
immunosuppression, 155
impairments, ix, 9, 14, 22, 45, 56, 77, 79, 88, 124, 212
impulses, 82, 84, 88, 91, 215
impulsive, 91, 166, 169
impulsivity, 165
in vivo, 159
incidence, ix, 9, 44, 97, 103, 115, 143, 149, 188
independence, 4, 10, 11, 22
independent variable, 170
individual differences, viii, ix, 2, 22, 35, 79
individual perception, 13
induction, 26
infarction, 108, 111
inferences, 133
information processing, 5, 8, 24, 27, 84, 116
informed consent, 118
inhibition, ix, xii, 20, 62, 76, 79, 85, 87, 88, 90, 91, 93, 95, 106, 148, 149, 153
inhibitor, 193
initiation, 56, 107
insane, ix, 26, 97, 103, 234
insecticide, 100

insects, 100
insertion, 37, 39, 43
integration, 22, 25, 59, 71, 81, 93, 210
interference, ix, 7, 79, 87, 90, 95
internal environment, 133
internal processes, 2
interneurons, 150
interpersonal relations, 45, 69
interpersonal relationships, 45
intervention, 66, 91, 152, 173, 177, 180, 184, 190, 230, 231
intoxication, xiv, 219
intrusions, ix, 76, 79, 80, 82, 83, 84, 86, 87, 88, 89, 90, 91, 92, 94, 95, 129, 203
irritability, 154, 186, 189, 193
Islam, 173, 177
isolation, 17, 102, 133, 186, 187, 200, 205, 229, 230, 231
Italy, 163, 168, 170, 178, 207

J

Japan, 33
Jordan, 52, 59

L

laboratory tests, 148
landscapes, 98, 99, 105
language processing, 215
later life, 175
laterality, 28
LD, 160
LEA, 26, 27, 73
learners, 23
learning, 7, 118, 150, 159, 174, 178, 211
left hemisphere, 18, 214
lesions, 99, 103, 104, 105, 109, 111, 161, 220, 222
lethargy, xi, 147
LIFE, 37, 45
life experiences, 63
lifetime, 6, 44, 83, 116, 118, 126, 167, 169
limbic system, 14, 21, 23
Limitations, 23
localization, 99, 106
locus, 5, 12, 13, 14, 22, 23, 26, 28
longitudinal study, 125, 129, 137, 143, 144, 145, 175, 203
long-term memory, 21
lymphocytes, 155, 161
lysergic acid diethylamide, 149

M

macular degeneration, ix, 97, 99, 110, 111, 220
magical thinking, x, 9, 118, 131, 136, 197, 199

magnetic resonance, vii, 1, 20, 26, 27, 28, 30, 99, 105, 107, 218
magnetic resonance imaging, vii, 1, 20, 26, 27, 28, 30, 99, 105, 218
magnetic resonance spectroscopy, 107
magnetoencephalography, 106
major depression, 59, 73, 75, 98
major depressive disorder, 62, 187
majority, 84, 104, 138, 169, 170, 171
management, 98, 107, 109, 145, 174, 180, 188, 189
mania, 62, 71, 72
manic, 62, 72, 91, 94, 148
manic episode, 62, 72, 148
manipulation, 86
mapping, 18, 26, 191
markers, xi, 6, 15, 132, 137, 140
medication, xi, xiv, 35, 66, 70, 147, 153, 154, 155, 156, 168, 170, 172, 176, 183, 187, 189, 219, 226
MEG, 28, 106
melody, 38, 40
memory, vii, ix, 2, 6, 7, 8, 12, 18, 19, 20, 21, 23, 38, 40, 51, 58, 59, 62, 67, 77, 78, 79, 81, 84, 85, 86, 87, 88, 90, 91, 92, 93, 94, 95, 99, 124, 142, 148, 150, 211, 212, 214, 217, 218, 227
memory processes, 86, 87, 88
memory retrieval, 212
mental activity, 46, 48, 221, 223
mental disorder, viii, ix, xiv, xv, 33, 54, 79, 80, 89, 90, 174, 176, 195, 196, 225, 233
mental health, 27, 70, 177, 234
mental illness, xii, 63, 163, 227
mental image, vii, 1, 2, 5, 6, 7, 8, 9, 10, 11, 16, 19, 20, 21, 22, 23, 24, 25, 27, 28, 29, 30, 31, 32, 85, 126, 214, 217
mental imagery, vii, 1, 2, 5, 6, 7, 8, 9, 10, 11, 16, 19, 20, 21, 22, 23, 24, 25, 30, 31, 32, 126, 217
mental representation, 6, 85, 86, 89, 126
mental state, viii, 2, 6, 23, 65, 103, 110, 196
mental states, viii, 2, 6, 65
messages, 171
messenger RNA, 158
meta-analysis, 145, 175, 176, 188, 193, 200, 204
metabolism, 151, 160, 217
metacognition, 24, 71, 76, 95
methylphenidate, 183
modelling, 30, 69
modernism, 234
modification, 69, 133, 180
modules, 222
monitoring, viii, 5, 6, 12, 13, 14, 25, 33, 36, 45, 51, 56, 57, 58, 59, 62, 72, 74, 76, 81, 88, 93, 94, 139, 177, 211, 212, 214, 215, 230
mood disorder, xii, 62, 68, 163, 171

mood states, 231
morbidity, 64
mortality rate, 188
motivation, xi, 6, 147, 152, 155, 159, 177, 182
motor control, 52, 53, 54, 58, 59
motor system, 56, 106
MRI, 20, 26, 27, 30, 75, 99, 105, 217
mRNA, 159
multidimensional, 196, 197, 198, 211
multiple sclerosis, 111, 112
muscles, 133
music, 37, 38, 39, 40, 41, 42, 43, 62, 69, 183, 191
music therapy, 183, 191
mystical experiences, 139

N

narcolepsy, 17, 108
National Science Foundation, 127
natural killer cell, 161
nausea, 150
negative emotions, 51
negative feedback, 20, 150
negative reinforcement, 230
negativity, 28
nerve, 159
nervous system, 105, 111, 133, 160, 220
Netherlands, 110
neural network, 218
neural networks, 218
neuritis, 105
neurobiology, 156, 222
neurodegenerative diseases, 148, 222
neurodegenerative disorders, 149, 219
neurofibrillary tangles, 182, 193
neuroimaging, ix, 14, 19, 22, 31, 64, 81, 93, 97, 99, 104, 105, 107, 108, 220, 222
neuroleptic drugs, xi, xii, 147, 152, 153, 154, 155
neuroleptic malignant syndrome, 149, 150, 155
neuroleptics, xii, 147, 148, 149, 150, 153, 221
neurons, xi, 147, 148, 150, 151, 154, 161, 193, 221
neurophysiology, 26
neuropsychiatry, 218
neuropsychology, 27, 56, 73, 76, 94, 128, 142, 216, 217, 222, 223
neuroscience, 141, 142, 144
neuroses, 90
neurotransmission, 157, 158, 221
neurotransmitter, 12, 106, 157, 192
New Zealand, 137, 143, 146, 204
nightmares, 221
NMDA receptors, 150, 151, 152
NMR, 28
noise, 9, 99, 133, 139, 165, 181

non-clinical population, 8, 9, 15, 32, 56, 80, 125, 145, 204, 218
norepinephrine, 161
normal aging, 85, 93
normal development, 141
normal distribution, 36, 125
North America, 145, 178
nucleus, 104, 106, 107, 111, 152, 159, 160, 221
nurses, 102
nursing, xiii, 100, 177, 179, 180, 181, 182, 183, 184, 185, 186, 188, 189, 190, 191, 192, 193
nursing home, xiii, 179, 180, 181, 182, 183, 184, 185, 186, 188, 189, 190, 191, 192, 193

O

obsessive-compulsive disorder, ix, 80, 82, 93, 95, 233
occipital lobe, 27, 104, 108, 111
occipital regions, 19
occlusion, 105, 109
occupational therapy, 183
OCD, 82, 83, 89, 91, 92
olanzapine, 108, 149, 152, 155, 157, 172, 175
old age, 222
olfaction, 125
openness, 51
optic neuritis, 105
orbit, 99
organ, xiv, 2, 34, 219
organic disease, 80, 91, 133
oscillations, 25, 220
oscillatory activity, 220
outpatients, 178
overlap, 148, 186
ownership, 44, 53, 58

P

pain, 181
pairing, 68
panic attack, 66
panic disorder, 76, 82, 95, 203, 233
parallel, 53, 91, 159, 209
parallelism, ix, 80, 84, 87
paralysis, 39, 228
paranoia, 43, 48, 56, 58, 68, 72, 142, 143, 202, 232
paranoid schizophrenia, 18
parietal cortex, 27, 53, 104
parthenogenesis, 99
path analysis, 42, 50
path model, 36, 42, 43
pathogenesis, ix, 97, 98, 99, 105, 132, 214, 215
pathology, 99, 103, 105, 203

pathophysiology, 11, 12, 97, 104, 105, 109, 148, 149, 150, 156
pathways, 27, 52, 72, 98, 104, 105, 106, 107, 108, 109, 111, 128, 221
PCP, 150, 151
perceived control, 68, 173
percentile, 119
perceptual processing, 81, 216
performance, 10, 30, 36, 55, 57, 84, 87, 88, 90, 91, 94, 160
perfusion, 106, 182, 191, 213, 214, 215
permeability, 160
permission, iv, 3, 24, 181, 184, 185
persecutory delusion, 28, 46, 83, 128, 129, 142, 172
perseverance, 115
personal communication, 102
personal life, 199
personal qualities, 148
personality characteristics, 230
personality disorder, xv, 37, 39, 43, 55, 58, 80, 128, 171, 225
personality inventories, 58
personality scales, 45
personality traits, 37, 39, 48, 50, 54, 116, 128, 136
personality type, 51
PET, 5, 157, 158, 216, 217
pharmacological treatment, 17, 187, 210, 230
pharmacology, 128
pharmacotherapy, xii, 148
phencyclidine, 150
phenomenology, viii, ix, 2, 4, 33, 34, 61, 62, 68, 71, 128, 223
phenotype, x, 32, 131, 140, 145
phenylalanine, xi, 147
physical abuse, 184, 185
physical activity, 46, 48, 190
physiopathology, 111
pilot study, 77, 176, 178, 217
placebo, 152, 193
plasma levels, xi, 147
plasticity, xii, 148, 156
pleasure, 186, 187
polarization, 210
police, 101
polymorphism, 184, 192
polymorphisms, 192
poor performance, 88, 91
population group, 117
positive correlation, 51, 123
positive reinforcement, 229, 230, 233
positron, 17, 18, 28
positron emission tomography, 18, 28
posttraumatic stress, xiii, xv, 74, 92, 195, 225

post-traumatic stress disorder, ix, 75, 80, 83
poverty, 148, 210
predicate, 7
predictive validity, 137
prefrontal cortex, 81, 151, 152, 157, 158, 159, 220, 221, 223
pregnancy, 160
prejudice, viii, 33
prevention, xi, 23, 70, 129, 132, 140, 176, 177
preventive approach, 145
primary visual cortex, 31, 99, 104
primate, 154
prior knowledge, 6
prisoners, 28, 57, 203
proactive interference, ix, 79, 87, 95
probability, 20, 58, 83, 106
problem behavior, 189
problem behaviors, 189
problem solving, 143
processing biases, 116
processing pathways, 52
processing stages, 7
prodrome, 72, 144, 145, 203
prognosis, xiv, 30, 207, 208, 210, 216
programming, 189, 191
project, 24, 100, 104, 148
prolactin, xi, 147, 154, 155, 160
promax rotation, 37, 39, 46, 119, 121, 122
propagation, 106
prophylactic, xi, 132
proposition, 105, 124
protein kinase C, 157
psychiatric diagnosis, 138, 233
psychiatric disorders, 40
psychiatric illness, x, 15, 27, 97, 98, 113, 211
psychiatric institution, 103, 226
psychiatric patients, 4, 26, 27, 172, 176, 203
psychiatry, 27, 74, 103, 141, 142, 144, 218
psychoactive drug, 200
psychological distress, 115, 126
psychological phenomena, 24, 140, 233
psychological problems, 138
psychological processes, 23, 89
psychological states, 116
psychological stress, 133
psychological variables, 139
psychologist, 119
psychology, 2, 142
psychopathology, viii, 2, 4, 22, 23, 44, 58, 95, 114, 116, 139, 143, 190, 202, 210, 232, 233, 234
psychoses, 30, 71, 142, 208, 216, 217
psychosocial functioning, viii, 2, 22
psychotherapy, 70, 127, 152

psychotic symptoms, x, xiii, 8, 9, 12, 13, 22, 24, 29, 30, 62, 63, 66, 73, 89, 94, 95, 129, 131, 132, 134, 135, 136, 137, 140, 142, 143, 144, 149, 151, 152, 155, 165, 189, 193, 195, 203, 212, 225, 233
psychoticism, 74
PTSD, 62, 63, 74, 83, 89, 91, 92, 93
public health, xii, 163
punishment, 67, 82, 200, 230
pyramidal cells, 150, 151

Q

qualitative differences, 34
quality of life, 74, 182, 191, 210, 216, 222
questioning, 139, 228
quetiapine, 172

R

radio, 100, 138, 165
rating scale, 74, 155, 210
raw materials, 99
reactions, 51, 222
reactivity, 76, 178
reading, 95, 133, 165
reading comprehension, 95
reality, x, xiv, 2, 7, 10, 11, 12, 14, 18, 19, 24, 25, 29, 34, 57, 58, 61, 63, 71, 81, 93, 99, 131, 133, 135, 165, 172, 173, 199, 201, 210, 212, 219, 225, 232
reasoning, 6, 7, 67, 135, 143, 165
recall, 85, 86, 229
receptors, xii, 147, 149, 150, 151, 152, 153, 156, 157, 158, 159, 164, 184
recognition, viii, 18, 34, 44, 56, 104, 133, 145, 214
recommendations, iv, ix, 61
reconstruction, 214
recruiting, 118
recurrence, 102, 107
redundancy, 12
reflectivity, 198
regression, 105, 168, 170
regression analysis, 105, 168, 170
rehabilitation, 70, 92
rehabilitation program, 92
reinforcement, 30, 133, 229, 230, 233
reinforcers, 229
rejection, 227
relatives, 9, 10, 13, 65, 130, 138, 154
relevance, 4, 124, 135, 142, 169, 173, 197, 198, 199, 200, 212, 217
reliability, 35, 36, 37, 39, 43, 46, 47, 51, 190, 202, 225, 226
REM, 220, 221, 223
remission, 13, 66, 112
rent, 126

replacement, 184
replication, 145, 232
resistance, ix, 48, 51, 79, 84, 87, 133, 210
resolution, 20, 28, 218
risk factors, 57, 73, 75, 78, 98, 170, 171, 175, 176, 185, 186, 202, 222, 223
risperidone, 149, 172, 188, 189, 193
romantic relationship, 228

S

sadness, 51, 64, 65
SAPS, 210
Sartorius, 4, 30, 62, 77, 142
Saudi Arabia, 234
schema, 68, 70, 72, 102, 178
schizophrenic patients, vii, viii, ix, xiii, 5, 10, 11, 12, 13, 15, 25, 26, 31, 33, 34, 44, 45, 53, 56, 57, 75, 77, 79, 82, 85, 86, 88, 90, 117, 148, 149, 150, 151, 152, 155, 164, 165, 169, 170, 175, 196, 202, 210, 214, 216, 218, 221
schizotypal personality disorder, 37, 39, 43, 55, 58, 128
Schizotypal Personality Disorder, 37
schizotypy, x, 9, 10, 13, 26, 28, 29, 32, 39, 42, 48, 50, 53, 54, 55, 57, 58, 115, 118, 119, 128, 131, 139, 143, 144
sclerosis, 111, 112
scotoma, 102
screening, 21, 36, 55, 58, 171
second generation, 209
secondary students, 197
secretion, 161
sedatives, 108
seizure, 117, 124
selective attention, 7, 95
selective serotonin reuptake inhibitor, 222
self esteem, 68, 70
self monitoring, 12
self-awareness, 227
self-consciousness, 44, 51, 52, 56, 83, 227
self-control, 48
self-esteem, viii, 46, 48, 61, 68, 75, 77, 135, 145, 199
self-image, 58, 70
self-monitoring, viii, 13, 33, 36, 45, 51, 57, 59, 62, 74, 94, 139, 211, 212, 214, 215, 230
self-reports, 23, 83, 126, 191, 199
semantic memory, 85, 90
semantic processing, 216
sensation, 3, 4, 53, 119, 229
sensations, 2, 5, 20, 52, 65, 76, 119, 205
sensing, 81
sensitivity, 11, 103, 105, 111, 129, 130, 149, 153
sensitization, 76

sensors, 151
sensory experience, 2, 61
sensory modalities, vii, 1, 4, 7, 9, 21, 215
sensory modality, 5, 7, 80, 220
sensory perceptions, xiv, 2, 219
sensory systems, 4, 56
serine, 151
serotonin, xi, 147, 149, 152, 153, 154, 157, 159, 160, 161, 184, 187, 191, 192, 193, 222
sertraline, 189, 193
sex, 48, 166
sex differences, 48
short-term memory, 148
side effects, 70, 149, 150, 154, 155, 188
signals, 3, 6, 15, 81, 133
signs, 26, 72, 93, 149, 171, 228
silk, 98, 100
Sinai, 176
skewness, 36
skills training, 70, 170, 173, 176, 177, 230
skin, 155
sleep disturbance, 186
sleep stage, 221
SMS, 45, 48, 49, 51
sociability, 45
social activities, 47, 48, 51
social adjustment, 228
social behaviour, 23
social cognition, 44
social context, 45
social desirability, 23
social network, 70, 108
social roles, 69
social situations, 46, 48, 50, 51, 52
social skills, 70, 170, 173, 176, 177, 230
social skills training, 70, 170, 173, 176, 177, 230
social status, 68, 227
social support, xii, 164, 200
social withdrawal, 148
Socrates, 178
sodium, 100, 108
software, 155, 161
solitude, 100
Spain, 79, 131, 136, 195, 225
specialization, 102
species, 99, 154
spectroscopy, 25, 107
speech, viii, xii, 7, 12, 14, 29, 30, 31, 33, 34, 36, 37, 39, 43, 44, 51, 52, 53, 54, 57, 59, 62, 67, 68, 77, 81, 88, 89, 91, 93, 133, 148, 164, 165, 210, 211, 214, 216, 217, 218, 229, 233
speech perception, 57
speech processing, 14

standardization, 171
statistics, 120
stigma, 211, 216, 227, 229
stimulus, vii, xiv, 2, 6, 8, 13, 16, 80, 88, 215, 219
stomach, 65
storage, 7
streams, 104
stressful events, 51
stressors, 230
striatum, xii, 106, 111, 147, 148, 149, 151, 152, 153, 223
stroke, 105, 106, 188
structural changes, 15
structural equation modeling, 129
subjective experience, 44, 54, 62, 114, 158
subjectivity, 23, 228
substance abuse, xi, 132, 168, 170
substance use, 170
substrates, 2, 6, 31
suicidal behavior, 171, 174
suicidal ideation, xii, 70, 73, 164, 169, 174, 177, 187
suicide, vii, viii, xii, xiii, 61, 64, 73, 75, 163, 164, 165, 166, 167, 168, 169, 170, 171, 173, 174, 175, 176, 177, 178
suicide attempters, xii, 163
suicide attempts, xii, 164, 165, 166, 167, 169, 174
supernatural, 228
suppression, 67, 73, 85, 91, 92, 95, 106, 165
survey, 8, 45, 46, 58, 59, 65, 68, 69, 76, 116, 130, 144, 178, 183, 188, 222
susceptibility, xii, 163, 202
Switzerland, 113
synchronization, 220
syndrome, xiv, 4, 17, 18, 20, 30, 78, 98, 99, 103, 109, 112, 139, 141, 145, 149, 150, 155, 200, 207, 208, 210, 212, 219, 220, 221, 222, 223
synthesis, 153
systematic desensitization, 230

T

T lymphocytes, 155
takeover, 116
tangles, 182, 193
tardive dyskinesia, 172
television commercial, 38, 40
temperature, xi, 147, 152, 154, 155, 156, 161
temporal arteritis, 105, 111
temporal lobe, 108, 117, 124, 213, 221
temporal lobe epilepsy, 108
temporo-parietal cortex, 27
terminals, 159
territory, 105
testing, 25, 29, 87, 165, 173, 191

Index

thalamus, 64, 106, 107, 111
therapeutic agents, 148
therapeutic approaches, 151
therapeutic goal, 231
therapeutic intervention, 23, 233
therapeutic interventions, 23, 233
therapeutic relationship, 173
therapy, xi, 24, 55, 70, 72, 74, 75, 78, 92, 112, 126, 129, 141, 143, 147, 152, 158, 168, 173, 175, 183, 188, 189, 190, 191, 193, 201, 202, 217, 231, 232
thermoregulation, 155
thoughts, ix, 10, 12, 15, 23, 38, 40, 43, 47, 54, 67, 73, 79, 80, 81, 82, 83, 84, 85, 87, 88, 89, 91, 92, 93, 94, 95, 115, 129, 133, 138, 144, 187, 196, 197, 198, 200, 201, 214, 227, 229, 230, 231, 232
threats, xiii, 164, 229
three-dimensional space, 3
tinnitus, 69
tissue, 153, 220, 221
tonic, 105
traditions, 227
training, 23, 70, 78, 92, 173, 178
training programs, 23
trait anxiety, 46, 59
traits, 9, 25, 37, 39, 45, 46, 48, 50, 51, 52, 54, 55, 64, 116, 128, 136
tranquilizers, 155
transformations, 30
transfusion, 105
transition rate, 146
translation, 118, 127
transmission, xii, 148, 151, 153, 157, 222
trauma, xi, 63, 66, 68, 77, 83, 92, 116, 132, 138, 141, 143, 144, 202, 229
traumatic events, 83, 84, 87, 91, 138, 168
traumatic experiences, 83, 140
tremor, 149
trial, 73, 75, 85, 107, 129, 152, 154, 155, 157, 158, 167, 169, 173, 174, 177, 190, 217, 232
tricyclic antidepressant, 222
tricyclic antidepressants, 222
triggers, 67, 70, 101, 229
true/false, 37
tryptophan, 158, 159

U

UK, 55, 73, 141, 142, 144, 145, 177
umbilical cord, 161
underlying mechanisms, 66, 104
unhappiness, 228
uniform, 201
United Kingdom, 207, 226
unusual experiences, 55
unusual perceptions, 114, 116
unusual perceptual experiences, 118, 123, 136
unwanted thoughts, 85
updating, 86, 94, 95
urbanicity, xi, 132, 138, 143, 145

V

validation, x, 32, 108, 114, 117, 123, 124, 127, 128, 142
variations, 20, 158, 159
vegetables, 154
vehicles, 101, 102
vein, 91
venlafaxine, 222
victimization, xi, 132
victims, xii, 163
violence, 165, 166, 167, 169, 170, 171, 176, 178
vision, 26, 27, 31, 39, 98, 99, 100, 102, 104, 109, 110, 111, 112, 222
visions, 97, 98, 99, 101, 102, 110, 112, 226
visual acuity, 101, 105, 109, 110
visual area, vii, 2, 17, 18, 19, 21, 23, 29, 31
visual attention, 21
visual field, 111
visual images, 3, 20, 30
visual modality, vii, 2, 17, 22
visual stimuli, 104
visual system, 106, 220
vulnerability, xi, 78, 87, 91, 92, 114, 128, 132, 137, 139, 140, 145, 177, 196, 197, 222, 234

W

waking, 221, 223
water diffusion, 15
weight gain, 150, 152
white matter, 5, 15, 24, 27, 124
withdrawal, xiv, 4, 148, 149, 168, 186, 187, 219
working memory, 86, 90, 142, 214, 217
workplace, 228
worry, 198, 227

Y

yes/no, 118, 119
young adults, 118, 145

Z

ziprasidone, 172